EFFECTIVE TSUBO THERAPY

Simple and Natural Relief without Drugs

By Katsusuke Serizawa, M. D.

J P

Japan Publications, Inc.

Published by JAPAN PUBLICATIONS, INC., Tokyo and New York

Distributors:
UNITED STATES: *Kodansha International/USA, Ltd., through Harper & Row, Publishers, Inc., 10 East 53rd Street, New York, N. Y. 10022.* SOUTH AMERICA: *Harper & Row, Publishers, Inc., International Department.* CANADA: *Fitzhenry & Whiteside Ltd., 150 Lesmill Road, Don Mills, Ontario M3B 2T6.* MEXICO AND CENTRAL AMERICA: *HARLA S. A. de C. V. Apartado 30–546, Mexico 4, D. F.* BRITISH ISLES: *International Book Distributors Ltd., 66 Wood Lane End, Hemel Hempstead, Herts HP2 4RG.* EUROPEAN CONTINENT: *Fleetbooks, S. A., c/o Feffer and Simons (Nederland) B. V., Rijnkade 170, 1382 GT Weesp, The Netherlands.* AUSTRALIA AND NEW ZEALAND: *Bookwise, 1 Jeanes Street, Beverley, South Australia 5009.* THE FAR EAST AND JAPAN: *Japan Publications Trading Co., Ltd., 1–2–1, Sarugaku-cho, Chiyoda-ku, Tokyo 101.*

First edition: October 1984

LCCC No. 84–080646
ISBN 0–87040–581–0

Printed in Singapore

Effective

TSUBO THERAPY

By the Same Author:

TSUBO: Vital Points for Oriental Therapy
256 pp., 7¼ × 10¼ in., over 1,000 illus., paperback.
ISBN 0–87040–350–8

MASSAGE: The Oriental Methods
78 pp., 7¼ × 10¼ in., many illus., paperback.
LC 73–188762, ISBN 0–87040–168–8

Preface

During the more than forty years in which I have been working in this field, the word *tsubo*, which was very little known in the West in the past, has come to have considerable international currency largely because of an intensifying reevaluation of Oriental medicine inspired by the inability of Western medicine to deal with the numerous pathological conditions arising from stress generated by human relations and other factors in increasingly complex modern society. As a result of my own many years of clinical research on tsubo, I have become convinced that the three-thousand-year-old medical wisdom of the East is by no means mere superstition. In addition, it is often very precise in its terminology. For instance, the names of the tsubo themselves clearly indicate their location on the body, the therapeutic effects to be expected from treating them, and their clinical significance in connection with the theories of yin and yang and of the Five Elements.

Investigations of the possibility of their physical existence have led me to the conclusion that the tsubo and the meridians connecting them are less morphological and structural than functional entities. In other words, they may be interpreted as the places on the surface of the body where pain, stiffness, and other conditions most easily arise as reflections of irregularities in body organs and tissues. Tsubo therapy is a system based on experience for assisting in the treatment of illnesses by stimulating the tsubo on the surface of the body and thus evoking reflex responses in the internal organs.

Fundamentally, Oriental medicine strives to keep the body in good condition and to prevent the development of illness. Sickness itself is the condition resulting when the body grows excessively tired or weak and when this condition becomes chronic to the extent that normal physiological functions are impossible and pathological symptoms emerge in the organs and tissues. Oriental medicine attempts to catch this process in the early stage when only fatigue has manifested itself and then to take suitable measures to prevent illness and keep the body fit.

People today are constantly subjected not only to physical fatigue, but also to weariness caused by psychological stress. Often people are too busy to get the rest and sleep that would set matters right. It is for such people that this book explains therapy based on specially effective tsubo.

In Part One, important widely clinically used tsubo on fourteen meridians have been selected. Location, applicability, and name derivation are given for each. Part Two introduces the most effective methods of dealing with fatigue conditions by treating ninety-one selected tsubos. Ordinarily, in the clinic, we rarely treat only one or two tsubos in dealing with symptoms. But, for the purposes of this book, I have minimized the number of tsubos and have combined them in such a way as to create the simplest and most efficacious treatment methods.

As I explain in the opening part of the text, the tsubo do not exist as definite points on the body like the ones shown in the figures. Tactile examination of the skin in an area about two centimeters in diameter, will locate muscles. In the text I have explained that tsubos are to be found certain centimeters from these muscles. But actually it is impossible to give exact measurements because of individual differences. The important thing is to follow the instructions, discover the locations of the required tsubo in accordance with the figures, and then stroke the skin in that area. Locating tsubo is explained in detail in the introduction. The reader should study this text carefully.

Although I am often asked about number of times and durations of pressure applications on tsubo, this too is impossible to give. As far as the treatment in this book is concerned, it is time to stop when the pressing or kneading of a tsubo brings a sense of relief and comfort. Of course, overdoing the pressure produces no good effects.

I shall be very happy if this book helps people today effectively recover from fatigue in its early stages and to find the comfort and good health to enable them to survive the stresses of modern living.

In conclusion, I should like to express my deep respect and gratitude to Stephen S. Brown, who patiently translated my text into English; to Iwao Yoshizaki, president of Japan Publications, Inc., who devoted great energy to the publication of this book; and to Yotsuko Watanabe for her editorial cooperation.

Katsusuke Serizawa

Contents

Introduction: Tsubo and Oriental Medicine

Tsubo Changed the Course of History

What comes to your mind when the word *tsubo* is mentioned? In Japan people often speak of "hitting the *tsubo*," and this phrase is used as an analogy to describe how something important has been pinpointed. As indicated by this expression, in a word, tsubos are places of special importance on the body. On occasion tsubos are referred to as "vital points." Since the location of these tsubos, unlike the eyes or nose, are not clearly visible, they have to be located by exercising special sensitivity. Thus, in Japan tsubo has become synonymous with something difficult to hit perfectly, but also something remarkably effective when a person finally succeeds.

The Chinese character for tsubo (壺) represents an earthenware vessel or jar, and this use is not entirely without reason. The tsubos discussed in this book are, of course, tsubos on the human body, and obviously there are no hollow places in the body like that of a jar. Tsubos here refer to invisible points on the surface of the body which are vital points where various physical symptoms can be alleviated by pressing, rubbing or massaging, and otherwise by acupuncture or moxibustion treatments.

Ashi-San-Ri 足三里 (ST-36) happens to be one of the most well-known tsubo with mention of it as "burning moxa on San-Ri," in the writings of the master poet of Japan in the seventeenth century, Matsuo Bashō. San-Ri is famous because fatigue in the legs can be effectively relieved by burning moxa on it, or by applying finger pressure. San-Ri will be discussed in greater detail later, but it is worth noting that it has a long history of use as a popular folk remedy. For example, the family of Manpei, a Japanese farmer in the province of Mikawa, became famous in the Edo period (1603–1867) for their longevity, and they swore by applying moxibustion on San-Li and were all renowned for their strong legs. There is also a story during the Second World War that among the retreating Japanese army there were those who knew about this tsubo and applied moxibustion and finger pressure on it. Supposedly, only those troops which used this tsubo were able to escape and return alive.

While tsubos have played a key role in Oriental medicine as will be discussed later, through its long history spanning several thousand years, tsubos have had an influence in even the West. Perhaps you know about Heinrich Himmler (1900–1945), the head of the Nazi secret police who served alongside Adolf Hitler (1889–1945), the Nazi dictator responsible for plunging the world into the tragic Second World War. Himmler was a staunch believer in Nazi principles and some of his methods were the height of cruelty. But this same Himmler suddenly began to change after a certain point, and he turned into an opponent self-critical of the tyrannical methods of the Nazis. The man who held the key to this sudden change in Himmler is said to be his masseur.

Himmler was actually a very nervous man, and perhaps for the same reason, he often experienced painful gastrospasms from which he suffered a great deal. Yet, because he was always in fear of being poisoned, he refused to take any form of medication at all. This is where the masseur became useful. Every time Himmler would have a gastrospasm, his masseur apparently firmly pressed the right tsubo to quickly cure the gastrospasm. Therefore, this masseur quickly became indispensable to Himmler. The masseur who received the special favor of Himmler found occasion to touch on the subject of his cruel methods and advised Himmler to reconsider them. Probably the masseur did not go as far as pressing tsubos inside Himmler's head to change him, but Erich Kästner (1899–1974) who wrote about this masseur in his book, *The Miraculous Hands*, credited him for massaging and bring about changes in not only Himmler's body, but his mind as well.

More recently, astounding results in the application of tsubo have been announced in China such as acupuncture anesthesia, and it has received worldwide attention. I have worked with tsubo for thirty-five years and have treated countless patients, but the tendency today seems to be for patients to come for help because they know of no other place to find relief. In many cases, stubborn symptoms which have troubled patients for years are relieved in a matter of two or three months. Many medical specialists who hear of this just dismiss it as "a mere coincidence," or "just a case of natural recovery." For this reason, I wish to remove the veil of mystery which has so far covered the subject of tsubo, and to discuss in this book how the invaluable experience of Oriental medicine over thousands of years can be put to practical use in our lives today.

The Roots of Oriental Medicine

When hearing the term Oriental medicine even Japanese have a preconceived notion that it is something very old-fashioned where old people concoct herbal remedies out of Korean ginseng or *Geranium nepalense*. The origins of Oriental medicine will be discussed here briefly so that the tsubo can be understood in true perspective.

Obviously, Oriental medicine was developed in the Orient. Yet the Orient includes a truely staggering land mass. Oriental medicine as known today in Japan was developed in China and subsequently made its way into Japan. Oriental medicine is also called *Kampō* 漢方 (the Chinese way) in Japan, but there are actually two main branches to *Kampō* consisting of that which developed in the Yellow River basin and that from the Yangze River basin. The former kind is acupuncture and moxibustion which includes *anma* or Oriental massage, and this variety is what has been widely disseminated as folk medicine in Japan.

As you may already know, the land in the Yellow River basin is not very fertile and there are very few large plants. About the only plants there are mugwort and other short plants growing close to the ground. Therefore, people who lived in this region came up with the folk remedies of using sharp stones to drain pus whenever a cut became infected, and to use dried mugwort leaves to burn the skin when they were not feeling well. This is how acupuncture and moxibustion got its start around the Yellow River. The *anma* massage technique was another folk remedy which resulted from the life-style of people in the Yellow River basin. *Anma* has now developed into a specialized massage technique in which stiff and sore areas are pressed and rubbed to remedy numbness and chilling in the extremities. Thus, people around the Yellow River used acupuncture, moxibustion and *anma*, which is to say, they used physiotherapy or manual methods to provide cures. Thus, through the years they learned the location of the most effective points on the body for treatment. These points are what are called tsubos. This branch of Chinese medicine is also referred to as "Northern medicine."

Opposed to this, the Oriental medicine which originated south of the Yangze River is Chinese herbal medicine which also happens to be experiencing a resurgence of popularity in Japan. The people who lived in the Yangze River basin where land was fertile and lush with vegetation learned to collect the roots of plants and the bark of trees for concocting herbal remedies to treat illness. This variety of Oriental medicine is also referred to as "Southern medicine."

Thus Chinese medicine originated from two entirely different sources; acupuncture, moxibustion and *anma* 按摩 originated around the Yellow River, and herbal medicine originated in the south. When China was unified under the Han Dynasty these two different forms of medicine were integrated and systematized. This is the so-called Oriental medicine of today and is what many Japanese refer to as *Kampō*.

It was not until the beginning of the sixth centrury (the Asuka period) when these methods were brought to Japan. *Kampō* reached its peak of popularity in the Edo period. Nevertheless, with the advent of the Meiji restoration (A.D. 1868) and the modernization of Japan, German and Dutch medicine eclipsed *Kampō*, and because herbal remedies were often ineffective in surgery or in perventing contagious diseases, it fell out of the mainstream. In the Edo period before the restoration, the Shogunate decreed that blind persons assume the job of masseur and acupuncturist as a welfare measure, so this type of therapy began to diverge from the original methods and became distorted. As a result, the word *anma* in Japan acquired some stigma as a lowly profession. Furthermore, many people think that all a person has to do in herbal medicine is to buy Korean ginseng or *Geranium nepalense* in stores and concoct these to use in their own way. To correctly make use of herbal medicine, however, one must receive a physical examination from a specialist and follow his directions carefully to take a prescription which is a precise combination of a variety of herbs.

In this way, opposed to Western medicine which was imported from the Western countries during the Meiji period, Oriental medicine which came to be called *Kampō*, became wrapped up in various misconceptions in Japan. Be that as it may, these are nothing more than misunderstandings about Oriental medicine, and as seen in China, where the government policy is to have Eastern and Western medicine on an equal footing, Oriental medicine has a theoretical framework backed by a long tradition of empirical knowledge from successful treatments. This basic framework is the concept of "six *zang* 臟 and six *fu* 腑."

The Six *Zang* and Six *Fu*

When a person has symptoms such as a fever, a headache, stiffness in the back of the neck and shoulders, a cough, an oppressive feeling in the chest, palpitation, pain in the joints, insomnia, general fatigue, or numbness and pain in the legs, generally in contemporary medicine, an attempt is made to match the symptoms up and identify some disease, be it the common cold or valvular heart diseases. Groups of symptoms are even organized into syndromes to arrive at the appropriate treatment. On the other hand, in Oriental medicine all the symptoms are categorized according to the basic principle of six *zang* and six *fu*.

Oriental medicine follows the principles of nature almost to the point of seeming simplistic. For example, all manifestations in nature are largely divided into either yin or yang. Thus, all phenomena such as day and night, or light and dark are classified as being yin or yang. In addition, nature is considered to consist of the five basic elements of plants, heat, earth, minerals and liquids. All things are therefore classified as either wood, fire, earth, metal or water. Thus, all of nature is seen as being related to one or more of these elements. These concepts make up the yin-yang and five element principles.

Human beings also come under the above-mentioned principles of nature, and these principles are applied to all aspects of the human body. For example, man is yang and woman is yin, and the organs in the human body are all either yin (*zang*) or yang (*fu*), and are organized in relation to the five elements. Therefore, just as trees and plants in nature put out a shoot, come into blooms, bear fruit and eventually wither away, human beings are born, live out their life and pass away as part of nature. Just as in nature where balmy spring days never last forever, and rain pours and storms rage from time to time, the body is also regarded as having its good and bad moments in addition to the cycle of growth and decline. The basic approach in Oriental medicine is to capture all these changes as part of a natural process, and this is an important feature which Western medicine does not have.

Then what is the key factor in sustaining the life force which is present within man which is yang and woman which is yin? It is the interaction of the five elements in nature—that of wood, fire, earth, metal and water—as mentioned earlier. These elements are each associated with a yin organ and a yang organ contained within the microcosm of the human body. The five essential organs are the liver, which is associated with wood, the heart, which is associated with fire, the spleen, which is associated with earth, the lungs, which are associated with metal, and the kidneys which are associated with water. When the word liver or spleen is used in Oriental medicine, often people assume that these are the same liver and spleen referred to in medicine today. Actually, however, even though these organs of Oriental medicine may bear some resemblance to their Western counterparts, they do not always mean the same thing. The reason for this is because in the East, modern medicine inherited the names for various organs from Oriental medicine while there remained a significant difference in their meaning.

The life of man is not sustained totally by the five essential organs (five *zang*).

There are also yang organs which form paired relationships with the above yin organs to each aid the work of its partner to maintain life functions. For example, the liver and gallbladder form a yin-yang combination. The gallbladder is the yang organ (*fu*) which supports the liver, the yin organ (*zang*). Viewed even from the standpoint of modern medicine, the liver and gallbladder are very closely connected. The gallbladder is attached to the bottom of the liver and stores bile which is produced in the liver.

In Oriental medicine the heart is paired with the small intestines, and the spleen is paired with the stomach. The spleen in Oriental medicine is not the same as that in contemporary medicine, instead it refers to the pancreas. The pancreas is located right behind the stomach, and these organs form an inseparable pair even from an anatomical standpoint. Further, in Oriental medicine the large intestines aid the work of the lungs, and the urinary bladder aids the work of the kidneys. The above mentioned combinations are called the five *zang* and five *fu*.

There is one more *zang-fu* combination in Oriental medicine. The yin organ in this pair is the heart constrictor. Since the heart is a crucially important organ which has to function continuously throughout one's life, the idea came about that the heart had to be securely protected by a sack-like covering, and this was named the heart constrictor. The yang organ paired with the heart constrictor is the triple heater. The concept of the triple heater was likewise derived from the idea that since the body was always warm while alive, there had to be a source or location for the production of this heat.

The last pair of organs may seem somewhat odd from the standpoint of modern medicine, but as mentioned before, the conceptual framework of Oriental medicine differs completely from that of Western medicine. Instead of each organ existing as an independent anatomical entity, the organs serve to hypothetically express the various functions needed to support the life of an individual within his natural environment. While the explanations provided by Western medicine concerning the organs are very rational and clear cut, everything must fit within its framework of careful reasoning, and those facts which do not fit within this framework are relentlessly discarded. Today, however, when the rational approach of the West has advanced to its limit and the world has become dominated by this approach, the problems of pollution and drug side effects have surfaced. The truth is, even those organs of our body which seem relatively easy to comprehend are full of unknown and mystifying features which cannot be fully explained by the rational Western approach even when examined very closely. An attempt is made in Oriental medicine to render these "mysteries of life" just as they are. Therefore, the body is not cut open any more than is absolutely necessary and every organ is not cut to pieces for the sake of examination, and moreover, logical theories are not conceived to explain the mutual relationship between organs. A much simpler approach is embraced with the yin-yang and five element principles, and this also applies to the concept of the six *zang* and six *fu*.

To summarize the foregoing discussion, the six *zang* are the liver, heart, spleen, lungs, kidney and heart constrictor, and the six *fu* are the gallbladder, small intestines, stomach, large intestines, urinary baldder and triple heater. The *zang* are the yin organs and the *fu* are the yang organs, and the six *zang* and six *fu* each are in a yin and yang, or interior and exterior relationship so as to coordinate and function in mutual support. Since the body is wholly under the control of the six *zang* and six *fu*, even if a problem occurs in just one of these organs, the condition of the whole body is upset, and the human individual comprising the microcosm is deprived of both physical and mental energy.

The Meridians Coursing through the Body

Thus, the six *zang* and six *fu* in Oriental medicine play a vital role in the life of a human being, but just how are these organs related to tsubo? Why is it that symptoms are alleviated and diseases are cured when tsubos are massaged or pressed, or otherwise when acupuncture and moxibustion are applied?

In Oriental medicine it is postulated that there is a circulatory system which courses through the six *zang* and six *fu* to suppy them with vital energy. These channels are called meridians and they comprise that fundamental conceptual framework for treatments in Oriental medicine. The meridians run in the vertical direction while the collaterals run in the horizontal direction (the general meaning of meridian includes collaterals). So in other words, a circulatory system of vital energy supplying the six *zang* and six *fu* flows horizontally and vertically from the top of the head down to the tip of the toes. Each one of these channels is named after the *zang* or *fu* it controls. The following then are the names of the twelve meridians.

(1) lung meridian, (2) large intestine meridian, (3) stomach meridian, (4) spleen meridian, (5) heart meridian, (6) small intestine meridian, (7) urinary bladder meridian, (8) kidney meridian, (9) heart constrictor meridian, (10) triple heater meridian, (11) gallbladder meridian, (12) liver meridian.

The above twelve meridians are called the "twelve regular meridians," and these twelve meridians begin at the lung meridian which circulates through the lungs. Each meridian passes through its corresponding organ and one cycle is completed at the liver meridian which flows through the liver. This flow of energy then begins another cycle by circulating through the lung meridian which controls the lungs. If vital energy is flowing properly through all these meridians, then it means that a person is healthy. From time to time, however, there is an overflow of energy from this circulation system.

There are eight additional meridians aside from those just mentioned which work to regulate the amount of energy overall, and they flow vertically, horizontally and diagonally. These are called the "eight extraordinary meridians." Among the extraordinary meridians, the conception vessel traveling through the median line on the front of the body from the middle of the face to the center of the chest and stomach, along with the governor vessel flowing through the median line on the buttocks up the back, the neck, and the back of the head and around to the middle of the face, is regarded as serving an especially important function. In a sense, the conception vessel and governor vessel work to constantly adjust the amount of energy circulating in the twelve regular meridians, and these two vessels function to supply all the organs with the appropriate amount of energy.

The energy which flows through these meridians and vessels is referred to as *ki-ketsu* 気血 (*ki* and blood), *ei-e* 栄衛 (defensive and nourishing *ki*) and *kei sui* 経水 (meridian fluid). The reason *ki-ketsu* was thought to flow through the meridians is probably because the ancient people regarded the air inhaled into the body as *ki*, and the blood flowing out when wounded as *ketsu*, and presumed that these supplied energy to all organs.

In Oriental medicine, among the twelve meridians, those that are associated with the six *zang* are yin and those associated with the six *fu* are yang. The symptoms related to each type of meridian is referred to as either yin symptoms or yang symptoms. Further, in this symptom classification system, when symptoms appear on the anterior abdominal area, yang symptoms are called sunlight yang and yin symptoms are called great yin. In a similar manner, when symptoms are manifested on the side of the body or the flank region, yang symptoms are called lesser yang and yin symptoms are called absolute yin. Furthermore, when symptoms appear on the posterior side or the back, yang symptoms are called great yang and yin symptoms are called lesser yin. Thus, the stomach meridian which is associated with one of the six *fu*, because its symptoms appear on the front of the body, is referred to as the sunlight yang stomach meridian. The twelve regular meridians are also divided by those which flow primarily on the arms and reach their corresponding organ, and those which flow primarily on the legs to reach their corresponding organs. Thus, the full name of meridians reads like the great yin lung meridian of the arms, or the lesser yang triple heater meridian of the legs, and the full names indicate the position of the meridian.

Tsubo to Find out Which Meridian Is Abnormal

Now that a basic knowledge concerning the system and concepts underlying Oriental medicine have been discussed, the question of where the tsubos are located on the body, and which tsubos to apply pressure on for which symptoms, and how to do so, will be answered. Before this, however, the question of why symptoms are alleviated just by applying pressure on the appropriate tsubo will be addressed briefly.

Occasionally one comes across a magazine which features some tsubos which are supposed to be effective for such things like stomach trouble and the location is shown by placing a black dot on a picture of the body. But these points do not always prove effective when pressure is applied on them as shown. It is only to be expected that such treatments do not work because even though a person may think that he is pressing the right point, he often misses the tsubo completely. It is not so easy to pinpoint a tsubo at first, but it is relatively simple once you get the knack.

Just as there are 365 days in a year, there are said to be 365 tsubos on the body. The meridians are the result of organizing these tsubos into lines. Since each meridian is associated with a *zang* or *fu* respectively, if there are any physical problems, a red warning lamp lights on one of the meridians. Therefore, even when locating tsubo for the sake of treating a specific symptom, the priority always lies in finding out which tsubo on which meridian is indicated. This is because even for just a headache, the tsubo to be used differs according to the nature of the pain and whether it is the result of a lung disfunction or a liver problem.

The figure below shows the tsubo for locating abnormalities among the tweleve meridians as well as their corresponding *zang* and *fu*. Examine the twelve tsubos shown on the front of the body (*bo* 募 points) and the twelve tsubos shown on the back (*yu* 俞 points) by lightly massaging, pinching, or pressing them. If there is a

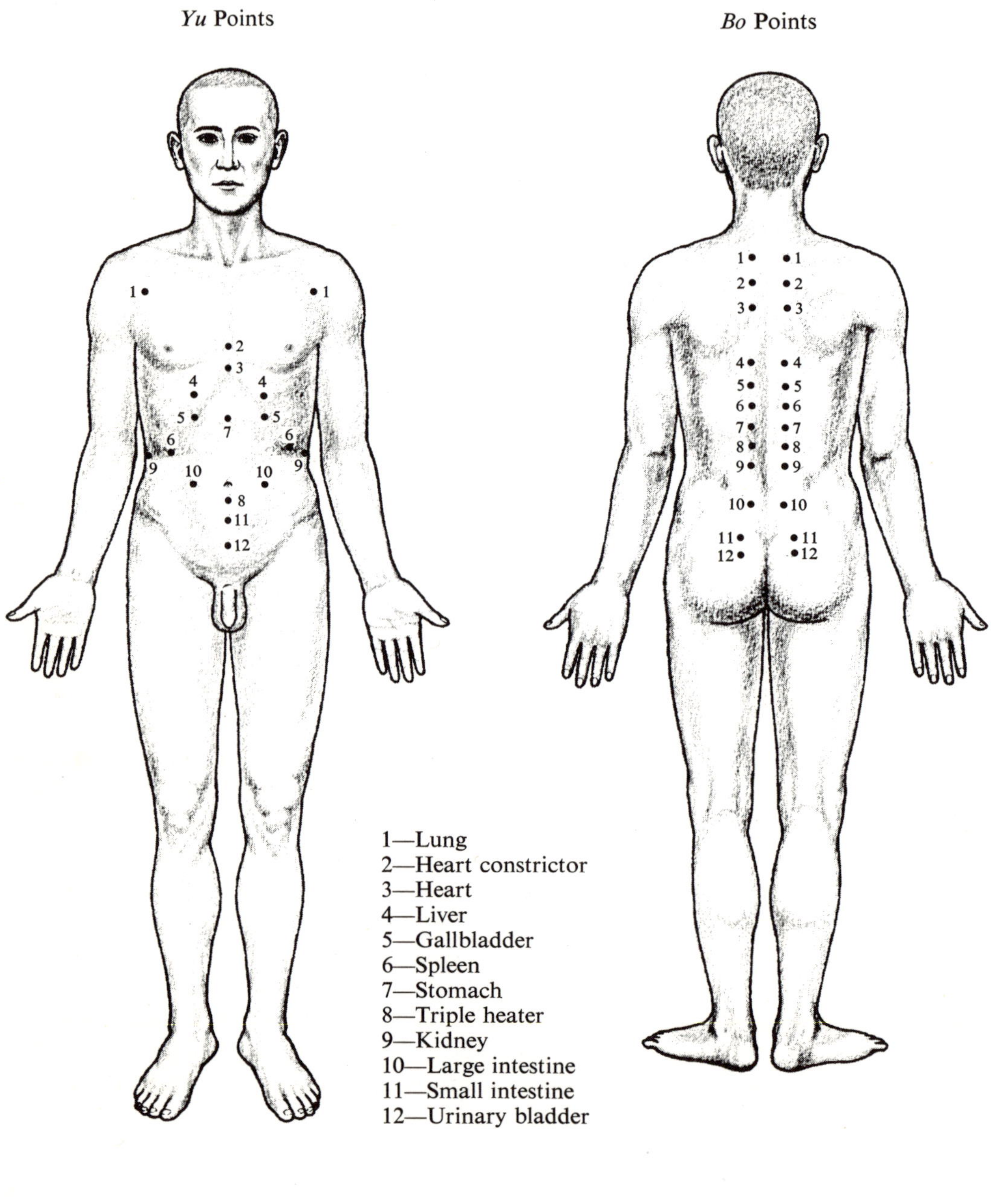

stinging sensation, pain or hardness in any of these points, an abnormality is indicated in the meridian and organ associated with that tsubo.

In order to determine whether there was any scientific basis to this tsubo diagnosis derived from long years of experience I conducted a clinical experiment comparing a group of fifty normal subjects against the same number of patients with various diseases. Data including the skin's electrical resistance at tsubos, electromyographs and pulse waves were studied, and although there were some individual differences, it was confirmed that changes in the state of the skin and muscles were indeed concentrated around the associated tsubo in the fifty patients.

Once you have determined which meridian and *zang* or *fu* is abnomal, begin by lightly pinching along the course of that meridian which is shown at the beginning of the section for that meridian. For example, if point 1 is found to be sore on both the front and back, pinch along the lung meridian, and if point 2 is sore, turn to the figure at the beginning of the section for the heart constrictor meridian and probe for tsubos along the line of that meridian. The location of tsubos in this book are often stated as being so many centimeters from a certain place, but this is not a precise distance. What is intended is that the tsubo be located around that point. The exact location varies according to each individual and his condition, so one must lightly pinch or press the approximate area to locate the exact point. There should be a point which feels somehow different, or even sore, though it is pinched or pressed in the same way as other places. A point that is slightly harder and quite sensitive can be felt by pressing in slowly here, and this often causes a dull pain. This is the tsubo which will relieve your pain, or your symptom.

Anatomical diagrams have been included in pages 25 and 26 of this book for your reference and they should be a help in locating the tsubos presented by their meridians.

Tsubos Are Neither Mysterious Nor Miraculous

Let us briefly consider why changes occur at the tsubos when there is an abnormality in our body, and why treatment at these tsubos can cure illnesses.

In Oriental medicine all diseases and their symptoms are regarded as being the result of problems in the circulation of *ki-ketsu* or vital energy. When the function of the six *zang* and six *fu* are impaired, the flow of energy in meridians begins to slow down just as if a hose of running water were being stepped on. The tsubos are located along the meridians and are places where the flow of energy becomes easily obstructed. The flow of energy through these tsubos is therefore stimulated by rubbing, pressing and massaging, or otherwise by acupuncture and moxibustion, to alleviate all types of symptoms. This is a basic principle in Oriental medicine, and tsubos are also called acupuncture points. These are points which show various changes as a result of obstructions in energy along the meridians. Of course, with the advancement of medical science today, there are few people left who think that the *zang* and *fu* as well as the meridians mentioned above actually exist in the body. Even the practitioners of traditional medicine including me regard these principles as a conceptual framework for physical phenomena which is very useful in diagnosis and treatment.

The principles of Chinese medicine have always given priority to phenomenology, while modern medicine has relied on the study of pathology based on anatomy and physiology, or the detailed study of the structure and function of the human body. Diagnosis and treatment is considered only after this in Western medicine. In contrast to this, the methods to treat the phenomenon at hand took precedence in Oriental medicine, and the concepts of *zang* and *fu*, and of meridians were conceived to explain the effect of these methods.

As an example, it becomes apparent by closely examining the tsubo which is sore, hardened, cool, hot, or depressed, that the skin there is very rough. Normally skin is slightly moist with the proper excretion of skin oils and sweat. When this excretion is impaired, however, the skin becomes rough. This is evidence that the autonomic nervous system which controls the function of all organs including those of the circulatory, respiratory, digestive, excretory and reproductive systems has become disturbed. This is because the nerves which control the skin's excretion of oil and sweat are also autonomic nerves. Therefore, by examining which tsubo the rough skin area is closest to, one can learn which organ's function related with the nerves going to that particular skin area has been adversely affected.

This fact has been proven by medical science. An English neurologist, Sir Henry Head (1861–1940), stated "disfunctions in the tissues and organs of the body produce various changes in muscles and skin through nervous networks with a deep connection to the brain and spine," and thus founded the theory of "skin segments," or areas of "referred pain" from organs to the skin. These skin segments were coined "Head's zones." Oriental medicine with its perspective of the *zang-fu* and meridian principles has systematized these zones into the twelve meridians and the acupuncture points. In Western medicine skin segments are designated according to the spinal nerves to form lateral cross sectional segments, and pain and hardness is said to occur in relation to these segments. Therefore, if we regard the point which becomes sore and stiff and the easiest point within a skin segment to have referred pain as being a tsubo, the observed phenomenon becomes the same from both the Eastern and Western medical standpoints.

It could just be a matter of a difference in the way people in the East and West view the world. It is interesting to note some differences between the East and West, for example, in the West, words are written sideways and among human relationships the husband-wife relationship is held to be of prime importance, while in the East, writing often goes from top to bottom and importance is placed more on the filial piety of children to their parents.

My patients who suffer from hemorrhoids are often mystified when they receive acupuncture or moxibustion treatments on tsubo of their head. Yet, because tsubos are points where the stagnation in a meridian associated with a particular organ is most easily manifested on the skin surface, it is entirely reasonable to treat a problem in the buttocks area by using a tsubo on the head. Furthermore, the reason pain or numbness is relieved with acupuncture, shiatsu or massage is because a form of interference is provided by the administration of a different form of stimulus on a location completely different than where the pain or numbness is relaying signals to the central nervous system, and this has the effect of counterbalancing the abnormal pain signals. Experiments in electrophysiology have proven that such stimulation acts to normalize the signals transmitted to the control centers in the brain.

Also, by examining physical phenomena such as chilling or hotness, or the circulation and muscular movements in the areas where stiffness occur, using electromyographs, photoelectric plethysmographs and measurements of the skin's electrical resistance, it can be seen that these symptoms are alleviated by skin stimulation. Such studies are conducted on a daily basis at our research center and it has become clear that when abnormalities in the tissues and organs become manifested as various changes in the muscles and skin. These changes can be reversed and the normal functioning of organs can be restored by applying stimulation to the appropriate tsubo. Moreover, it has recently been confirmed that, even when giving injections, the effect is more pronounced if a tsubo is located and the injection is given at that point. Quite a number of pain control clinics at university hospitals which serve as research facilities, as well as other institutions of medical research are now beginning to undertake research concerning tsubo. From the above points it can be seen how Oriental medicine is neither mystifying nor miraculous, but that it is instead a scientific method of treatment based on experience.

The Most Effective Way to Press Tsubo with Fingers

Finally, some explanation will be given concerning the methods of treatments using tsubo. Among the ways to stimulate a tsubo, there is massage, shiatsu, acupuncture and moxibustion, but the easiest methods by far are massage and shiatsu where nothing else but the use of one's fingers is required.

(1) Rubbing and stroking

As mentioned before *anma* is one of the therapeutic methods of Oriental medicine along with acupuncture and moxibustion. In *anma* the overexcitation of the nerves and muscles are sedated by "an" which means to press, and deterioration in the functional integrity of physical systems is normalized through "ma" or rubbing. The latter technique is referred to as "normalization through rubbing." To do this one palm is placed firmly against the skin surface with a moderate amount of pressure to rub and stroke the body. In this case, it does not matter if the whole palm is used to do the rubbing, or if only the thumb or the four fingers are used to do the rubbing.

(2) General massage

In this technique the whole palm, the thumb and the four fingers are moved together to draw small circles and knead the muscles along meridians. Do not move just the fingertips, but instead leave the palm and fingers firmly in place to massage with the action of the wrist and elbows. If only the fingertips are used to massage, the patient's skin may become irritated and this could make things worse than before the treatment. The main aim here is to massage and knead out the tension in muscles.

(3) *Localized massage*
This method is used to remove tension and stiffness right around the tsubo. The trick here is not to vary the pressure of the hand, thumb and four fingers from beginning to end. The ideal amount of pressure against the skin is three to five kilograms, and this can be learned by measuring the pressure on a gauge or pressing on a scale variously with your hand, thumb and four fingers. The correct amount of pressure can be learned by the reading on the scale. When massaging a person, carefully rub along the line of the meridian and massage mainly around tsubo. Use mostly the thumb and index fingers, and sometime all four fingers to locate the hardness and stiffness which appear as lumps or lines of tension. Apply strength gradually in a soft and gentle manner.

(4) *Pressure*
This is what is commonly known as shiatsu or acupressure and this emphasizes the "an" portion of *anma*, and is a manipulative technique which has incorporated aspects of *Judo* and *Dō-in*. This method is simple enough and all one has to do is to use the thumbs, four fingers, or the whole palm to apply pressure gently at first and then gradually increase the amount. Press each point three to five seconds. This is a very effective way to quiet pain and muscular spasms caused by the over-excitation of nerve and muscle function. Further effectiveness can be obtained by varying the pressure by going light at times and heavier at other times, and otherwise by varying the speed of pressing from fast to slow.

The above methods are all manipulative techniques, but there are other ways to stimulate tsubo such as using a hairdrier to apply hot air, or using any of a wide variety of devices which have become available recently. These are all valid methods for stimulating tsubo so you should keep them in mind as alternative tsubo treatments.

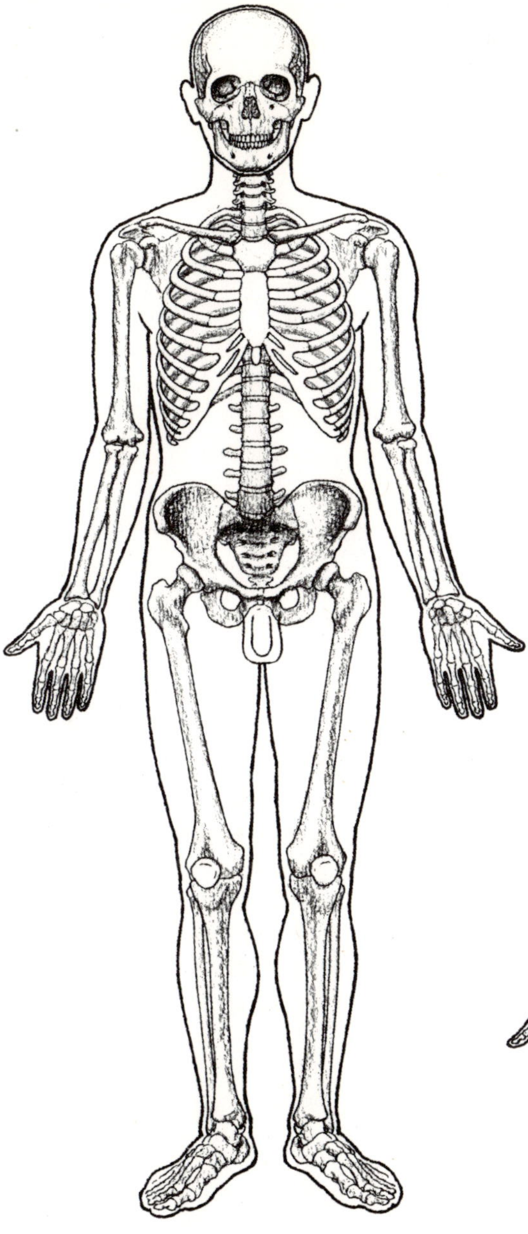
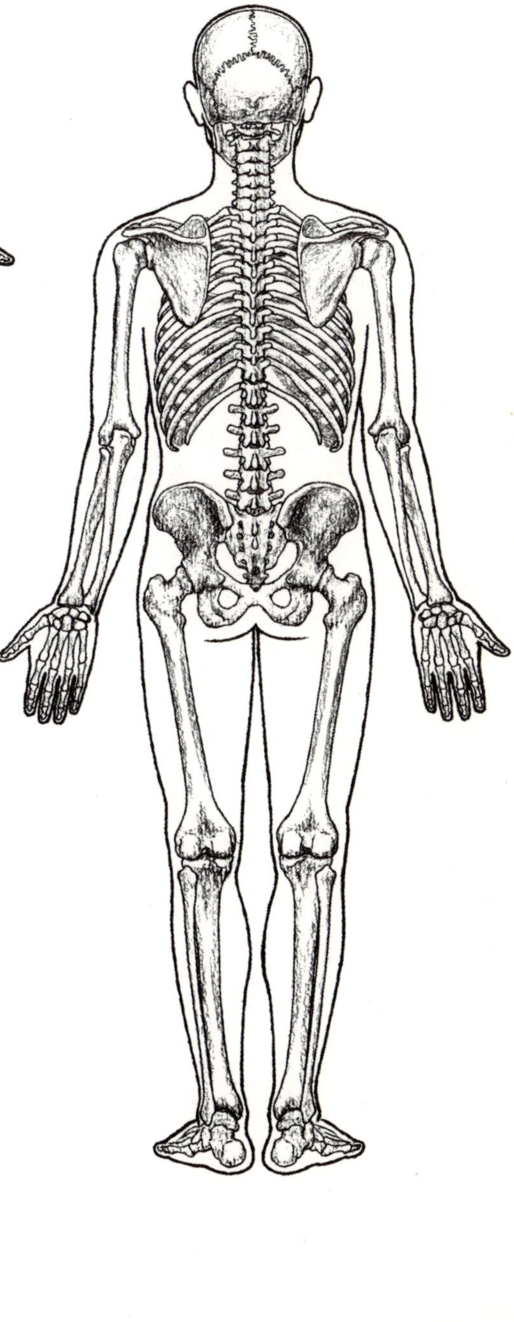

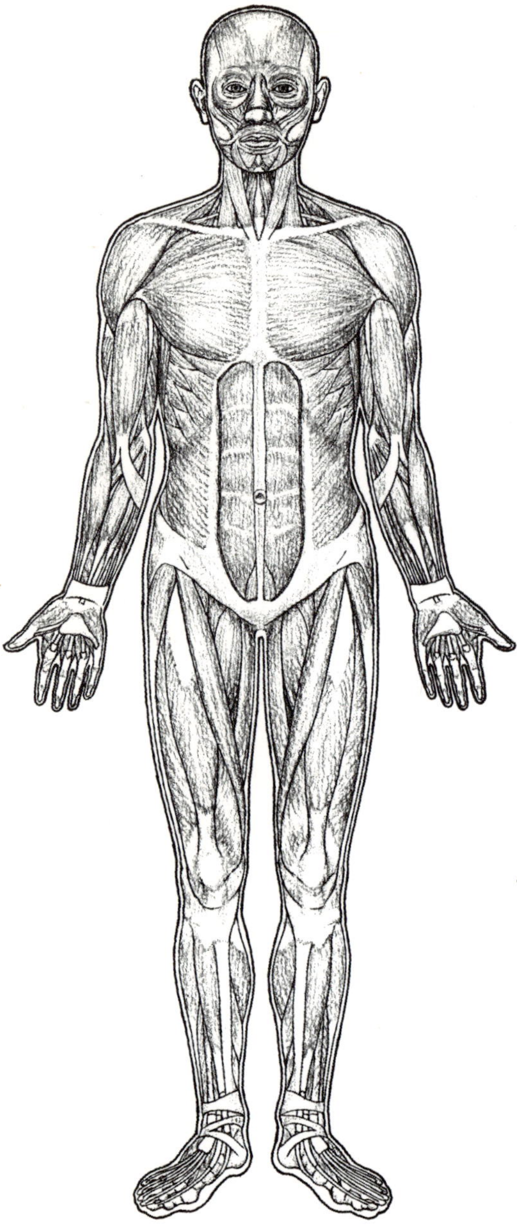
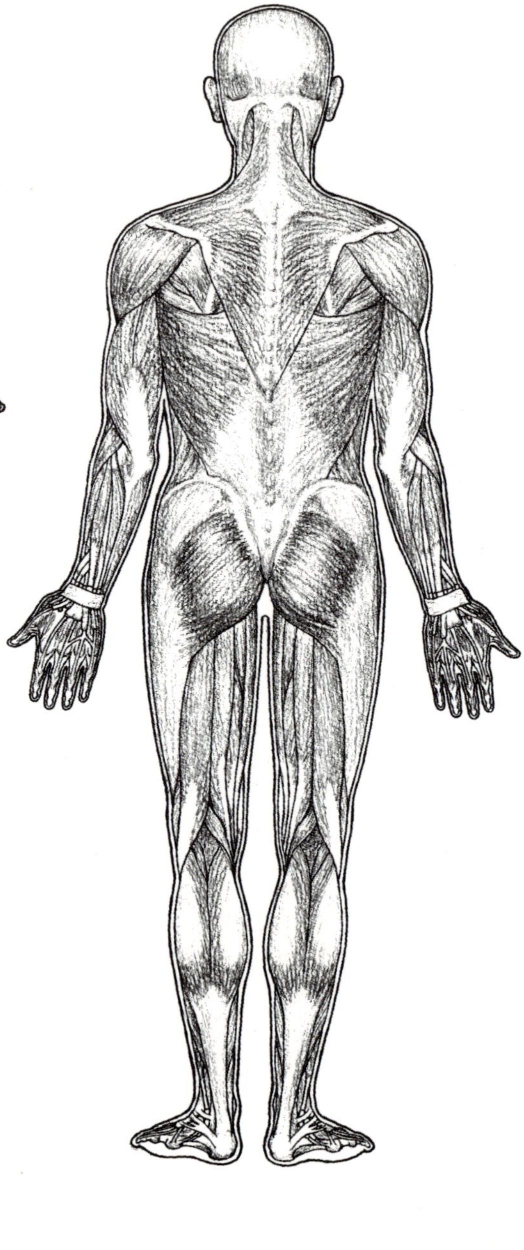

Part One:

Location of Tsubo by Meridians

1. Lung Meridian

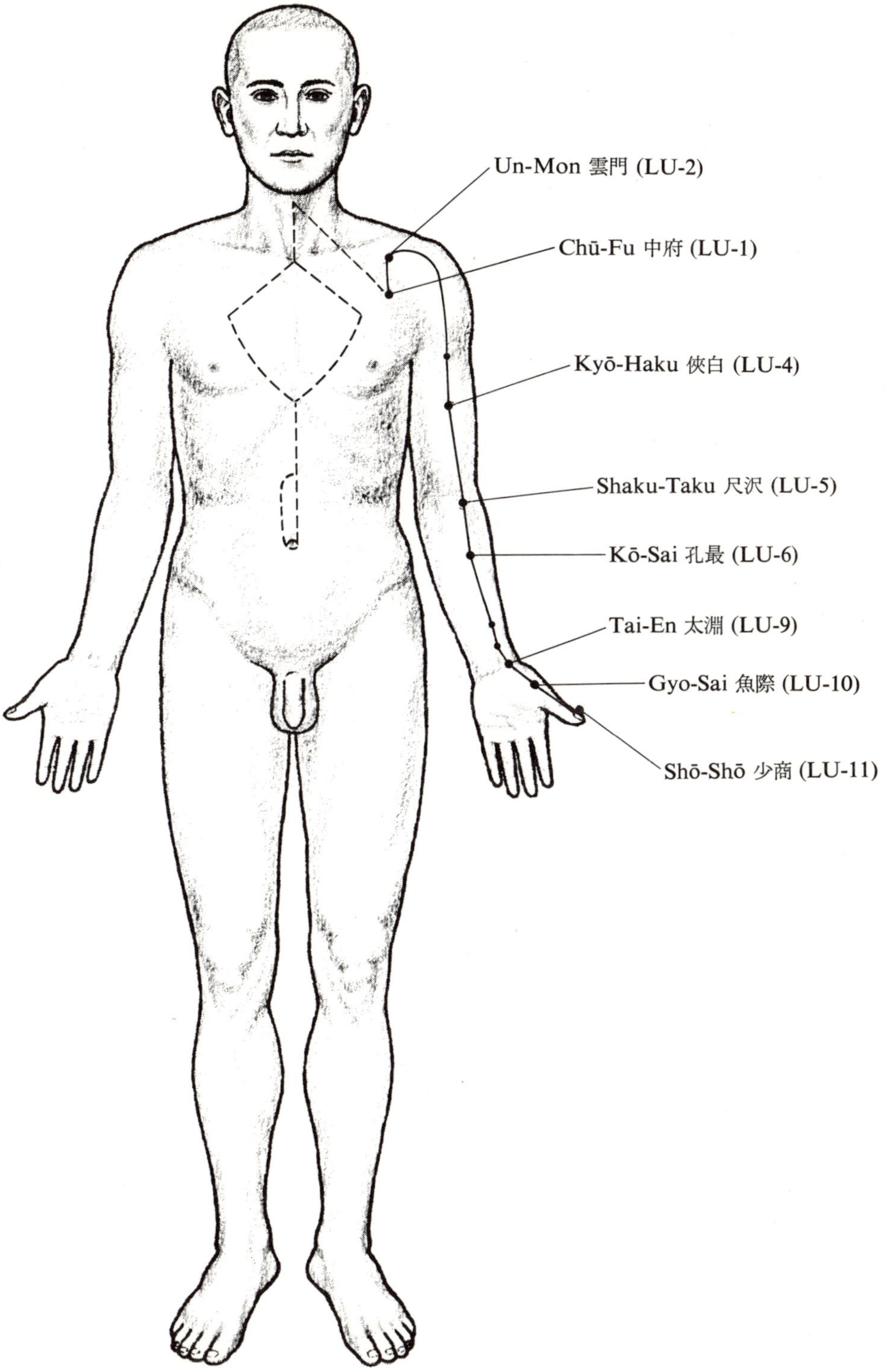

The discussion on tsubo will begin with the lung meridian which circulates through the lungs. The lung meridian, as shown in the preceding page, is the meridian which comes out of the lung area and courses down from the chest to the arms, and passing the inside of the forearm, ends at the outside base of the thumb nail. Along the course of this meridian are tsubos which are effective in relieving various symptoms associated with lung problems. The lungs are the uppermost among the five essential organs and they cover the other organs like an upside-down lotus flower. The lungs work to distribute the vital energy taken in from the atmosphere evenly among the essential organs. Like the gaseous exchange which takes place in internal respiration, the lungs work to take in an ample supply of air and then return the unused portion back to the atomosphere. When this essential function of the lungs becomes impaired, naturally, the flow of energy along the lung meridian is impeded. In such cases the function of the lungs can be normalized by massaging and pressing the tsubo on the lung meridian to improve its flow. Tsubos are points where the flow of energy in meridians most easily becomes obstructed or stopped up, so tsubos are stimulated to restore this flow.

What are the major symptoms which appear when the function of the lungs are impaired? First of all, the face becomes flushed, the mouth gets dry and the chest feels obstructed. Symptoms of coughing, palpitation, and shortness of breath appear. As additional symptoms, pain and numbness occur between the shoulder and the wrist, and the palms of the hand begin to feel hot. One's voice becomes raspy or high pitched and the skin becomes dry and loses its luster and turns white. Since the lungs which take in air from the atmosphere are weakened, one loses vigor and in others' eyes one may appear weak willed and unreliable. One's tastes will change away from greasy foods to more digestible food like fish. Also sometimes a person will acquire a taste for hot spicy foods.

If you get such symptoms, you can be quite sure that the function of your lungs has weakened. Massage or press the tsubo along the lung meridian in this case, or apply acupuncture or moxibustion to improve the flow along the lung meridian and remove the above symptoms. It must be noted here that the lung in Oriental medicine is not exactly the same organ as understood in modern medicine. The mention of a lung condition here does not necessarily refer to something serious like tuberculosis or pneumonia, but usually indicates a much broader range of problems in the respiratory system.

The lung meridian has eleven tsubos from the chest down to the base of the thumb nail. If the aforementioned symptoms are present, at least one of these tsubos should show special sensitivity when rubbed or pressed. The tsubo to be used, however, varies according to the symptom, so be sure to choose the most appropriate tsubo. In this chapter eight of the most commonly used tsubos among the eleven on the lung meridian will be discussed in detail.

1. Chū-Fu 中府 (LU-1)——*Tsubo for asthma attacks*

When wearing a knapsack, the straps go across the bones above the chest which are called clavicles. Apply light finger pressure to the points four or five centimeters below the outer edge of the clavicles on the right and left sides equally. There is usually a slightly hard spot where the right side is sore but the left side is not, or vice versa. This is the tsubo Chū-Fu 中府 (LU-1).

In the olden days *Fu* 府 used to be the central location in a province where people gathered, and even today there remain numerous towns in Japan named Fuchū 府中. The tsubo Chū-Fu also happens to be the most important tsubo in the lung meridian, and when there is a lung problem, all types of symptoms are said to gather here. To determine whether there is any obstruction in the lung meridian, rub, press or massage this tsubo to see if it is sore. *Chū* 中, among other things, means to hit the mark, so the tsubo Chū-Fu when hit squarely can dispell the cause of disease gathered there.

When there are symptoms such as a feeling of oppression in the chest, difficulty in breathing, or coughing, quietly pressing these points will relieve these symptoms. Also it is worth keeping in mind that this tsubo is used often in case of colds.

2. Un-Mon 雲門 (LU-2)——*Tsubo for frozen shoulders (periarthritis)*

In Oriental medicine the area above the clavicle on the body is referred to as the "heaven section," the area from the clavicle down to the navel is the "man section," and the area below the navel is the "earth section." This notion came from comparing the microcosm of the human form to the macrocosm of nature where life exists between heaven and earth. Un-Mon 雲門 (LU-2) is located right below the clavicle and its name denotes the "cloud gate" lying between the heaven section and the man section. Un-Mon lies right above Chū-Fu 中府 (LU-1) and it is effective not only for frozen shoulders which many middle-aged people suffer from, but it also is good for nose colds, sore throats and hoarseness. Even from the modern anatomical perspective both Un-Mon and Chū-Fu are important points where nerves and blood vessels form a complex web.

What do you suppose happens if these tsubo are pressed continuously even though a person does not have any problems? Recently there has been an increase among young women of the strange condition called "backpack paralysis" where their arms become numb and chilled and immobile because they carried too heavy of a load in hiking or backpacking. These symptoms came about as a result of their unknowingly applying pressure on Un-Mon and Chū-Fu. When this occurs, most people rub and massage their arms and hands, but the numbness and loss of circulation can be restored much easier by lightly stroking the tsubos Chū-Fu and Un-Mon which were the original cause.

3. Kyō-Haku 侠白 (LU-4)——*Tsubo for coughing and shortness of breath*

Sumō wrestling, the national sport of Japan, incorporates many ancient traditions which have things in common with Oriental medicine. For instance, the *sumō* mound with its four corners is symbolic of the five elements. The mound itself is earth and yellow, the blue corner represents wood, the red corner, fire, the white corner, metal, and the black corner, water. In Oriental medicine the human form is regarded as being a microcosm within the macrocosm of nature so all things large and small are correlated with the five elements. Thus, of the *zang* and *fu* in the body the liver and gallbladder are associated with wood (blue), the heart and small intestine, with fire (red), the stomach and spleen, with earth (yellow), the lung and large intestine, with metal (white) and the kidney and urinary bladder, with water (black). *Haku* 白 of Kyō-Haku 侠白 (LU-4) means white which is the color representing the lungs.

It has been known since the old days that the skin was not nourished properly when the lungs were afflicted, and that this made a person's complexion appear white. There was a time when some women with pulmonary tuberculosis were regarded as beauties because of their fair white skin. In any case, the lungs have traditionally been associated with the color white, and this seems to appear most in the complexion. Kyō-Haku means tsubos located on either side of the lungs (on the arms). They are highly effective for symptoms like shortness of breath and coughing—especially coughing fits. To locate Kyō-Haku stand up straight with the arms hanging down and probe for the tsubo in the biceps brachii muscle at the height of the nipples.

4. Shaku-Taku 尺沢 (LU-5)——*Tsubo for pain and numbness in arms*

Shaku-Taku 尺沢 (LU-5) is an important tsubo located on the inside of the elbow. It is especially effective in relieving pain and numbness in the arm and the feeling of heat in the palms. Bend your elbow slightly as if to receive something from someone, and a very hard tendon will appear in the center of the inside elbow. Lightly pinch or press this area with your fingers. The point toward the outside which can make the tip of your hand feel slightly numb is Shaku-Taku. This tsubo is approximately thirty centimeters above the wrist.

The name *Shaku-Taku* means the bank of a river where the grass and water meet. In Oriental medicine this tsubo is seen as the banks for the flow of energy along the meridian. This tsubo is located in the depression between bone and muscle where the meridian forms a sort of a creek. When this tsubo is pressed hard, it reduces circulation to cause the tips of the fingers to become numb. When there is pain or numbness in the hands, it presumably means that the flow of energy is stopped up at Shaku-Taku without it being pressed. Pressure and otherwise acupuncture or moxibustion are applied here to improve circulation and stop the numbness. Since this tsubo belongs to the lung meridian, it goes without saying that it is effective for lung symptoms such as dryness in the mouth, oppressive feeling in the chest and palpitation, just like the other tsubos of the lung meridian.

5. Kō-Sai 孔最 (LU-6)——*Tsubo for colds*

Recently, due to air pollution there has been a large increase in the number of people suffering from symptoms similar to asthma. Children and old people seem to be the most affected. Kō-Sai 孔最 (LU-6), aside from use in colds, is very effective in quieting coughing fits which occur in the middle of the night, or early in the morning.

To locate Kō-Sai, face your palm upward and find the place one third the distance to the wrist from the elbow and lightly pinch toward the outside of the arm using your fingers. There is usually a slight tingling pain here and applying some pressure can be enough to cause a person to cry out.

The character *Sai* 最 is used to add emphasis to some expression, and in Kō-Sai, it means that the harmful energy in the lung meridian readily accumulates here. It is a *geki* 郄 point where muscles and bone intersect. A formula in Oriental medicine says, "treat acute symptoms using the *geki* point." Sudden coughing spells are, in fact, relieved just by pressing Kō-Sai. When the symptoms are very severe, applying pressure in addition, to the tsubo on the back on either side of the third thoracic vertebra (Hai-Yu 肺兪: UB-13), is even more effective. Aside from coughing spells, Kō-Sai is used to relieve symptoms such as chronic asthma, a constant oppressive feeling in the chest, phlegm discharge and various types of coughs.

6. Tai-En 太淵 (LU-9)——*Tsubo to check for abnormalities in the lungs*

In Oriental medicine, as mentioned many times already, all symptoms and diseases are regarded as being the result of an obstruction in the flow of energy along a meridian. The character *En* 淵 in Tai-En 太淵 (LU-9) means a deep pool, such as that found under a waterfall, where the water flow tends to collect and come to a stop. All the harmful energy of the lung meridian is said to accumulate here at Tai-En. In other words, you do not have to bare your chest to check whether a symptom is related to the lung meridian. You can find out right away just by checking this tsubo. Tai-En is thus one of the most important tsubo on the lung meridian.

Spread your fingers wide apart and look at your wrist and you will see a thick tendon in the wrist at the base of the thumb. Tai-En is the place on the wrist to the outside of this tendon that is sensitive to light pressure. This tsubo is used often to cure coughing fits and sore throats, as well as all other symptoms related with the lung meridian. In Japan there used to be a folk remedy where children with asthma would receive mild moxa treatment on the outside corner of their wrists. Although this may seem like a strange practice, it is a very sound way of relieving asthma attacks because burning moxa on Tai-En is based on the empirical knowledge of Oriental medicine.

7. Gyo-Sai 魚際 (LU-10)——*Tsubo for diarrhea*

In the Orient the muscle at the base of the thumb on the palm is said to resemble the belly of a fish. The tsubo Gyo-Sai 魚際 (LU-10) is on the inside edge of the thumb bone above the wrist. To locate this tsubo pinch the muscle there and find the point that is the most sensitive.

Gyo-Sai is used to cure intestinal trouble. When a person gets diarrhea as the result of eating or drinking too much, just touching this tsubo will cause a blue streak to appear. Pressing this tsubo for a while, however, will make the blue streak disappear. This should also serve to give relief from diarrhea. From times past in Japan it has been said that if there was intestinal trouble blue veins appeared on the belly of the fish, and that Gyo-Sai was the tsubo to use for improving the condition of the stomach. The reason a tsubo of the lung meridian is used for the stomach is because, as explained earlier, both the lung and large intestine meridians are associated with the element metal and they form a yin-yang relationship.

When a person gets very tired, this can cause the palms to feel quite hot, and Gyo-Sai is one of the tsubo which works to correct this. If a person works more after already being tired out, a simple cold can turn into bronchitis or pneumonia, and the very first signs of this appears at Gyo-Sai.

8. Shō-Shō 少商 (LU-11)——*Tsubo for curing a raspy voice*

The last tsubo of the lung meridian is Shō-Shō 少商 (LU-11) which is located on the outside of the base of the thumb nail. The first character Shō 少 means small, or otherwise an end point. This refers to Shō-Shō being at the very end of the meridian. The second character *Shō* 商 refers to the fourth note in the Chinese music scale correlated with the five elements—*kaku* 角, *chi* 徵, *kyū* 宮, *shō* 商 and *u* 羽. This scale was used by the court orchestra and corresponds to the elements wood, fire, earth, metal and water in nature. *Shō* corresponds to metal which means it is related with the lung and large intestine meridians. Thus, just the name *Shō-Shō* indicates that the tsubo is located at the end of either the lung or large intestine meridians. In this manner, most names for the tsubo have a special meaning which reveals something about its location or remedial effects.

The note *shō* in court music is a squeaky high pitched note, and in fact, when the lungs are ailing a person's voice tends to become raspy and high pitched. In other words, the note *shō* is the sound caused by lung diseases. Shō-Shō is also effective in relieving the feeling of hotness in palms which comes from fatigue.

2. Large Intestine Meridian

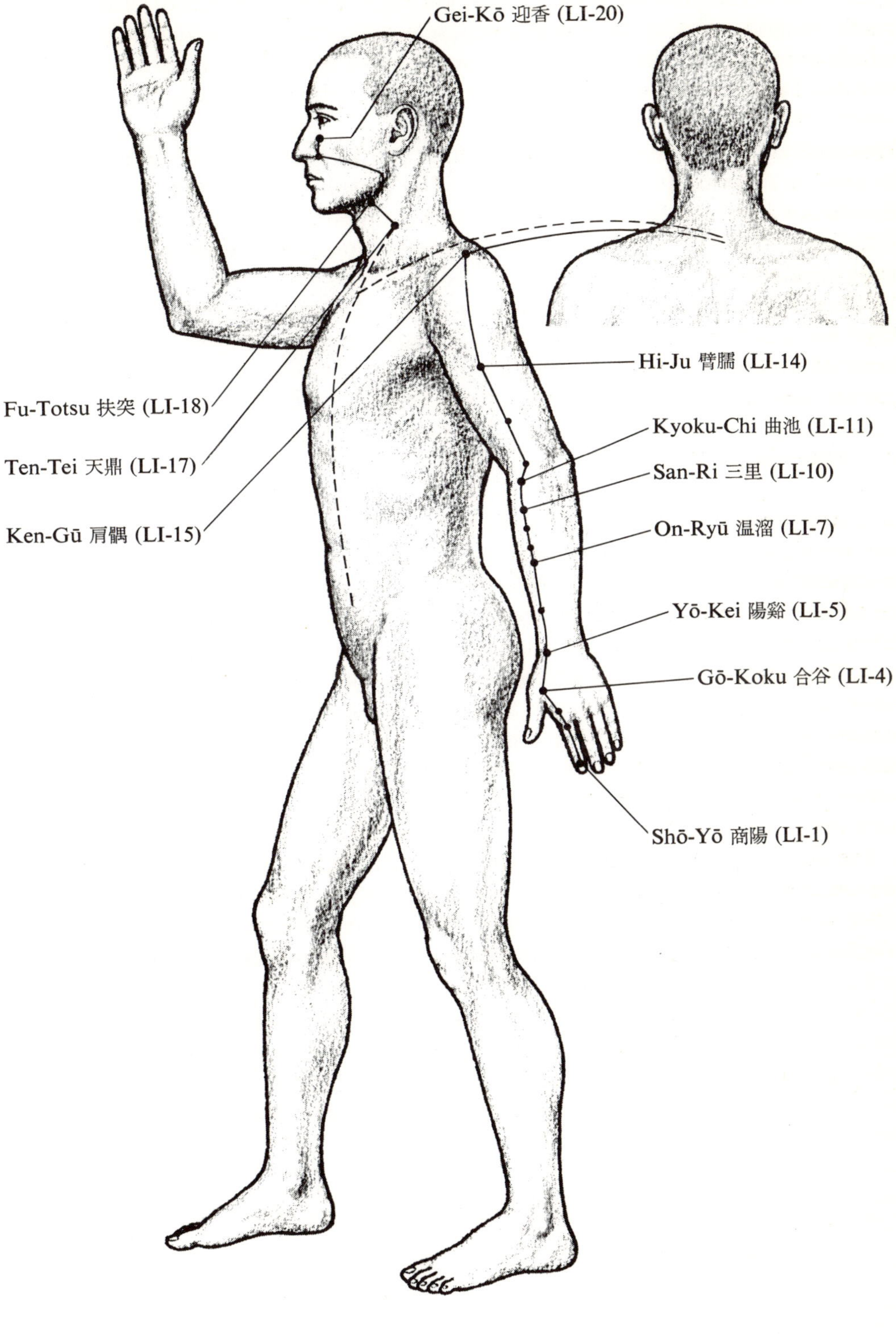

The large intestine meridian is closely connected with the lung meridian. As one evidence of this, when there is a problem in the lung meridian, one's nutritional condition deteriorates and the skin begins to appear transparent. Further, when the function of the respiratory organs are impaired, the same poor state of nutrition results. In such cases, if the function of the large intestines involved with digestion is strengthened, one's physical condition will improve of its own accord, and the functional state of the lungs and other respiratory organs will be restored.

According to medical science the large intestine is a section of the digestive tract about one and a half meters in length which lies between the small intestines and the anus, and consists of the cecum, the colon and the rectum. According to Oriental medicine the large intestine starts from the small intestines at the height of the tsubo Sui-Bun 水分 (CV-9) located about three centimeters above the navel. It subsequently winds around and stacks over itself sixteen times before it reaches the anus through the rectum. Supposedly, digested materials are separated into liquid and solid wastes at Sui-Bun and the large intestine is the organ which carries the solid wastes out of the body.

When problems arise in the large intestine and the meridian passing through it, the following symptoms may occur. First of all the eyes turn yellowish; toothaches, nasal congestion and occasional nosebleeds occur; there is dryness in the mouth, swelling and soreness of the throat and neck pain. Also, pain travels down the shoulders and arms, and in particular, down to the index finger so that at times this finger cannot be used. In such cases, if a person is examined closely there will be a hardened and tense area on either side of the navel (this is the tsubo Ten-Sū 天枢 (ST-25) introduced with the stomach meridian) as well on both sides of the vertebrae right below where the belt goes across (Dai-Chō-Yu 大腸兪: UB-25). When these points are lightly pinched or pressed and this causes a characteristic sensation which cannot be felt anywhere else, it is a warning from the large intestine, so rub or otherwise apply pressure to the appropriate tsubo of the large intestine meridian right away. Also, try thermal stimulation from time to time.

The large intestine meridian begins at the base of the nail on the index finger. As shown in the figure, starting at the index finger, this meridian goes straight up the forearm in line with the thumb, and going past the elbow and upper arm, it goes around and reaches the backbone. After meeting at the base of the neck, this meridian travels through the supraclavicular fossa (the hollow area above the clavicle) and goes inside the chest and down to the lungs. After passing through the lungs, this meridian enters the large intestine to circulate there, where it comes to an end. The other branch of this meridan which separates at the supraclavicular fossa travels up the neck to the cheeks and goes through the lower teeth and around the mouth to reach a point right between the nose and the lips. The meridian from the right and left cross over here and end at either side of the nose. The tsubos of the large intestine meridian are all located along the meridian just described, and there are a total of twenty tsubos. Eleven of the most commonly used tsubos among these will be presented here.

9. Shō-Yō 商陽 (LI-1)——*Tsubo for mild diarrhea*

The large intestine meridian begins at Shō-Yō 商陽 (LI-1). This tsubo is located on the outside corner at the base of the index finger's nail. The name *Sho-Yō* indicates that the lung meridian which traveled from the base of the neck down the arms to Shō-Shō 少商 (LU-11) at the tip of the thumbs switches over to the large intestine meridian at this tsubo. As explained earlier, in Oriental medicine the meridians are all associated with either a *zang*, which is yin, or a *fu*, which is yang. The name Shō-Yō came about because Shō-Shō of the yin meridian transfers over to the yang (*Yō* 陽 in Japanese) large intestine meridian. The first point or terminal point of each meridian is called the "well point," and these are held to be a very important point.

Among all the points of the large intestine meridian Shō-Yō is especially effective for diarrhea resulting from intestinal trouble. This tsubo is effective not just for ordinary diarrhea, but for that which occurs during a cold when a person has a fever. As you may well know, the intestines and colds are not entirely unrelated. When people have a cold, quite often their bellys have been chilled, so along with the cold symptoms such as a fever and a headache, there is griping stomach pain and diarrhea. In these cases this tsubo will have the effect of killing two birds with one stone.

10. Gō-Koku 合谷 (LI-4)——*Tsubo indicating stomach condition*

Gō-Koku 合谷 (LI-4) is also called *Ko-Kō* 虎口 (tiger's mouth). This is because it is on the back of the web between the thumb and index finger, and the shadow made by opening and closing the thumb against the fingers resembles a tiger's mouth. The most important tsubo in any meridian is the *gen* 原 (source) point, and the *gen* point of the large intestine meridian is Gō-Koku. In other words, one can find out at a glance, or rather, by a touch, whether there is a problem in the large intestine meridian. Lightly pinch or press this tsubo and you will find a hard spot which moves around a bit. If there are any symptoms caused by problems in the large intestine this point will be very sensitive.

Lightly press this tsubo without tensing this area between the finger and thumb. Note how this feels and then stretch out your legs and lie on your back to check the hardness of your belly. If the hardness is similar to that of Gō-Koku, it means the condition of the stomach and intestines are good, while if there is a difference in consistency, it means their functions are impaired. In abdominal diagnosis of Oriental medicine a hard abdomen is called a *jitsu* 実 (excess) condition and a soft abdomen is called a *kyo* 虚 (deficient) condition.

Aside from this, Gō-Koku is highly valued for its effectiveness against sore throats, pain in the gums and teeth, eye fatigue, tinnitus (ringing in the ears) and especially facial furuncles (boils).

11. Yō-Kei 陽谿 (LI-5)——*Tsubo for wrist pain*

The character *Yō* 陽 in Yō-Kei 陽谿 (LI-5) is the same as the one in Shō-Yō 商陽 (LI-1) and shows that it belongs to the yang large intestine meridian. Also, it shows that this tsubo is on the back of the hand since generally tsubos on the back of the hand are yang, and those on the side of the palm are yin.

To find this point, extend your thumb as far out as it will go. This will cause two tendons to appear at the outside base of the thumb, and Yō-Kei is located in the hollow area between these tendons. The character *Kei* 谿 is used because this tsubo is likened to a canyon surrounded by steep mountains. Other tsubos located in hollow places or in a crevice between bone and muscle where the meridian energy flows are also given names with the character *Kei*.

The effectiveness of this tsubo for toothaches, sore throats, tinnitus and minor hearing problems has been proven since the old days. Also, this tsubo has a direct effect on various problems of the wrist joint because of its being located right on the wrist. It is the ideal tsubo when there is pain in moving the wrist, or when wrist movement feels hindered and is not smooth.

12. On-Ryū 温溜 (LI-7)——*Tsubo for acute large intestine symptoms*

The name *On-Ryū* 温溜 (LI-7) comes from "pathogenic heat" (*On* 温) which produces harmful energy that collects (*Ryū* 溜) at this tsubo. Harmful energy refers to various causes of diseases such as "pathogenic wind." Since On-Ryū is the *geki* point of the large intestine meridian, it is especially effective for acute symptoms.

On-Ryū is located right at the midpoint between the wrist and elbow, in line with the thumb. If you carefully massage and press this area between the wrist and the outside of the elbow, lightly pinching up the skin there, you will find a muscle which is harder than the others. When this muscle is pressed straight down, it causes a surprisingly sharp pain.

This tsubo has traditionally been regarded as being effective for "exterior heat" of the large intestine, and today it is used most often for acute intestinal catarrh (inflammation), upset stomachs accompanied with fever, and febrile diarrhea. Otherwise On-Ryū is commonly used for muscular pain in the arms and legs, as well as for toothaches, just as Gō-Koku 合谷 (LI-4) and Yō-Kei 陽谿 (LI-5) are. It goes without saying that using a combination of tsubos effective for the same symptom usually increase the effect.

13. San-Ri 三里 (LI-10)——*Tsubo for calming irritation*

There is a tsubo named *San-Ri* 三里 (LI-10) also on the legs. To distinguish this tsubo, it is referred to as the San-Ri of the arm, or the upper San-Ri. It is located on the forearm in line with the thumb and about six centimeters from the outer crease of the elbow. If the skin here is pinched up lightly or pressed firmly from the outside of the elbow toward the thumb, there will be something similar to a tendon which is sensitive, and when pressed strongly the sensation may reach down to Gō-Koku 合谷 (LI-4), the tsubo mentioned earlier. Right below San-Ri on the same meridian are the tsubos Jō-Ren 上廉 (LI-9) and Ge-Ren 下廉 (LI-8). The name *San-Ri* (three villages) came about because it was likened to the third village along the same path.

Aside from calming down emotional excitement, San-Ri has long been used for people whose throats get sore and tonsils become swollen by the slightest infection, and otherwise for diarrhea. Also, if a person has a bad case of acne and pimples, pressing this tsubo will cause great pain. In this case, either thermal stimulation, or massaging with light pressure is highly effective. This tsubo is also used for hemiplegia and brachial neuralgia.

14. Kyoku-Chi 曲池 (LI-11)——*Tsubo for headaches and diarrhea*

The tsubo located at the outside of the elbow's crease is Kyoku-Chi 曲池 (LI-11). *Kyoku* 曲 means bend, and it is right where the elbow bends. The character *Chi* 池 (pond) was added to make the name because harmful energy in the body tends to collect here. When harmful energy collects here like waste water, it means that the organ supplied by this meridian (the large intestine) is somehow malfunctioning.

This "pond" rather than being a nuisance by collecting waste water, is an important point where the condition of the large intestine can be examined by the amount of harmful energy present there. The symptoms caused by the large intestine can all be removed by cleaning out this "pond" and making sure that the water (energy) flows unobstructed.

Among the symptoms associated with the large intestine, this tsubo is especially effective for diarrhea, headaches and heaviness of the head which results from large intestine problems, and conditions where the skin gets hot and feverish. The harmful energy when one has a fever is called "pathogenic heat." For such cases, apart from Kyoku-Chi, also use San-Ri 三里 (LI-10) and Gō-Koku 合谷 (LI-4) listed earlier. Other applications for Kyoku-Chi include that for hemorrhoids and pain or numbness in the arms.

15. Hi-Ju 臂臑 (LI-14)——*Tsubo for brachial neuralgia*

In Oriental medicine the forearm from the wrist to the elbow is called *Hi* 臂 and the upper arm from the elbow to the shoulder is called *Ju* 臑. Hi-Ju 臂臑 (LI-14) got its name because it is effective for symptoms of both the upper and lower arm. The location of this tsubo is approximately twenty-two centimeters from the previously mentioned Kyoku-Chi 曲池 (LI-11), to the outside of the upper arm. There is no need to worry about the exact distance since this varies from person to person. This tsubo is just where the deltoid muscle of the shoulder turns into a tendon on the outside of the upper arm.

When receiving an injection, ideally, the hypodermic needle goes into the deltoid muscle from below the shoulder, but occasionally when the needle is placed farther down toward the middle of the arm, it can cause paralysis in the hand.

This is because a nerve right beneath Hi-Ju, the radial nerve which controls the thumb and index finger, is damaged accidentally. It can be understood from this how important this tsubo is in maintaining the proper functioning of the arm. Therefore, its effects are most pronounced for pain resulting from brachial neuralgia or frozen shoulders.

16. Ken-Gū 肩髃 (LI-15)——*Tsubo for frozen shoulders*

The deltoid muscle on the end of the shoulder becomes large when the arm is raised to the horizontal position. When this muscle is felt with the arm raised, there is a cleft toward the front. This cleft is where Ken-Gū 肩髃 (LI-15) is located. Press the index finger into this cleft and move it back and forth until you find a big tendon. When this tendon is pressed hard by applying force from the elbow, there should be a point which causes a dull pain reaching all the way down the arm, especially to the index and middle fingers.

Often, company managers around the age of fifty complain that their shoulders get stiff and sore from doing the same work. Ken-Gū is most effective tsubo for such symptoms of shoulder pain, often referred to as "frozen shoulder." Try relaxing during a break from work and apply finger pressure to this tsubo alternately to both sides. A person should be able to obtain simple relief from frozen shoulders in this way without the need for strong massaging or vigorous movement of the arms. This tsubo is also very effective for pain and numbness in the arms.

Thermal stimulation is especially effective on this tsubo. Place a ball of moxa as large as the end of your thumb on this tsubo, and light it and let it burn down until the heat is felt; then quickly remove it. Repeating this four or five times in a row will warm up your shoulder and relax it considerably.

17. Ten-Tei 天鼎 (LI-17)——*Tsubo for high blood pressure*

To locate Ten-Tei 天鼎 (LI-17), first turn your head as far as you can to the left. This will cause a tendon to appear at the front base of the neck. Following this muscle upward, you will find that it ends at a protrusion in the skull behind the ears. This muscle is the sternocleidomastoid muscle. The trapezius muscle goes from the side of the neck to the tip of the shoulder. The clavicle lies below to the front of both these muscles. A triangle is formed between the clavicle and the trapezius and sternocleidomastoid muscles. Ten-Tei is located close to the top of this anatomical triangle, behind the sternocleidomastoid muscle.

Tei 鼎, the second character of this tsubo, represents a ceremonial vessel, a three legged vase, which was used for such things as burning incense. This tsubo probably got this character from being at the top corner of a triangle. To the inside of the sternocleidomastoid muscle, where this tsubo is located, lies blood vessels which connect the heart and brain, as well as numerous nerves, so it is a very vital area. It is also a very important location for regulating blood flow, and when there are abnormalities in circulation caused by high blood pressure, a hardened spot or knot forms close to this tsubo. Ten-Tei is stimulated to relax this hard spot. Aside from this, Ten-Tei is used for sore throats, toothaches and pain in the tonsils.

18. Fu-Totsu 扶突 (LI-18)——*Tsubo for lowering blood pressure*

Fu-Totsu 扶突 (LI-18) is located about ten centimeters to either side of the Adam's apple, and it is effective in relieving the previously mentioned stiffness in the sternocleidomastoid muscle, as well as symptoms of the throat such as asthma, coughing, and difficulty in breathing.

The character *Fu* 扶 in China means the width of four fingers. Try placing four fingers—the index finger, middle finger, ring finger and little finger—vertically on your throat next to the Adam's apple. The finger toward the back will reach the sternocleidomastoid muscle which goes from the back of the ear to the top of the chest. Fu-Totsu is located in this sternocleidomastoid muscle.

If you feel back from the Adam's apple, you will find a place where the carotid artery is pulsating. Fu-Totsu lies just to the back of this artery, so it is a tsubo which has a great deal of influence on circulation around the throat and through the neck. This tsubo, along with Jin-Gei 人迎 (ST-9) of the stomach meridian and Ten-Chū 天柱 (UB-10) of the urinary bladder meridian, has long been known as an indispensable tsubo for lowering blood pressure. Fu-Totsu also lies in the path of the vagus nerve which is responsible for symptoms such as belching, nausea and upset stomachs, as well as the sensation of hunger. Tsubos along this path are commonly used for improving the condition of the stomach.

19. Gei-Kō 迎香 (LI-20)——*Tsubo for nasal obstruction*

Among the classifications of the five elements, there is what is called the "five odors." These are the five basic aromas chosen and categorized according to the five elements as well as the shape and color of their corresponding organs. These five ordors are, rancid (臊), burned (焦), fragrant (香), fishy (腥) and putrid (腐). Matching these odors up with the five elements and the organs (meridians), rancid corresponds to wood and the liver and gallbladder, burned corresponds to fire and the heart and small intestine, fragrant corresponds to earth and the spleen and stomach, fishy corresponds to metal and the lungs and large intestine, and finally, putrid corresponds to water and the kidney and urinary bladder. Thus, according to the five odors, the stomach and spleen are associated with fragrance. Gei-Kō 迎香 (LI-20) (welcome fragrance) means that the large intestine is coming to an end and is switching over to the stomach and spleen meridians.

The location of this tsubo is right beside the nose, or to either side of the wings of the nose. Gei-Kō is effective for nasal obstruction, facial paralysis on one side and facial neuralgia.

3. Stomach Meridian

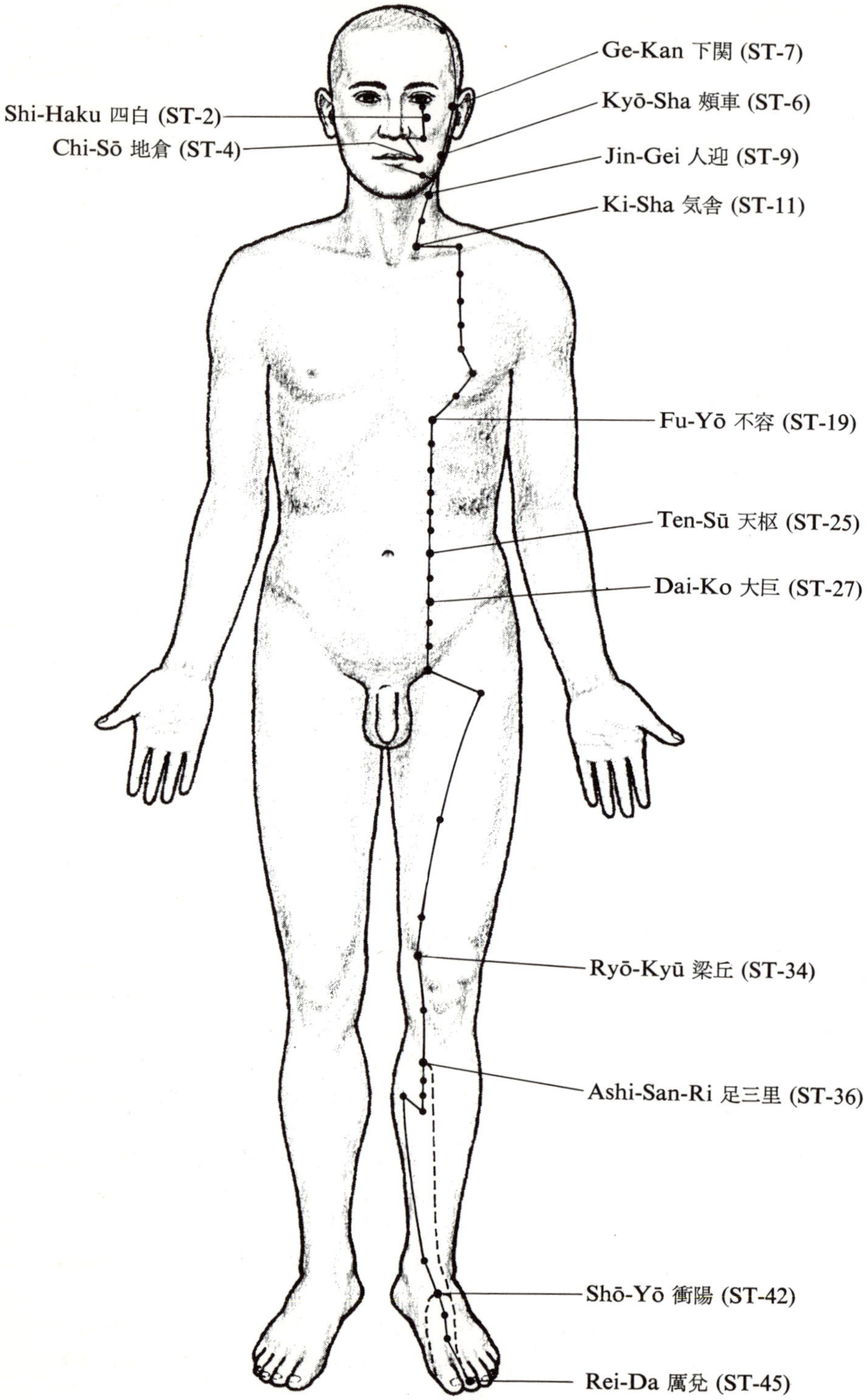

As you may well know, the stomach is an organ under the diaphragm lying beside the liver, and serves an indispensable role in digestion. Therefore, this meridian has a large number of tsubos and covers a large area of the body from head to toe. It begins from Gei-Kō 迎香 (LI-20) and travels up the side of the nose to cross over to the inner corner of the eye on the other side and from there it goes down and flows through the upper teeth and crosses over once more at the lower lip. The stomach meridian then divides at the side of the chin and one branch goes up the side of the face to the middle of the forehead, and the other branch goes to the supraclavicular fossa where it divides again into two branches. The surface meridian travels down the chest and stomach while the internal branch circulates through the stomach and spleen (pancreas). The surface meridian goes over the inguinal region down the outside of the thigh and divides again further down to terminate at the ends of the second and third toes.

As to the symptoms for which the tsubos of the stomach meridian are known to be effective, firstly a very common place symptom, the headache, can be raised. These tsubos are especially effective for headaches extending from the forehead to the back of the skull. These tsubos also work for nasal obstruction, occasional nosebleeds, sores around the mouth due to poor stomach condition, swelling of the throat, neck pain, tension in the stomach area, as well as fatigue, numbness or pain in the thighs, knees, lower legs and back of the legs, and down to the tip of the second toe. It goes without saying that tsubos of the stomach meridian are effective for symptoms caused by stomach trouble, but aside from this, these tsubos are good for people whose blood tends to rush to their head.

People with the above mentioned symptoms are easy to spot. First of all their face and skin lack luster and appears either yellow or greyish. Their lips are usually thin and chapped and wrinkled. Their voice is generally cheerful and melodious, but their pronunciation is unclear. They get worried about things easily and tend to succumb to the summer heat. They like sweet things, but they usually prefer bland food to strongly flavored food. For these people, standing for any length of time, or sitting still for a long period causes cramps. There are many people like this around.

Lie on your back and lightly press in the area between your navel and solar plexus using both hands with your left hand placed over your right. Is there any oppressive pain? Next, stand up straight with your arms straight down to your side. The elbows are usually at the height of the twelfth thoracic vertebra, so apply pressure there on either side of the spine. Do you find any hard spots or pain there? If these signs are present, it can be stated with certainty that there is some problem with the stomach.

The stomach meridian has forty-five tsubos on each side. Detailed explanation will be provided here for thirteen particularly important tsubos among these.

20. Shi-Haku 四白 (ST-2)——*Tsubo for eye fatigue and facial neuralgia*

Touching right below the eyes you can feel the hard skull bone. Going down about three centimeters from there to press the area next to the nose, a dull pain can be felt which sometimes reaches the eyes. This is the tsubo called *Shi-Haku* 四白 (ST-2). The character *Haku* 白, aside from white, means empty or hollow. This probably refers to the hollow area below the eyes.

This tsubo is very effective when people cannot close their eyes and when they cannot laugh due to facial paralysis, as well as when there is pain in the upper cheeks due to facial neuralgia. The nerve affected in facial neuralgia (the trigeminal nerve) comes from the base of the brain and one of its branches comes out to the upper rim of the eyes to reach the forehead, and another branch comes through the skull at Shi-Haku to extend under the eyes, to the nose, the cheeks, the area in front of the ears and the upper jaw. So try applying firm finger pressure at this tsubo in cases of facial neuralgia where the right half of the face is in real pain, especially around the eyes, nose and upper jaw. Such a treatment is often enough to relieve spasmodic pain in the upper jaw. Pressure should be applied to this tsubo also for facial spasms which cause occasional involuntary winking. Shi-Haku is also known as being effective for eyestrain.

21. Chi-Sō 地倉 (ST-4)——*Tsubo for sores at the corner of the mouth*

Chi-Sō 地倉 (ST-4) is among the commonly used tsubos in the stomach meridian. It lies on either corner of the mouth. This is a place where sores and small eczema form easily due to stomach problems. It has been substantiated in modern medicine also that this point serves as a barometer for knowing the condition of the stomach. When sores form in this area, also the mouth takes on a bad odor.

As to the origin of the name *Chi-Sō*, *Chi* 地 is earth of heaven and earth, or otherwise, the "energy of earth." In Oriental medicine the vital energy breathed in through the nose and then breathed out—what we call air—is called the "energy of heaven." In contrast to this, the "energy of earth" refers to food, or the five grains of the Orient which corresponds with the five elements—rice, oats, foxtail millet, Chinese millet, and common millet. This "energy of earth" is taken in from the mouth and reaches the stomach. The stomach is also called *Tai-Sō* 大倉 (large storehouse). So the energy of earth was thought to pass through the mouth and reach the "large storehouse." This is why the corners of the mouth came to be called *Chi-Sō*.

This tsubo is effective for stomach problems and various facial symptoms arising from stomach trouble, as well as distortion of the mouth and difficulty in speech caused by high blood pressure.

22. Kyō-Sha 頬車 (ST-6)——*Tsubo for pain in lower jaw and teeth*

One of the most commonly used tsubo in the stomach meridian is Kyō-Sha 頬車 (ST-6) on the cheek. The character *Kyō* 頬 (cheek) indicates the location of the tsubo. *Sha* 車 is a wheel, and means the place where the jaw pivots as if it were the hub of a wheel. In other words, it refers to the joint of the jaws. When the jaw is opened and closed, a lump forms to the front of the ear. Kyō-Sha is located right below this lump on the outer corner of the jaw where it pivots. This tsubo has long been known to relieve pain in the teeth and gums.

The area in front of the ear is full of muscles for chewing and one of these in front of the ear can be felt by gritting your teeth. Sometimes this muscle goes into a spasm. Just applying pressure at Kyō-Sha is very effective when this muscle is twitching. This tsubo is also very effective for facial neuralgia where the pain runs from in front of the ears down to the lower jaw and the tip of the chin. It is especially effective when relatively strong thumb pressure is applied from the back of the jaw below the earlobe toward the front, and also when massaged in small circles with the fingertips.

23. Ge-Kan 下関 (ST-7)——*Tsubo to stop tooth- and earaches*

Take your fingers from just in front of the ears and feel along the cheek bone to the highest point. This is called the zygomatic arch. Press the bottom rim of this bone from the ear toward the nose. The first big depression is the tsubo Ge-Kan 下関 (ST-7), and strong pressure here will cause a penetrating sensation in the jaw. The character *Kan* 関 of Ge-Kan means to separate. In other words, this tsubo is located where the cheek bone divides the cheek and temple. *Ge* 下 means that this tsubo is *under* this bone.

This tsubo is effective for relieving toothaches and earaches, and also it is used along with the previously mentioned Kyō-Sha 頬車 (ST-6) for neuralgia affecting the area between the lower eyelid and the upper jaw. There are times when taking a nap in the summertime with the fan cooling just one side of the face causes half of the face to become paralyzed. Then the eyes cannot be closed, the cheeks cannot be puffed out, the mouth is drawn to one side and saliva escapes. These symptoms are called Bell's palsy or facial paralysis. In such cases, stroking, rubbing and massaging around Ge-Kan, and making faces in front of the mirror will eventually cure the problem without any special treatment. In Oriental medicine this disease is known as *Kō-Gan-Ka-Sha* 口眼過斜 (mouth and eyes very slanted) which aptly describes the symptoms.

24. Jin-Gei 人迎 (ST-9)——*Tsubo for lowering blood pressure*

To locate Jin-Gei 人迎 (ST-9), place your thumb and index finger on either side of your throat. You will find a pulsating artery about five centimeters behind the Adam's apple. This tsubo is located on one of the most important areas of our body, the neck, which connects the head and the trunk. This vital area is called Jin-Gei in Oriental medicine, and the pulse here is referred to as the "Jin-Gei pulse." There is a traditional method of diagnosing a person's physical condition by comparing the pulse at Jin-Gei to that of the wrist (radial artery).

First of all, Jin-Gei is very effective in reducing blood pressure, and is highly valued by people with hypertension. There is an important nerve receptor which controls blood pressure right around Jin-Gei, so blood pressure can be lowered by stimulating this tsubo without having to resort to drugs. This tsubo is remarkably effective also for asthma and inflammation caused by chronic bronchitis, as well as Hashimoto's disease, a chronic hyperthyroidism on the increase lately among Japanese women.

25. Ki-Sha 気舎 (ST-11)——*Tsubo for stomach symptoms*

Why are tsubos of the stomach meridian located on the neck? Many readers may think of Oriental medicine as being very peculiar in some respects, but the neck is, in fact, very closely associated with the stomach and intestines. When problems arise in the visceral organs, at times there is a definite sensation of pain, and at other times there is great discomfort although there is no pain. The discomfort may range from nausea, a feeling of hunger, to the tense feeling caused by a full bladder. These are called organic sensations, and are picked up by the vagus nerve which comes out of the brain and passes through the sternocleidomastoid muscle at the side of the neck and reaches all the way down to the visceral organs. Just recently it has become widely recognized that tsubos around the sternocleidomastoid muscle are good for abdominal discomfort. Ki-Sha 気舎 (ST-11) is located right in this important area.

Ki-Sha 気舎 (energy lodge) means the place where harmful energy collects. This tsubo is located right next to the top button of the shirt, and is on the top corner of the sternum (breast bone) and above the inside tip of the clavicle. This is right next to the lymph nodes in the supraclavicular fossa which have a deep connection to the functioning of the digestive organs. Therefore, this tsubo is effective for various symptoms of the stomach as already mentioned. Unfortunately, it cannot cure stomach cancer, but it can serve as an aid in early detection. Also, since this tsubo is located on the neck, it is good for such things as "a crick in the neck."

26. Fu-Yō 不容 (ST-19)——*Tsubo for a chronically weak stomach*

The character *Fu* 不 originally meant beginning, while *Yō* 容 means container, and thus Fu-Yō 不容 (ST-19) means the tsubo on the very top of the stomach. This tsubo is located at the tip of the eighth rib, just to either side of the pit of the stomach. When there are stomach problems, there is usually pain and a distended feeling around the pit of the stomach and below the ribs, and just light pressure on this area feels painful. Fu-Yō is the most efficacious tsubo for relieving various stomach symptoms. This includes continuous pain and discomfort in the stomach area, occasional sharp colic pain, belching, heartburn, food setting in the stomach, a feeling of oppression as if the stomach was being pressed in and the retention of liquids in the stomach. These symptoms caused by diseases such as gastrasthenia, chronic gastritis, gastroatony and gastroptosis are alleviated to a great extent just by applying pressure to Fu-Yō. Also, aside from stomach symptoms, this tsubo is good for intercostal neuralgia where pain extends along the ribs from the spine. This pain can be relieved by rubbing along the affected rib and massaging this tsubo. In addition, Fu-Yō is used for mitigating coughing and breathing difficulty caused by asthma.

27. Ten-Sū 天枢 (ST-25)——*Tsubo for upset stomach*

There is a very important tsubo located three finger widths to either side of the navel which is good for all manner of stomach problems. There is a slight difference in the location according to each person, but Ten-Sū 天枢 (ST-25) lies approximately five or six centimeters to the side of the navel. When the stomach is upset and there is diarrhea or constipation, apply finger pressure here. This tsubo is effective not only for stomach trouble, but also for gynecological problems, so women should learn the location of this tsubo because it could come in handy.

In cases where there is a feeling of lassitude, a tendency to become tired easily, work is just a drag, and there is a lack of motivation, press Ten-Sū along with Kō-Yu 肓兪 (KI-16), a tsubo of the kidney meridian, which lies just to the inside of Ten-Sū, and it will likely cause a deep pain. In this case, usually there is a hard spot in the soles of the feet. This is called a "deficiency of kidney energy" in Oriental medicine, and is a sign that the physical condition is deteriorating. Acupuncture and moxibustion at Ten-Sū are also very effective ways to treat this condition.

In Oriental medicine the body is also divided at the navel into two halves, and the top half is called "heaven" and the bottom half, "earth." Ten-Sū got its name because the level of the navel which divides heaven (*Ten* 天) and earth is axial (*Sū* 枢) in the body.

28. Dai-Ko 大巨 (ST-27)——*Tsubo for menstrual problems*

Dai-Ko 大巨 (ST-27) is located about six centimeters below the previous tsubo mentioned. It is regarded as one of the main places where signs of diseases in the lower half of the body appear, so it is also called *Eki-Mon* 腋門 (fluid gate). The tsubos Katsu-Niku-Mon 滑肉門 (ST-24) and Dai-Ko together number four points right and left, and these are referred to as the "four spirit points," and they are of special importance among the tsubos on the abdomen.

When constipated and somewhat lacking in appetite, finger pressure to Dai-Ko will amazingly facilitate bowel movements and make the stomach feel much better. Dai-Ko on the left side, in particular, has been used for centuries to check for "stagnation of blood" in women, and to clear this obstruction. "Stagnation of blood" is another term for menstrual disorders, and this can become the cause for symptoms such as blood rising to the head, low back pain, tension in the lower abdomen and chilling of the feet. Therefore, along with the previously mentioned Ten-Sū 天枢 (ST-25), Dai-Ko is a precious tsubo for women.

Far below Dai-Ko, to the outside of where the thighs join the trunk, there is a tsubo by the name of Hi-Kan 髀関 (ST-31). We will not dwell on this tsubo, but it is very effective for low back pain coupled with a neuralgia-like pain to the outside of the thighs, so it should be kept in mind.

29. Ryō-Kyū 梁丘 (ST-34)——*Tsubo to stop gastrospasms*

When the knee is straightened out a groove will form to the outside of the kneecap. Lightly trace this groove upward and it will come to an end about seven centimeters from the top of the patella (kneecap). This is the location of Ryō-Kyū 梁丘 (ST-34). Among the various kinds of stomach pain, some are just psychosomatic, while others occur when there is actual stomach trouble. Ryō-Kyū is effective in stopping stomach pain especially of the former type, known as gastrospasm, where there is a sharp constrictive pain. Applying finger pressure to this tsubo over a period of time will make the stomach pain go away almost mysteriously.

There may be people who wish to know more specifically which diseases Ryō-Kyū is effective for, instead of just stomach pain in general. Names of diseases, however, are a question for Western medicine. In Oriental medicine symptoms are given the greatest attention and the question is always how to cure the symptoms. In any case, this tsubo gives direct results in relieving knee pain or swelling in the legs.

30. Ashi-San-Ri 足三里 (ST-36)——*Tsubo for health and longevity*

Ashi-San-Ri 足三里 (ST-36) is located on the outside of the lower leg about ten centimeters below the kneecap, just to the outside of the shin bone.

Moxibustion on Ashi-San-Ri has been practiced in Japan from centuries past as a way to health and logevity. The farmer Manpei in the province of Mikawa who supposedly lived to the age of 242 during the Edo period is said to have done this every day along with all the rest of his family. Also the renowned poet Bashō recorded in his work—*Okuno Hosomichi*—how he burned moxa on San-Ri during his travels. Further, there is a story of how the defeated Japanese troops in the Second World War, making a hasty retreat both by day and night, cut up pieces of their shirt to burn on San-Ri to help them make it back alive after marching for hundreds of miles.

San-Ri, with a host of stories about it from times past, is a tsubo effective for a wide variety of symptoms. It is used first and foremost for stomach problems and trouble with the digestive organs including problems of the liver and gallbladder, as well as various symptoms associated with diabetes such as general fatigue, loss of weight and excessive thirst. It is also effective for neuralgia, of the brain softening and fatigue of the legs coming from cerebral apoplexy (strokes). Further, San-Ri is good for problems with the respiratory organs causing discomfort in the chest, coughing, blood rising to the head, hotness or chilling of the feet and psychosomatic nose diseases.

31. Shō-Yō 衝陽 (ST-42)——*Tsubo for allergic constitutions*

It occasionally happens that nervous people with allergic constitutions complain of digestive problems and unconsciously poke the back of their feet with the tip of a pen or a pencil, or otherwise massage the highest point between the second and third toes. People with such constitutions often develop hard spots on the back of their feet, and their feet feel more comfortable after they are massaged on the back and also this causes the condition of their stomach to improve. Somehow these people unknowingly manage to press just the right tsubo. This place on the back of the foot where a pulse can be felt is Shō-Yō 衝陽 (ST-42), a tsubo which is considered very important among specialists of Oriental medicine.

Aside from the type of people with allergies as mentioned above, this tsubo is good for those who have a poor appetite and those with emotional problems. Shō-Yō has a deep connection with Ashi-San-Ri 足三里 (ST-36) mentioned before. People with allergic constitutions, especially those with digestive problems, will have a band of tension and hardness along the stomach meridian which extends from Ashi-San-Ri down to Shō-Yō. Giving thorough finger pressure and massages along this area with small circular movements will give relief and the stomach symptoms should ease.

32. Rei-Da 厲兌 (ST-45)——*Tsubo for gastric neurosis*

The very last tsubo of the stomach meridian is Rei-Da 厲兌 (ST-45). It is located just to the outside of the base of the second toenail. It has been known since the old days as being very effective for diabetes. Aside from this, it is used for toothaches and digestive disorders. Among stomach symptoms, Rei-Da is especially efficacious for cases of psychosomatic stomach trouble known as gastric neurosis. In this case, there is no real problem with the stomach, but irritation and stress cause an oppressive and heavy pain in the stomach along with nausea and an upset stomach.

The character *Rei* 厲 of Rei-Da means to advance or to encourage, and *Da* 兌 means to change. So in other words, Rei-Da facilitates the function of the stomach and changes over to the next meridian.

It is very significant in itself that a tsubo on the tip of the foot is effective for treating problems in the digestive organs like the stomach. This is because the tsubos were systematized through centuries of clinical experience. The principle in circulation of blood by modern physiology verifies that circulation through the hands and feet rely on an extremely delicate mechanism. When the circulation through peripheral vessels and capillaries is normal, the hands and feet stay warm. Further, when tsubo on the hands and feet are stimulated, it serves to facilitate circulation through the whole body, especially the abdominal area, and this in turn acts to alleviate a wide variety of symptoms.

4. Spleen Meridian

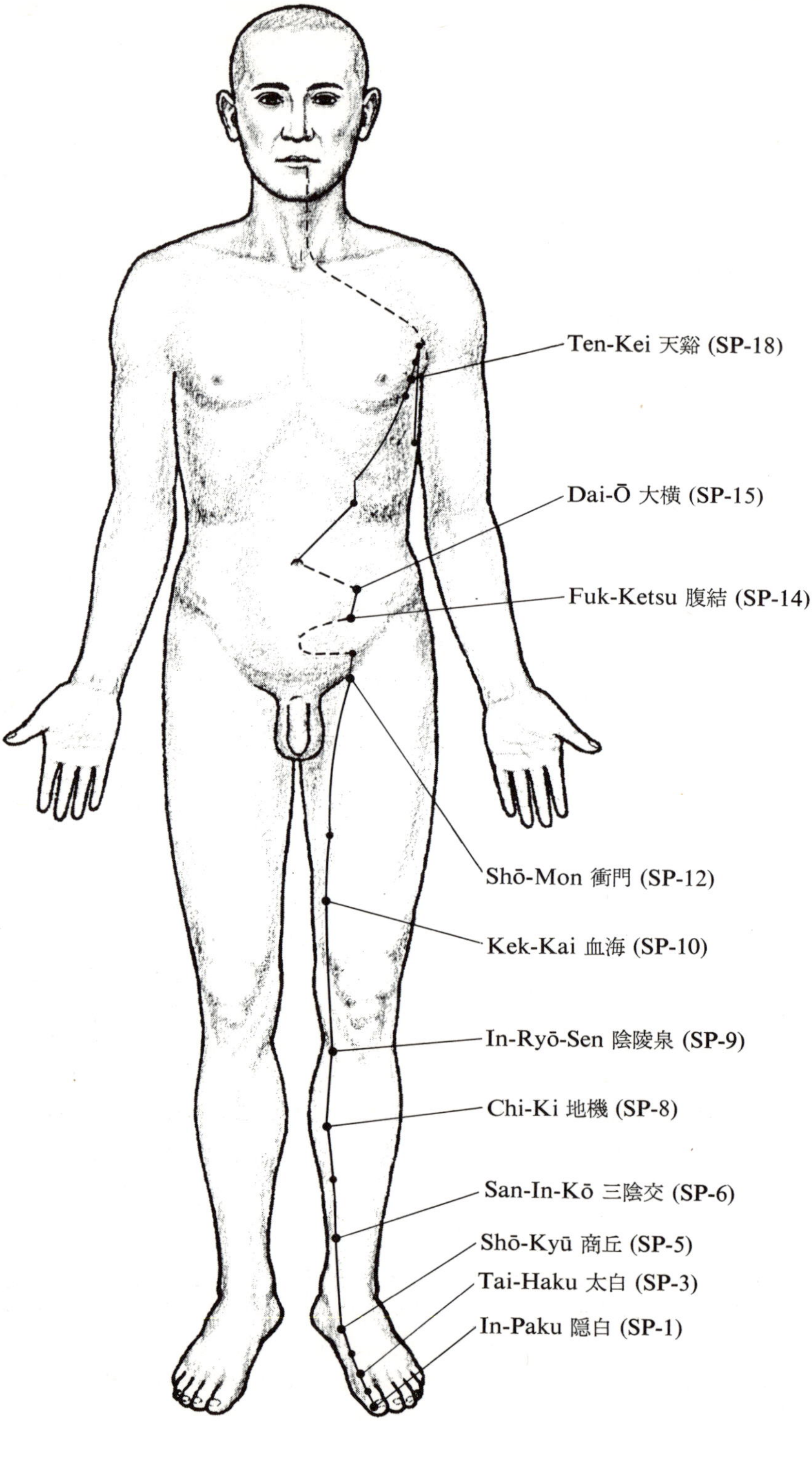

The spleen meridian is the meridian which circulates through the "spleen." The "spleen" in modern medical terms is the pancreas. The pancreas is a leaf-shaped yellow and greyish gland lying sidewise behind the stomach, and it secretes pancreatic juice. Pancreatic juice acts to further digest the food coming from the stomach. Also the pancreas produces and secretes a hormone called insulin which facilitates the metabolization of sugars and serves to maintain the appropriate level of sugar in the muscles and other tissues throughout the body. If the quantity of sugar absorbed in digestion is excessive, this is stored in the liver in the form of glycogen. When a shortage of sugar occurs in the muscle tissue, glycogen is converted into readily usable glucose to supply the area.

In Oriental medicine the function of the "spleen" is regarded as, warming the essential organs, covering the stomach and constantly working to digest and absorb the solid and liquid contents of the stomach. The digested materials were thought to go from the stomach directly to the "spleen" where this was distributed among the organs to nourish the whole body, fill out the physical frame and supply the skin and hair. The "spleen" is considered as being yin, and the stomach, yang. These yin and yang organs form an inseparable pair to facilitate the function of digestion and absorption.

What symptoms appear when the function of the "spleen" is impaired? First of all, the tongue becomes tied, there is an oppressive feeling or pain in the pit of the stomach accompanied with nausea and belching. Sometimes it becomes hard to swallow or to get food down, and either diarrhea or constipation becomes a problem. On top of this, the feet tend to get chilled and standing for long periods causes the knees and thighs to swell up. Additional symptoms may include insomnia and the whole body feeling run down. When tsubos of the spleen meridian are used in these cases, the symptoms can be relieved or cured completely.

The spleen meridian begins at the tsubo In-Paku 隠白 (SP-1), located close to the inside corner at the base of the big toenail. From there it goes to the inside ankle bone and goes up its front and travels upward passing on the inside of the shin bone. Next, it passes through the inside of the kneecap and goes up the inside front of the thigh and goes past the inguinal region and onto the belly. This meridian travels straight up the lower abdomen past the navel, and from there enters into the viscera to circulate around the "spleen" and reach the stomach. The surface branch of the meridian goes up onto the chest and passes to the outside of the nipples and ends up below the windpipe. A branch off the main channel travels through the stomach and goes to the heart where it connects with the heart meridian. The spleen meridian has twenty-one tsubos, and among these, eleven of the most used tsubos will be introduced.

33. In-Paku 隠白 (SP-1)——*Tsubo for convulsive fits in children*

Other names for In-Paku 隠白 (SP-1) include *Ki-Rui* 鬼塁 and *Ki-Gan* 鬼眼 and it is used commonly for children with convulsive fits, or those in overexcited states. It has been said since the old days that tsubos with the character *Ki* 鬼 (demon) in it were very good for calming a person down. *Ki* originally meant spirit, and a modern interpretation of this would be "mind." Thus, the other names of In-Paku probably indicate the effects of this tsubo on the mind.

People these days seem to become irritated over the slightest of things, but applying strong pressure to this tsubo next to the base of the big toenail should help relieve this irritation. This should be a much better way of relieving stress than finding diversion in drinking and gambling. Aside from calming a person down, In-Paku works to relieve the feeling of fullness in the stomach, nausea, chilling and numbness of the feet, as well as a feeling of fullness in the chest together with a mild fever. This tsubo is also used when there is the menstrual problem of excessive bleeding.

This tsubo got the name *In-Paku* because the outside of the foot is yang and the inside (the big toe) is yin in Oriental medicine, and since the arch of the foot is called *Haku-Niku* 白肉 (white flesh), they came to call this tsubo located next to the inside base of the big toenail *In-Paku* (yin white).

34. Tai-Haku 太白 (SP-3)——*Tsubo to check condition of "spleen"*

When the big toe is pulled upward and back, a thick tendon appears under the large joint of the big toe. Tai-Haku 太白 (SP-3) is located just above this tendon right in back of the bone protruding from the joint of the big toe. This is one of the most important tsubos in the spleen meridian.

The character *Tai* 太 is a honorific term similar to *Dai* 大 as used in the words captain or minister, and *Haku* has another meaning as a wine cup. So *Tai-Haku* means a big wine cup and it probably got the name from being in a hollow area like a *sake* cup. Also, as mentioned before, the skin on the arch of the foot is called "white flesh" and the name *Tai-Haku* also means that it is a prominent tsubo among those located on the boundary between the skin on the top and bottom of the foot. Applying light pressure or massaging Tai-Haku will produce a sharp pain when there are symptoms such as cold feet or stomach problems. This tsubo is very effective for relieving pain in the shins and cramps in the calf muscles. Another reason this tsubo is important because it is a *gen* point used to check the condition of the spleen and the stomach meridian. One rule of diagnosis in Oriental medicine states "the condition of the five essential organs are manifested around the four joints." This means the many important tsubos are located either to the front or back of the major joints including the wrist, ankles, elbows and knees. It is held that all diseases of the internal organs can be treated here.

35. Shō-Kyū 商丘 (SP-5)——*Tsubo to relieve stomach tension*

In a condition traditionally called *Ri-Kyū-Kō-Jyū* 裏急後重 (tenesmus) the large intestines are affected and there is a strong urge to defecate, but the bowel movements do not come. The stomach is filled with gas which produces rumbling sounds and the stomach feels tense and distended. *Ri-Kyū-Kō-Jyū* (interior rushing, rear heavy) means the interior or the digestive organs are trying to expel, but the bowels are heavy and slow to move. Shō-Kyū 商丘 (SP-5) is very effective against this kind of tenesmus. It is located to the front and bottom of the inner ankle bone, and just light pressure here can relieve a person of this condition.

Shō 商 means a high pitched melancholy note, and among the five elements it is related to metal which is associated with the lungs. Shō-Kyū therefore has a similar significance to the important tsubo Shō-Shō 少商 (LU-11) of the lung meridian. It can be understood from this that Shō-Kyū is also effective for various symptoms related to lung problems. It is even called the "lung metal point" of the spleen meridian, and the rule is to use this tsubo when an ailment of the spleen is accompanied with that of the lungs. This tsubo is also commonly used for pale complexions, coughs, gastrasthenia (weak stomach) and when the whole body feels tired and run down.

36. San-In-Kō 三陰交 (SP-6)——*Tsubo for fatigue in knees and legs*

As the name *San-In-Kō* 三陰交 (three yins cross) indicates, this is an important tsubo where three yin meridians (the great yin spleen meridian, the absolute yin liver meridian and the lesser yin kidney meridian) converge. San-In-Kō 三陰交 (SP-6) is located about ten centimeters above the inner ankle bone (medial malleolus) on the inside edge of the shin bone (tibia). Just remember this tsubo as being four finger widths above the top of the inside ankle bone.

In Japan there is a phrase "essential as the liver and kidneys," and this shows just how important the liver and kidneys are among the organs. When the body is divided in two at the navel, the liver is in the upper half (heaven section) and the kidney is in the lower half (earth section). The liver has traditionally been said to house courage and the kidney is thought to be the source of motivation. Therefore, people with courage and strong motivation who are also considerate and well mannered are regarded as having a strong liver and kidney—a sure sign of health. The "spleen" joins this vital pair to meet at the tsubo San-In-Kō where three yin meridians come together.

This tsubo is said to be good for fatigued legs and knees, as well as obesity, or loss of weight. Aside from this, it is used for low back pain and to calm down overexcitement. It is also said that acupuncture to this point during pregnancy can cause the fetus to die. There is even a story about how unscrupulous acupuncturists during the Edo period, in order to cover up the mischief of the ladies in the palace, induced abortions by placing needles in this tsubo. San-In-Kō, along with Gō-Koku 合谷 (LI-4) of the large intestine meridian, is famous for causing miscarriages. In actual practice, however, this effect is not so pronounced.

37. Chi-Ki 地機 (SP-8)——*Tsubo to increase appetite*

Lack of appetite, swelling of legs, infrequent urination and tension in the abdomen are all symptoms associated with the "spleen." Tracing up the inside edge of the shin bone from San-In-Kō 三陰交 (SP-6), you will reach a hard spot about fifteen centimeters below the knee which feels like a lump, or a tendon. Apply light pressure here and it should cause a deep pain which almost makes one cry out. This is the tsubo Chi-Ki 地機 (SP-8) and it is the *geki* point of the greater yin spleen meridian. *Geki* 郄 means crevice or cleft, and here it means a groove between muscle and bone. In Oriental medicine acute symptoms are treated at the *geki* points, and these points are traditionally held to be very important. Along with Tai-Haku 太白 (SP-3), mentioned earlier, Chi-Ki is a tsubo where symptoms like chilling or swelling of the feet, lack of urination or poor stomach conditions can be detected very easily. When such symptoms exist, rubbing, massaging or applying hot compresses on this tsubo will alleviate the symptoms.

38. In-Ryō-Sen 陰陵泉 (SP-9)——*Tsubo for knee pain*

Not too long ago, the "miracle of Chinese medicine" was publicized where brain surgery was conducted under acupuncture anesthesia, and this caused a big sensation throughout the world. In-Ryō-Sen 陰陵泉 (SP-9) happens to be one of the tsubos used in this procedure. In the classics of Oriental medicine it is listed as being "under the medial condyle." In-Ryō-Sen is generally used for such symptoms such as chilling or pain in the knees, stomach pain, lack of appetite, oppressive pain in the flank region, shortness of breath, blood rushing to the head and low back pain.

In *Ling Shu*, the oldest work on Oriental medicine, it is written, "For symptoms of the interior up high use the Ryō-Sen (hill spring) on the yin side, and for symptoms of the exterior up high use the Ryō-Sen on the yang side." Symptoms "up high" refers to symptoms above the navel such as headaches, dizziness, ringing in the ears, stiff shoulders, coughing, palpitation and shortness of breath. Symptoms of the interior refers to those caused by cooling, while symptoms of the exterior mean symptoms caused by over heating and are represented swelling. Therefore, In-Ryō-Sen is used often even for symptoms in the upper part of the body, such as cases where chilling during the night causes stomach trouble. On the other hand, for headaches caused by a sunstroke, Yō-Ryō-Sen 陽陵泉 (GB-34), located on the opposite side of the leg from In-Ryō-Sen, is used. Yō-Ryō-Sen is also one of the points used in acupuncture anesthesia.

39. Kek-Kai 血海 (SP-10)——*Tsubo for menstrual disorders*

Traditionally, it is said that the "spleen" controls blood, and that the tsubo Kek-Kai 血海 (SP-10: blood sea) is supposed to remove the stagnation of blood and facilitate its flow. It is effective especially for the "discharge of blood," or various problems associated with menstruation in women. This tsubo is commonly used for menstrual irregularity, as well as for beauty purposes. It is also used for tension in the lower abdomen and swelling in the legs related to menstrual problems. In Oriental medicine, the symptoms which occur as the result of menstrual problems such as knee pain, low back pain, tension in the lower abdomen, stiff shoulders and headaches, all come under the "stagnant blood" syndrome.

The condition of "stagnant blood" is treated at Kek-Kai. It is the one tsubo which should be learned by women who suffer from menstrual cramps.

Kek-Kai is located in the muscle about six centimeters above the inside top corner of the kneecap where a hollow spot forms when the leg is straightened. About five centimeters under the navel there is a tsubo by the name of Ki-Kai 気海 (CV-6) which is supposed to nurture vital energy. Lying on your back with your legs opened to sixty degrees forms a right triangle between the Kek-Kai of both legs and Ki-Kai as the apex. In Oriental medicine both *ki* 気 (energy) and *ketsu* 血 (blood) are said to circulate through the meridians. The three tsubos of Kek-Kai and Ki-Kai work to remove stagnation in the flow of this energy and blood. Kek-Kai is well known as a tsubo for discharging old blood and also as being effective for symptoms of anemia.

40. Shō-Mon 衝門 (SP-12)——*Tsubo to stop blood rushing to head*

Have you ever experience dizziness, right after coming out from a bath or being exposed to heat, that is accompanied with pain that runs up from the navel to the pit of the stomach? This symptom is most common among women past their menopause. It is a problem in the autonomic nervous system and the dizziness results from blood rushing to the head. In Oriental medicine this is called *Jō-Shō* 上衝 (upward thrust), and the name *Shō-Mon* 衝門 (SP-12) comes from this concept. This tsubo has long been known as being effective against blood rushing to the head.

This tsubo is located on the outer corner of the pubic bone where the femoral artery is pulsating strongly in the fold where the thighs join the trunk (inguinal region). Furthermore, Shō-Mon is about fifteen centimeters under Dai-Ō 大横 (SP-15), which is located twelve centimeters to the side of the navel, so Shō-Mon is straight below this, around where the pubic hair begins.

Aside from stopping blood from rushing to the head, Shō-Mon is effective in diminishing pain and hard areas in the abdomen caused by chilling. Further, it is used for convulsive fits in children, and also, it is often used during pregnancy when the fetus moves up and places pressure on the mothers's solar plexus area to cause difficulty in breathing.

41. Fuk-Ketsu 腹結 (SP-14)——*Tsubo for enterogastritis*

If the intestines become filled with gas, the lower abdomen becomes distended and a hard area forms around the navel. People who tend to jump to conclusions often get worried about the possibility of cancer and run in far a checkup, and have x-rays taken, but usually nothing shows up. This is a common symptom for those who are chronically constipated, and light pressure on Fuk-Ketsu 腹結 (SP-14) is usually sufficient to give relief. Fuk-Ketsu is located about four centimeters below the next tsubo, Dai-Ō 大横 (SP-15), which is about twelve centimeters straight to the side of the navel.

The above mentioned symptoms are typical of enterogastritis. When there is diarrhea and a rumbling sound around the navel, it is an indication of enteritis. Inability to defecate despite the urge to do so is a sign of colitis. Stomach pain accompanied with nausea can be regarded as a possible sign of gastric catarrh. Fuk-Ketsu is effective for all these conditions, and otherwise it serves to indicate the presence of digestive disorders when there are hard sports here. In this case, a thorough massage and finger pressure should improve the condition.

42. Dai-Ō 大横 (SP-15)——*Tsubo for diarrhea and constipation*

In Japan, the navel was once also called Shin-Ketsu 神闕 (CV-8), and was regarded as a very important place. The ancient people thought that the body with the hands raised could be divided in equal halves right at the level of the navel. Thus, the navel was regarded as a central point. Dai-Ō 大横 (SP-15: big side) is an important tsubo about twelve centimeters straight to the side of the navel. Lying on your back with your legs straight out and trying to sit up in this position causes two muscles to appear vertically on both sides of the navel, and these muscles stretch from the solar plexus to the pubis. The spleen meridian passes to the outside of these muscles, so Dai-Ō is located on the outer edge of these muscles. This tsubo is regarded as being important for checking whether the condition of the upper half of the body is in balance with the condition of the lower half. This tsubo is specially effective for symptoms associated with impaired function of the intestines such as diarrhea and constipation.

There is a tsubo named Fu-Sha 府舎 (SP-13) about thirteen centimeters below Dai-Ō (two centimeters above Shō-Mon 衝門, SP-12) and this tsubo is also used often for diarrhea and constipation. Therefore, it should be remembered along with Dai-Ō. The character *Fu* 府 indicates a place where harmful energy collects, also because Fu-Sha is located where the spleen and liver meridians meet, it is very effective in removing various symptoms asscociated with these meridians.

43. Ten-Kei 天谿 (SP-18)——*Tsubo to remove lumps in breasts*

Ten-Kei 天谿 (SP-18) will be the last tsubo of the spleen meridian to be discussed. This tsubo is located slightly above the fourth rib and about six centimeters to the outside and a little up from the nipples. The character *Ten* 天 indicates the "heaven section" or the upper half of the body, and *Kei* 谿 is a deep gorge. Ten-Kei thus means a depression like a ravine that connects with the lungs which draw in the "energy of heaven," and distribute this among all the organs.

This tsubo is especially effective in reducing swelling of the breasts in women. Sometimes a woman's breasts swell up after giving birth, and on occasion this is accompanied with fever. Instead of massaging the breasts at such times, Ten-Kei on the side of the breasts should be rubbed. When the fever is not very high and a hard spot can be felt there, lightly massaging this area after applying gentle finger pressure should reduce the swelling and fever. If there is a lump in the breast which is not painful when pressed, a medical specialist should be consulted because it could be a malignant tumor.

Aside from the above, Ten-Kei is quite effective for symptoms of the lungs (respiratory organs) and heart (circulatory system) as suggested by its name. In modern medicine the cross sectional strip of the body surface including the breasts and nipples is known as the skin segment of the fourth thoracic nerve, and the occurrence of prickling sensations, pressure sensitive points and hard sports have been noted in patients with circulatory disorders. Keep in mind that this tsubo is also used for shortness of breath, oppressive chest pains, palpitation and blood rushing to the head.

5. Heart Meridian

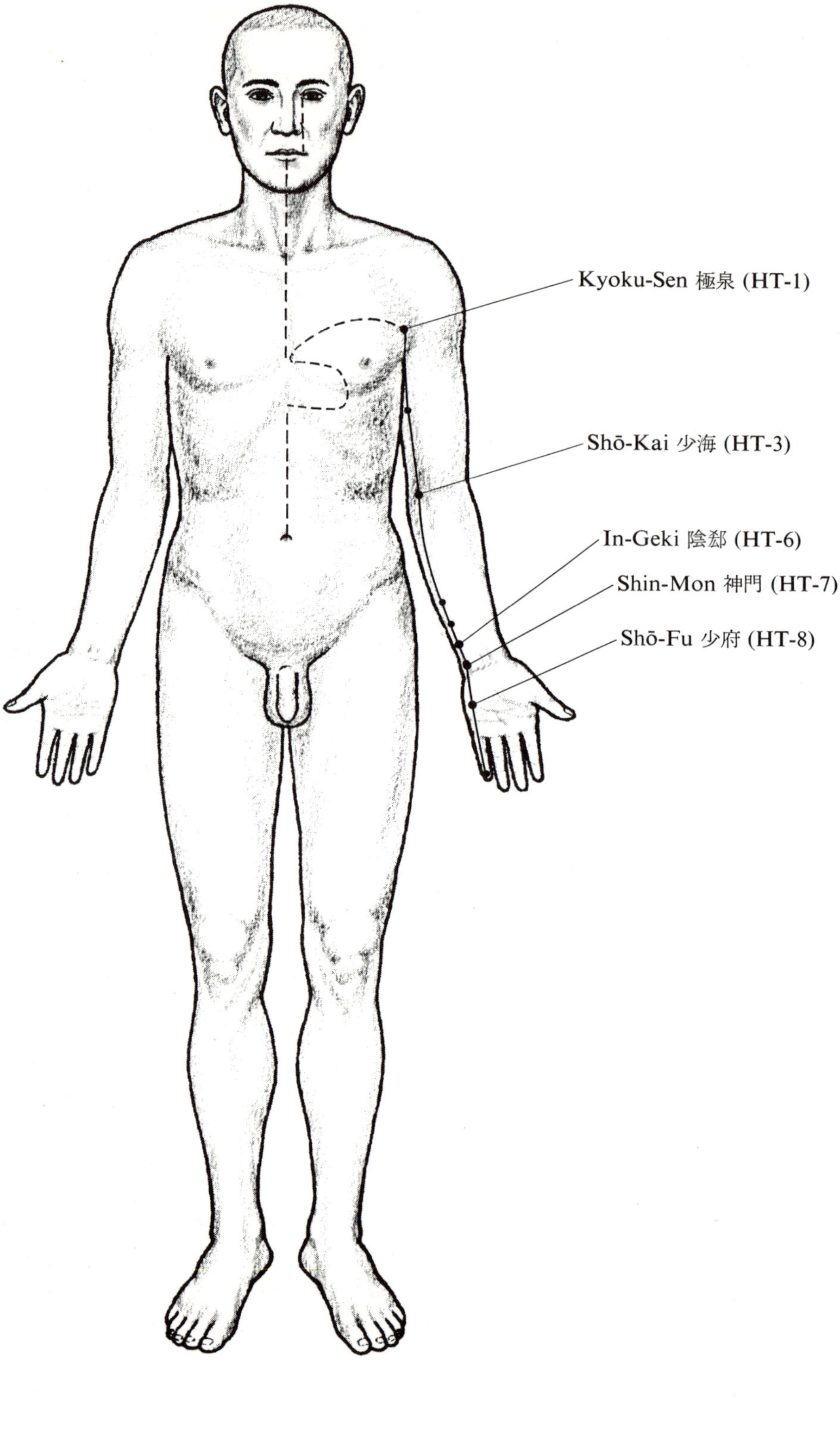

The "heart," one of the five essential organs in Oriental medicine, corresponds to the heart in modern medicine, and it is described as being shaped like a lotus bud and as being located above the diaphragm and under the lungs. It was believed to be firmly attached to the fifth thoracic vertebra. The heart meridian is the channel for the circulation of vital energy to the heart. When there is a problem with the heart, symptoms appear on tsubos of this meridian. Symptoms of the eyes are particularly common when there is a problem here, and there is especially a tendency for the eyes to become bloodshot. Other symptoms include excessive thirst, pain in the pit of the stomach, feeling chilled, pain or numbness down from the armpit to the elbow as well as on the inside of the forearm in line with the little finger. Occasionally, the palm of the hands become hot and painful. The above symptoms are clear signs that there is something wrong with the heart. All these complaints can be relieved by rubbing, massaging, pressing, or otherwise, acupuncturing the points listed below.

People with the above symptoms generally have flushed faces as if blood had risen to their head. Also, the pulse at their neck, wrist, stomach and feet can be felt very strongly. Such people have a very cheerful voice and are generally very enthusiastic, but they also tend to become over excited. Nevertheless, their personality is such that they share the joy of others on happy occasions and they worry together with someone when there is a problem. In short, they tend to have a great deal of empathy. People with heart conditions tend to succumb to the summer heat, and they prefer foods with a burned flavor such as toast or roasted fish. Also such people often complain that their eyes become tired easily when reading a book. When such people are examined, they most often have pain and hard spots at the tsubo Ko-Ketsu 巨闕 (CV-14) located in the pit of the stomach, and at Shin-Yu 心兪 (UB-15) to the side and slightly below the fifth thoracic vertebra between the shoulder blades.

The course of this meridian begins in the heart and goes down the center of the body passing through the diaphragm and goes to the small intestines. This is the interior meridian and a branch off of this goes up from the heart and passes to either side of the throat and reaches the eyes. The surface branch, on which the tsubo are located, starts from the heart and passes through the lungs and comes out at the armpit. Surfacing at the tsubo Kyoku-Sen 極泉 (HT-1), this meridian goes down the inside of the upper arm in line with the little finger and passes the elbow and goes down the forearm into the wrist joint. Further, this meridian goes between the base of the ring finger and little finger on the palm and ends up at the inside base of the little finger. The heart meridian has nine tsubos, and among these, five of the most commonly used tsubos will be introduced.

44. Kyoku-Sen 極泉 (HT-1)——*Tsubo for underarm odor*

Kyoku-Sen 極泉 (HT-1) is the first tsubo of the heart meridian. As indicated by the character *Kyoku* 極 which means the upper extreme, and *Sen* 泉 which means a spring, it is located at the very top of the heart meridian and is the spring from which the energy of the heart meridian comes forth. In other words, the meridian energy which branches off the internal channel flows out from this tsubo, and courses down the upper arm and forearm. Its location is under the armpit right where the arm attaches to the torso, or in the center of the fold of the armpit when standing with the arms down to the side. Also, this is the place where the pulse of the artery in the armpit can be felt.

This tsubo is used for cases of pain in the chest and side, but most commonly for strong underarm odor (hircismus). Some people have very strong underarm odor in the summertime. The traditional cure for this was to draw a slight amount of blood with a three edged needle. The skin was lightly pricked with a sharp needle with a three sided tip to draw a single drop of blood. This method was once used widely as being effective for removing underarm odor. Aside from this, Kyoku-Sen is used for pain in the pit of the stomach, chest pains with persistent strong palpitation, as well as palpitations caused by overexcitement or anxiety.

45. Shō-Kai 少海 (HT-3)——*Tsubo to remove pain in arms*

Shō-Kai 少海 (HT-3) is recorded as being "to the inside of the big bone of the elbow and half a *cun* 寸 from the inside of the elbow." So this tsubo is a point on the inside corner of the big bone to the inside of the head of the elbow. When the elbow is bent, a crease forms to the inside, and Shō-Kai is located on the inside end of this skin fold where a faint pulse can be felt. The traditional approach in locating tsubos was to look next to where pulses could be felt for the yin meridians, and next to bones for the yang meridians. Since the palm is considered to be yin and the back of the hand is considered to be yang, presumably, locations next to pulses should be found for tsubos on the same side as the palm.

The flow of energy in meridians is likened to the flow of water in Oriental medicine. Therefore, five points out of each meridian are given special names. The first point is called *sei* 井 (well), and is like the wellhead from which the energy first issues. The place where there is a small flow like a creek is called *ei* 栄 (spring). The place where the flow comes together as a body of water is called *yu* 兪 (stream). The place where the flow becomes great is called *kei* 経 (river), and finally, where this flow joins a large body of water, much as a river joins the sea, is called *gō* 合 (sea). *Gō* points are mostly located around the knee and elbow joints. Shō-Kai (lesser sea) is located right where the flow of the *lesser* yin heart meridian "enters the *sea*." In other words, Shō-Kai means the place where the energy flow of the lesser yin meridian goes inward to join the meridian's interior energy channel.

Shō-Kai is effective for eye fatigue, headaches, pain in the side, swelling of lymph nodes in the armpits, frozen shoulders and neuralgia affecting the arm on the side of the little finger.

46. In-Geki 陰郄 (HT-6)——*Tsubo to relieve angina pectoris*

Bend your wrist backward and twist your palm toward your little finger. This will cause a noticeable bump to appear at the wrist on the side of the little finger.

In-Geki 陰郄 (HT-6) is located about two centimeters above this bone. This tsubo, much like the previous tsubo Shō-Kai 少海 (HT-3), is used often for eye fatigue, pain in the armpits, pain down the upper arm to the elbow and on the inside of the forearm in line with the little finger, nasal obstruction and nosebleeds.

Attacks of angina pectoris, caused by such things as hardening of the arteries and often a forerunner to serious heart attacks, are characterized by a piercing pain which shoots down the course of the heart meridian on the left side, from the armpit to the little finger. In such cases, applying strong finger pressure to In-Geki along with the tsubos, Shin-Mon 神門 (HT-7) the next in line, Shin-Yu 心兪 (UB-15) located on either side of the fifth thoracic vertebra and Dan-Chū 膻中 (CV-17) in the middle of the chest between the nipples, will provide amazingly prompt relief.

In-Geki indicates that this tsubo is a *geki* point of the lesser yin heart meridian, and this means that this tsubo is a place in the heart meridian where the energy circulation system supplying the heart tends to become stagnated. Thus the flow of meridian energy can be improved by the stimulation of this tsubo by rubbing and finger pressure, and this in turn will help relieve the heart problem and the various symptoms resulting from trouble in the heart meridian.

47. Shin-Mon 神門 (HT-7)——*Tsubo to check condition of "heart"*

The name *Shin-Mon* 神門 (HT-7) originated from the Oriental concept that one's spirit and emotions come, not from the head, but from the six *zang* and six *fu*, particularly the heart. In other words, the heart was thought to be the seat of the spirit for man, the homo sapiens. The name *Shin-Mon* (spirit gate) was given because this tsubo connects to the "heart." This tsubo is the *gen* point of the heart meridian, and the presence of problems in the "heart" can be detected here without having to check along the whole meridian. Therefore, Shin-Mon is a very important tsubo in the heart meridian.

The location of Shin-Mon is recorded in the classic text *Su Wen* as being "on the edge of the sharp bone and on the artery to the outside of the wrist." It can be located easily at the front side of the wrist near the corner on the side of the little finger. This tsubo has been used since the old days to determine whether a woman was pregnant. Supposedly, the pulse here beats strongly once a woman becomes pregnant.

This tsubo is effective for eye fatigue, excessive thirst coupled with lack of appetite, strong palpitations, sense of oppression in chest, pain or numbness in the hands and the feeling of hotness in the palms.

48. Shō-Fu 少府 (HT-8)——*Tsubo to remove hotness in palms*

Bend your little finger and ring finger into your palm. They will touch the soft mound of flesh toward the little finger. The point between the tips of these fingers is the tsubo Shō-Fu 少府 (HT-8). Pressing strongly here with the thumb should produce a deep penetrating sensation.

Massaging this tsubo thoroughly is effective in relieving numbness in the little finger and ring finger as well as removing the feeling of hotness in the palms. In Oriental medicine the sensation of hotness in the palms is referred to as "pain and heat in the palms," and this is regarded as a sign of exhaustion, or of being very run-down. Sweating only in the palms is a sign of nervous tension, and nervous people tend to sweat a lot in their palms. The thing to do in such situations is to relax and take it easy, and to lightly press this tsubo on the palm and rest.

The palms are amazingly characteristic things and just touching the palm of the hands reveals the personality and physical condition of a person. For example, those with soft and warm palms are generally very kind hearted and are healthy, while those with pale colored palms that are cold and hard tend to be rational and cold hearted people, and also their body tends to be weak. Also, take note if the skin on the palms is dry because it is a sign that the chest and stomach are in poor condition.

6. Small Intestine Meridian

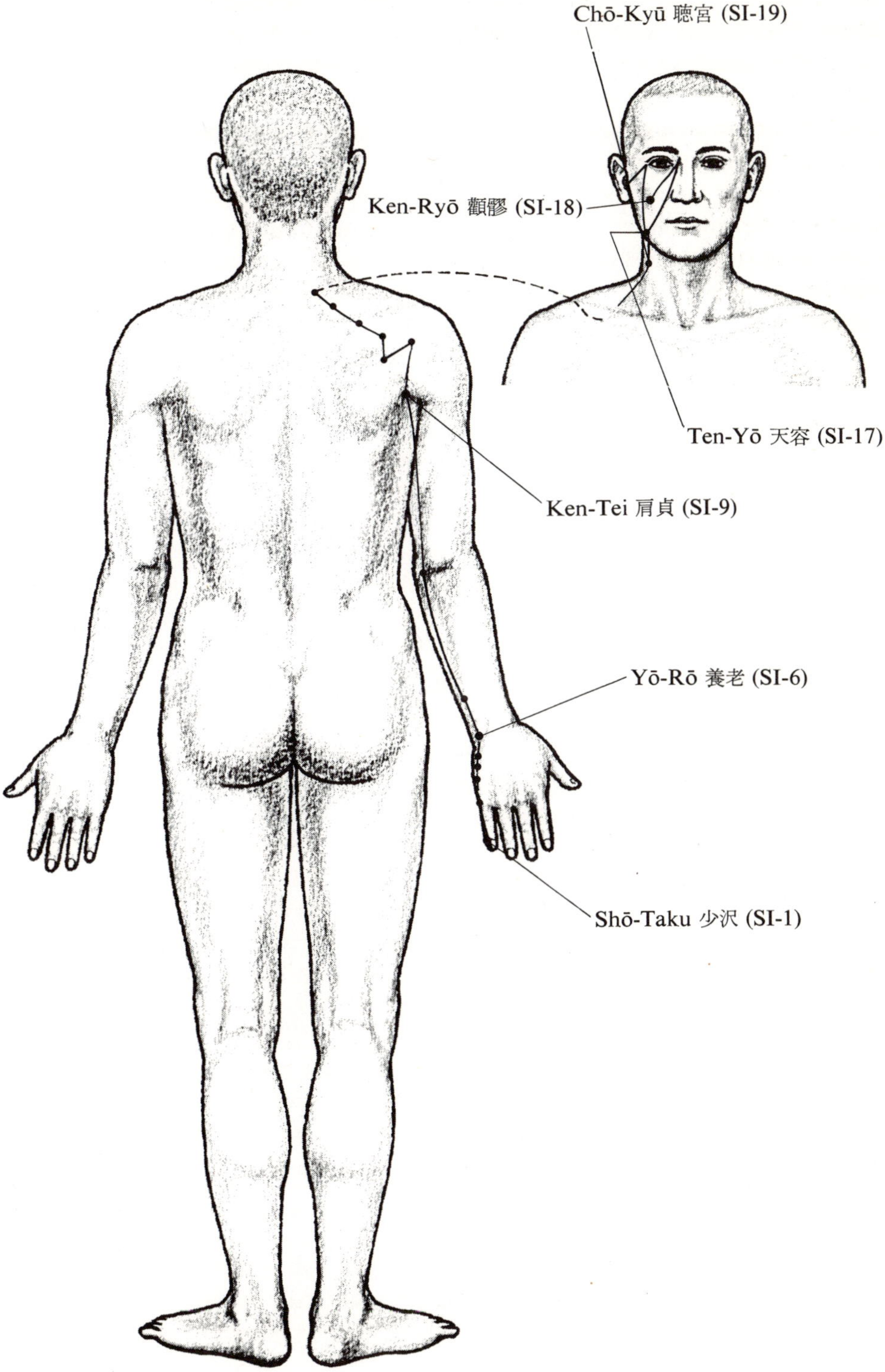

Most everyone knows that the small intestine is a part of the digestive tract between the stomach and the large intestine about from four to five meters in length. The small intestine consists of three parts—the duodenum, ileum and jejunum. These are all involved primarily in the physiological process of digestion and absorption. When there are symptoms of heartburn and stomach pain between meals, or when hungry, often people become concerned about the possibility of a duodenal ulcer.

The small intestine in Oriental medicine is described as follows: "The small intestine is three *jō* (about nine yards) and two *shaku* (about two feet) long, and folds around to the left sixteen times. The bottom opening of the stomach forms the mouth to the small intestine, and solid and liquid materials enter at this point two *cun* (about two inches) above the navel. The point one *cun* above the navel is Sui-Bun 水分 (CV-9) and this is the bottom opening of the small intestine. Here the clear and coarse substances are separated and the liquids go to the urinary bladder and the solids enter the large intestine."

In simpler terms, this means that the small intestine comes to an end beneath the tsubo Sui-Bun located about three centimeters above the navel, and connects to the large intestine. Of the digested material, the liquid waste goes to the urinary bladder and the solid waste material passes on to the large intestine and eventually reaches the anus.

Symptoms which appear when the function of the small intestine is impaired include, eyes becoming yellowish, hearing problems, swelling of cheeks, pain in the throat, heavy sensation in the head, and pain or numbness down the upper arm, elbow and forearm. When these symptoms are present, pain and hard spots appear at Shō-Chō-Yu 小腸兪 (UB-27) which is to either side of the vertebra below the belt right in the hollow area between the spine and the pelvis, and also at Kan-Gen 関元 (CV-4) about ten centimeters below the navel. The points on the small intestine meridian are effective in alleviating all of the above listed symptoms.

The small intestine meridian begins at the tsubo Shō-Taku 少沢 (SI-1) located at the base of the nail of the little finger, and travels up the outside of the arm past the elbow and the upper arm to curve around the back of the armpit and shoulder blade to reach a point under the seventh cervical vertebra. From here, one branch of the meridian goes to the front into the visceral organs, while another branch goes to the base of the neck in front and passes over the large muscle in the side of neck and around the cheek bone to enter the ear. Another branch separates at the cheek bone to go to the inner corner of the eyes. The small intestine meridian has nineteen tsubos in all, and the tsubos used most often are Shō-Taku 少沢 (SI-1), Yō-Rō 養老 (SI-6), Ken-Tei 肩貞 (SI-9), Ten-Yō 天容 (SI-17), Kan-Ryō 顴髎 (SI-18) and Chō-Kyū 聴宮 (SI-19). The details concerning which tsubos are effective for what symptoms will be explained below.

49. Shō-Taku 少沢 (SI-1)——*Tsubo effective for cataracts*

The small intestine meridian begins at this tsubo located just to the outside base of the nail of the little finger. As mentioned before, *Sho* 少 means an end point, so this character alone tells us that this tsubo is at the beginning end of this meridian. Concerning this tsubo it is written in the classics, "bleed slightly to cure clouding in the eyes." In today's language this means that it is effective for cataracts and glaucoma. Since clouding in the eyes can mean any hindrance in vision, drawing a drop of blood from Shō-Taku 少沢 (SI-1) is supposed to stop one from "seeing stars," aside from curing cataracts and glaucoma.

On the subject of drawing blood, this tsubos is also used in case of strokes. It is said, "the five tsubos at the tip of the fingers and toes cure hemiplegia." Therefore, drawing a bit of blood from the five tsubos at the base of the nails of the fingers and toes is considered to be very effective for paralysis and numbness. This is called the "ten well point venesection," and this procedure is performed on the fingers and toes of the left side when numbness affects the left half of the body, and on the right side when numbness affects the right half. When this does not prove effective, another rule of acupuncture is used where pain or numbness on the right side is treated on the left side and vice versa.

Aside from the symptoms mentioned above, Shō-Taku is commonly used for the feeling of fullness in the chest, elbow pain, coughs, pain from the head down the nape of the neck, blurred vision and headaches.

50. Yō-Rō 養老 (SI-6)——*Tsubo for carbuncles and facial furuncles*

Yō-Rō 養老 (SI-6) is located in a groove of the bone on the outside of the back of the wrist. This tsubo is often used in cases where carbuncles form on the back, or when furuncles form on the face. It is also remarkably effective in alleviating acute symptoms related to the small intestine meridian such as sharp pain which travels down from the shoulders to the elbows, or blurring of vision. *Yō-Rō* which means "well-being in old age," is also known as one of the moxibustion points for promoting health and longevity.

When boils on the back or the face become a problem, burning moxa on these tsubos directly is often more effective than applying only finger pressure on them. A cure can be effected even faster when this treatment is augmented with heat stimulation on the tsubos Gō-Koku 合谷 (LI-4) and San-Ri 三里 (LI-10) as mentioned in the section for the large intestine meridian.

To check for problems in the small intestine meridian, the tsubo Wan-Kotsu 腕骨 (SI-4) is used. This tsubo is located below the wrist in line with the little finger, just below the smaller bump to the outside of the wrist. When there are abnormalities in the small intestine meridian, just a slight amount of pressure on this tsubo will produce a strong pain. Wan-Kotsu is also known to be effective for headaches, ear problems, numbness in the fingers and convulsive fits in children. Nevertheless, since Wan-Kotsu is the *gen* point of the small intestine meridian, it is most important as the tsubo for checking the condition of the small intestine meridian.

51. Ken-Tei 肩貞 (SI-9)——*Tsubo for frozen shoulders*

The tsubo Ken-Tei 肩貞 (SI-9) is located right above the vertical crease at the back of the armpit when the shoulders are relaxed and the arms are hanging down to the side. This tsubo is directly behind the shoulder joint. Ken-Tei is highly effective for so-called frozen shoulders which is common among middle-aged people who complain of pain and stiffness in the shoulders. When using this tsubo to treat this condition, also use Ju-Yu 臑兪 (SI-10) located about six centimeters above for even better results. The character *Ju* 臑 means upper arm, and *Yu* 兪 means acupuncture point. Thus, Ju-Yu simply means acupuncture point on the upper arm. This tsubo is used when the upper arm is in pain and cannot be raised. It is also used for pain in the supraclavicular fossa, ringing in the ears, and numbness in the arms and legs.

Other tsubos effective for frozen shoulders include Ten-Sō 天宗 (SI-11) located approximately in the center of the shoulder blade, Ten-Chū 天柱 (UB-10) at the base of the skull on the nape of the neck, Kyoku-En 曲垣 (SI-13) above the inside corner in the spine (horizontal ridge) of the scapula (shoulder blade), Ken-Ryō 肩髎 (TH-14) on the top of the shoulder toward the back, Ken-Gū 肩髃 (LI-15) located to the front of Ken-Ryō, and Un-Mon 雲門 (LU-2) right below the clavicle. Whenever there is a strong pain in the shoulder area, massage and apply finger pressure on the above tsubos along with the first two mentioned.

52. Ten-Yō 天容 (SI-17)——*Tsubo to relieve throat pain*

Perhaps some of you have the experience of not being able to sleep because of a sore throat, and instinctively massaging the side of the neck below the ear and behind the corner of the chin to bring relief. This relief was obtained because the tsubo Ten-Yō 天容 (SI-17) is located in this area and it was stimulated. The location of Ten-Yō, more precisely, is to the front of the midpoint of the sternocleidomastoid muscle.

The character *Ten* 天 means the "heaven section" above the clavicle, and *Yō* 容 means to contain, wrap, fill, or otherwise use. Therefore, Ten-Yō means a tsubo used for various symptoms in the "heaven section" including chest pain, neck pain, toothaches, and ringing in the ears, not to mention sore throats.

There are many tsubos on the neck which have the character *Ten* 天 in their name. It is said in Oriental medicine that the "heaven section," including the neck and the head, have "seven orifices." These are, two for the eyes, two for the ears, two for the nose and one for the mouth. These orifices are likened to the "stars in heaven," and if they each retain their shine respectively, the microcosm of the human body is considered to be healthy. Conversely, if there is a problem in the clarity of one of these "stars," one's health is undermined. All the tsubos which start with the character *Ten*, including Ten-Yō, are for dispelling diseases from the "seven orifices."

53. Ken-Ryō 顴髎 (SI-18)——*Tsubo for facial neuralgia and beauty*

Ken-Ryō 顴髎 (SI-18) is located at the bottom of the cheek bone to the outside. In more specialized terms, Ken-Ryō is located below the bottom edge of the protuberance of the zygomatic bone. This tsubo is used to relieve facial pain caused by trigeminal neuralgia, swelling in the cheeks, fatigue of the eyes and toothaches. Also Ken-Ryō has the wonderful effect for women of making their face more beautiful. The primary enemy to facial beauty is wrinkles, such as those across the forehead, those on the outside corner of the eyes and those on the neck. These wrinkles are of special concern to middle-aged women.

The reason wrinkles form on the face in the first place is due to the structural properties of the face. Just pinching up the skin on an arm or chest will tell you that the skin and muscle tissue there are separate. In contrast to this, facial skin alone in the body is interwoven with muscle tissue to form a cohesive whole. This is the reason all manner of complex facial expressions such as laughing and weeping can be made by the contraction of the facial muscles. The lack of tone in these muscles, however, causes the skin to loosen and forms wrinkles. Therefore, even people without neuralgia should given light fingertip massages to the many tsubos on the face, including Ken-Ryō. Also press the tsubos on the forehead, around the eyes, cheeks, nose, ears and lower jaw. This should restore the tone and texture of facial skin.

54. Chō-Kyū 聴宮 (SI-19)——*Tsubo to stop tinnitus*

Ringing in the ears, apart from ear diseases, is often caused by emotional excitation and vascular obstructions. Sometimes it is a buzzing sound, and at other times it is a high pitched ringing sound. The buzzing type is called vibratory tinnitus and is relatively easy to cure. The ringing type is called nonvibratory tinnitus and is difficult to cure.

The tsubo used often for tinnitus is Chō-Kyū 聴宮 (SI-19), and it is located to the front of the tragus, the fleshy protrusion at the front of the ear which extends over the opening. The character Kyū 宮 means a very important place such as the emperor's palace, so the name *Chō-Kyū* (hearing place) indicates a very important tsubo which is effective for all types of ear problems. Aside from tinnitus, Chō-Kyū is very effective for hearing problems or deafness, facial paralysis, facial neuralgia, headaches, dizziness and weakening eyesight.

Recently, the account of how deaf children were made to hear with acupuncture treatments in Red China reached Japan and caused a big sensation. The tsubos used in this treatment included Chō-Kyū, Ji-Mon 耳門 (TH-21) and Chō-E 聴会 (GB-2), all to the front of the tragus, as well as Kaku-Son 角孫 (TH-20) to the top of the ear, Kyō-In 竅陰 (GB-11) to the back of the ear, and Ei-Fū 翳風 (TH-17) located in the hollow place behind the earlobe.

7. Urinary Bladder Meridian

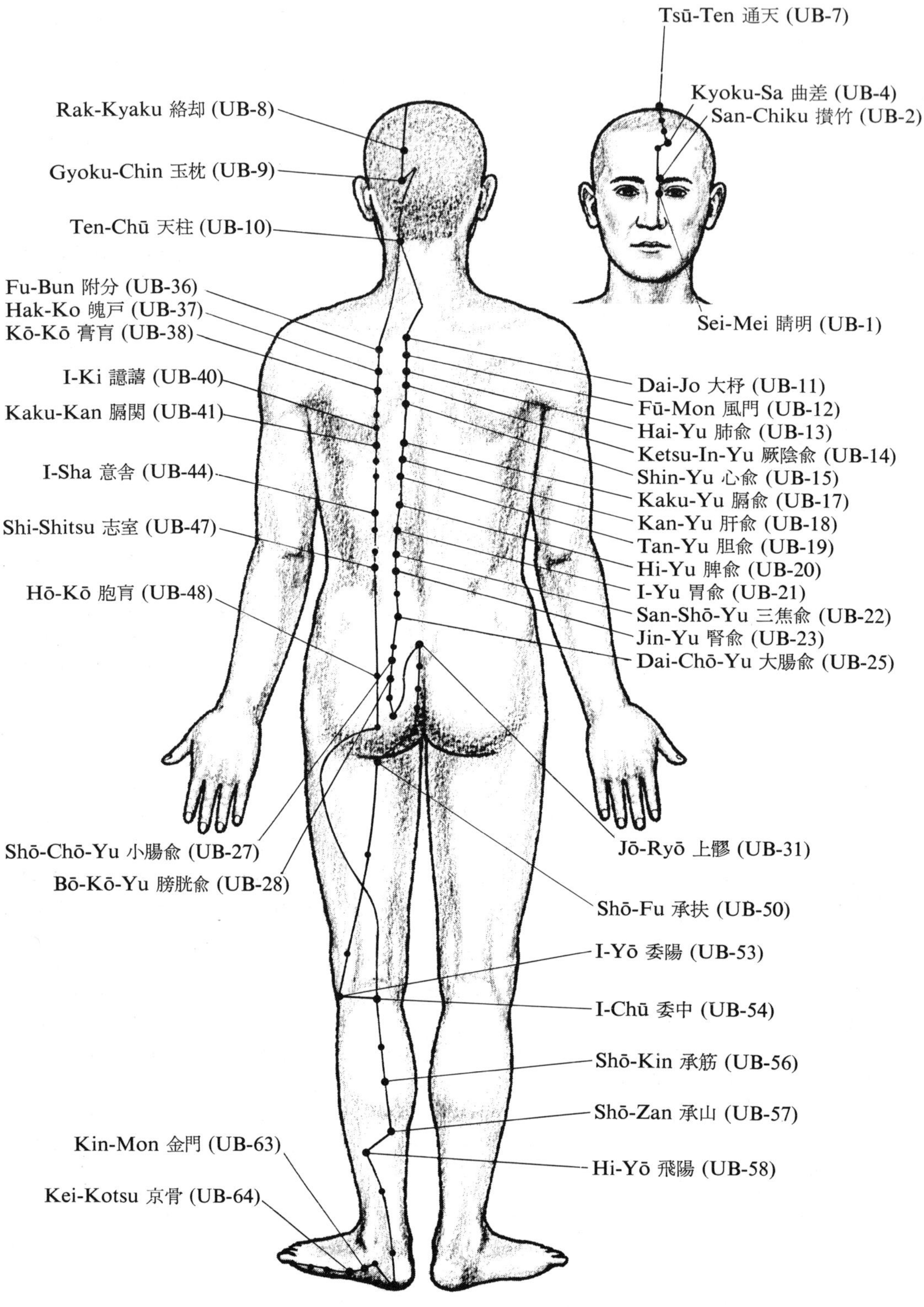

The urinary bladder meridian is the longest meridian among the fourteen major meridians and contains a very large number of important tsubos which will be discussed next. According to Western medicine urine is produced in the kidneys and comes through the ureter to collect in the urinary bladder. When the bladder becomes full, the urine is expelled through the urethra. The urinary bladder in traditional Oriental medicine differs slightly from this. Supposedly after the food which has reached the small intestines through the stomach is fully digested and absorbed, the unnecessary water, or "fluids," seep through the small intestines to collect in the urinary bladder.

As to the symptoms associated with the urinary bladder meridian, since it is a very long meridian running down from the top of the head to the shoulders, back, waist, sacral region, hips, thighs, and back of the lower leg to the tip of the little toe, the variety of symptoms is also very extensive. Since the path of this meridian is so long and complicated, refer to the figure to learn the precise course it follows.

Problems in the urinary bladder meridian are associated with symptoms such as pain and sensations of heaviness from eye fatigue, along with looseness of the scalp which is caused by poor circulation and congestion in the head. Other symptoms include nosebleeds and nasal obstruction, as well as pain in the joints and muscles along the course of the urinary bladder meridian which includes the neck, shoulders, back, waist, hips, back of knees, calf muscles, behind the outer ankle bone and down the little toe. Muscular pain down the back, waist and hips occurs more frequently as people advance in age. The spine begins to age and deform as people get older and the sponge-like structure between the vertebrae become hardened and this exerts pressure on the spinal nerves of the upper and lower back at the places they leave the vertebrae. This causes pain and numbness in the neck, shoulder, back, arms and legs. Aside from this, pain in the hip joint, sciatica, cramps in the calf muscle and hemorrhoids are also associated with problems in the urinary bladder meridian.

Furthermore, since the *yu* points (for diagnosis) of all organs lie on the path of the urinary bladder meridian, it is directly related with the respiratory, circulatory and excretory systems. When the above symptoms are present, or there is some organic disfunction (disease) the associated tsubo along the urinary bladder meridian must be checked carefully to find the most appropriate tsubo for treatment.

To determine whether there is any problem in the urinary bladder meridian itself, check the tusbo Chū-Kyoku 中極 (CV-3) which is straight below the navel and right above the pubic hair. Also use light pressure to check Bō-Kō-Yu 膀胱俞 (UB-28) which lies to either side of the middle of the sacrum above the coccyx. If there is pain or hard spots in these places, it means there is a problem in the bladder or the urinary bladder meridian. The urinary bladder meridian has sixty-seven tsubos in all, but only thirty-nine of the most important tsubo will be discussed in detail here.

55. Sei-Mei 睛明 (UB-1)——*Tsubo to make the eyes beautiful*

Everyone presses between the inner corner of the eyes and the bridge of the nose with their thumb and index finger now and then without being aware of it, after staying up late reading a book, or tiring out the eyes by doing needlework. This tsubo is located right above where eyeglasses rest on the nose. Finger pressure to these points seems to relieve tiredness of the eyes and so people end up pressing this tsubo unconsciously. This tsubo is Sei-Mei 睛明 (UB-1), and not only it is good for bringing relief to tired eyes, but it restores clear vision and bright eyes when vision has become blurred and the eyes have become bloodshot. The name *Sei-Mei* even means clear and bright eyes, so it is easy to understand how this tsubo has been used often through the years to treat various symptoms of the eyes.

In Japan, when children throw tantrums or cry for a long time, this is called *kan-no-mushi* (mad bug). It is not that a mad bug really gets into the child, but it describes a condition where the child has become hypersensitive. This word came from experience where children became very irritable when they were infected with parasitic worms, and it was thought that they went mad because of the bug. In any case, this condition in children can be taken care of by finger pressure or acupuncture at Sei-Mei.

56. San-Chiku 攢竹 (UB-2)——*Tsubo for trigeminal neuralgia and pain in the eyes*

The number of women between the ages of puberty and menopause who suffer from trigeminal neuralgia has been on the increase recently. The trigeminal nerve is the sensory nerve of the face, and it differs from the facial nerve which controls the movement of facial muscles, because it is in charge of the sense of touch and pain. When the trigeminal nerve is affected, therefore, symptoms arise such as, pain in the forehead and cheeks, pain behind the eyeballs, congestion in the eyes causing the eyes to water and become very bloodshot. San-Chiku 攢竹 (UB-2) is a tsubo commonly used for eye fatigue as well as all the symptoms described above. The character *San* 攢 of San-Chiku means to gather or to collect, while *Chiku* 竹 means bamboo, or a bamboo stick. This name presumably came from harmful energy *collecting* here and causing the eyesight to fail so that a *bamboo* stick was needed to find one's way around.

The location of San-Chiku is under the inside end of the eyebrows with the eyes closed. Gently probing in the upper rim of the eye socket with the soft part of your thumb, you will come across a thin muscle which moves back and forth slightly, near the bridge of the nose. This is the location of San-Chiku. Pressing this tsubo for a long time will cause a penetrating pain up the forehead even in those who are healthy. This tsubo should be pressed three to five seconds at a time, applying pressure gradually. Repeating this three or four times will help to relieve the discomfort.

57. Kyoku-Sa 曲差 (UB-4)——*Tsubo for headaches and nasal obstruction*

Kyoku-Sa 曲差 (UB-4) is located on the hairline straight up from the inside corner of the eyes. This tsubo is most often used for headaches, nasal obstruction and symptoms of a cold. The character *Kyoku* 曲 of Kyoku-Sa means bend, and *Sa* 差 means difference. The reason this tsubo got this name is because it is on a bend of the skull where the forehead ends, and it lies on the hairline which is a different place. The name thus indicates that this tsubo is on the borderline between the face and the scalp.

The problem exists in how to distinguish the face from the scalp because the difference is all but impossible to make out in people who are bald. In one method, the index finger, middle finger, ring finger and little finger are placed sidewise on top of the eyebrows and the forehead is everything covered by the fingers, and the rest is the scalp. However, the only method accurate from an anatomical standpoint is to decide from the structure of the facial skin and muscles. To do this, raise the eyebrows as far up as possible to form wrinkles on the forehead. The very top of these wrinkles is the border between the face and scalp. The reason this distinction can be made is because, on the face, the skin and muscle tissues are interwoven so that the skin wrinkles along with muscular contractions, but on the scalp, the skin and muscle tissues are separate, so no wrinkles form.

58. Tsū-Ten 通天 (UB-7)——*Tsubo for growths in the nose*

The tsubo Tsū-Ten 通天 (UB-7) is located to the back of the previous tsubo, Kyoku-Sa 曲差 (UB-4), and it is about five centimeters from the very top of the head. This tsubo is usually hard to find because there is a lot of hair here, so refer to the figure to locate the exact point. This tsubo is effective for symptoms of the nose such as growths in the nose called nasal polypuses which can impair one's sense of smell. This tsubo is also good for nasal obstruction which can cause difficulty in breathing through the nose, and headaches associated with this. Aside from symptoms of the nose, this tsubo has traditionally been used for migraine headaches and tension in the back of the neck.

The character *Tsū* 通 of Tsū-Ten means to pass or penetrate, while *Ten* 天 means heaven, or the very top of the head. This name comes from this meridian branching off at this tsubo to go to the top center of the head where it goes inside and circulates through the brain. Since it connects to "heaven," this tusbo is effective against headaches. This tsubo is also used to treat facial paralysis which often comes before a serious stroke. Headaches in the part of the head where the urinary bladder meridian passes is traditionally called headaches of the "greater yang area." In today's words, this means migraine headaches. Headaches in the "greater yang area" are treated using the tsubos of the urinary bladder meridian on the head. Also, aside from this, there is a rule in acupuncture called *En-Dō-Shi* 遠道刺 (distant path puncture) where a distant treatment point, such as Kon-Ron 昆崙 (UB-60) located behind the outer ankle bone, is selected.

59. Rak-Kyaku 絡却 (UB-8)——*Tsubo for tinnitus*

When a person has an ear disease or high blood pressure, the auditory nerve is adversely affected, and this causes tinnitus, or so-called ringing in the ears. Tinnitus also can occur when a person is overworked and exhausted, or when one is in a state of extreme emotional excitement. This tsubo, Rak-Kyaku 絡却 (UB-8), is very effective in such cases. Finger pressure is, of course, effective, but moxibustion using tiny pieces of moxa is indispensable for treating tinnitus.

Thus Rak-Kyaku is among the most important of the tsubo in the urinary bladder meridian on the head. It is located about five centimeters behind the previous tsubo Tsu-Ten 通天 (UB-7), which lies about ten centimeters behind the front hairline, and these tsubos are about five centimeters to either side of the center line. The character *Raku* 絡 of Rak-Kyaku means meridian, or those branches (collaterals) which connect sideways, while *Kyaku* 却 means to return. The urinary bladder meridian branches off from its main course at Tsū-Ten to circulate through the head and then once more returns to the main channel which runs parallel to the center line of the head. Thus, Rak-Kyaku got its name from the meridian branching off from the main channel to circulate elsewhere and once more returning to the main channel at this tsubo. Needless to say, this tsubo is also effective for headaches accompanying tinnitus.

60. Gyoku-Chin 玉枕 (UB-9)——*Tsubo to keep blood from rising to head*

In addition to the previously mentioned tsubos, Kyoku-Sa 曲差 (UB-4), Tsū-Ten 通天 (UB-7) and Rak-Kyaku 絡却 (UB-8), there is another tsubo called *Gyoku-Chin* 玉枕 (UB-9) which is used to alleviate symptoms of the head, eyes, nose and ears including, the feeling of heaviness and pain in the back of the head, dizziness, severe pain behind the eyes, tinnitus and blood rising to the head in women.

Gyoku-Chin is located about five centimeters behind Rak-Kyaku, or about nine centimeters up from the hairline at the back of the head. This tsubo is about four centimeters to either side of Nō-Ko 脳戸 (GV-17) which is right on the center of the bump behind the skull (external occipital protuberance). Actually, there are varying opinions regarding the exact location of these tsubos on the head. It is even written in one classic, "Since it is difficult to judge the exact distance of points from the hairline because the radius of the head at the center line differs from that of the lines on either side, tsubos should be located without so much attention to exact measurements."

All one has to do to locate Gyoku-Chin is to trace a straight line from between the eyebrows to the back of the head until the back end of the skull (the occiput) is reached. There is a big bump at the back center and Gyoku-Chin can be located about four centimeters to either side of this bony protrusion. Gyoku-Chin (jewel pillow) is remarkably effective in relieving headaches in the back of the head. So, in a manner of speaking, it is a tsubo that is precious as a *jewel* which is located where the head comes to rest on the *pillow*.

61. Ten-Chū 天柱 (UB-10)——*Tsubo famous for relieving headaches*

At the back of the head, going down from the nape of the neck to both shoulders, there are thick and hard muscles which are called the trapezius muscle. Ten-Chū 天柱 (UB-10) is located just to the outside of the very top of these muscles where they attach to the back of the skull. When the thumbs are used to press this tsubo near the hairline, it has the effect of clearing the eyes and generally making a person feel much better. This tsubo is especially effective in relieving headaches and eyestrain. It is also very effective in relaxing tension in the shoulders and the back of the neck.

It is thus written in *Ling Shu*, the oldest text of Oriental medicine; "When there is a fever which begins in the head and neck, acupuncture the greater yang on the nape of the neck; this will cause sweating and the fever will subside." What this means is that, when there is a fever and the head and the neck ache, the tsubo of the greater yang on the head (i.e., Ten-Chū of the greater yang urinary bladder meridian) should be treated, and that the fever will subside once the patient begins to sweat.

There is another rule in Oriental medicine which goes, "When energy accumulates in the head, use Ten-Chū and Dai-Jo 大杼 (UB-11)." In this way, all diseases of head and neck area can be treated with Ten-Chū and Dai-Jo, which is the tsubo which comes next. The character *Ten* 天 means the head or the area above the neck, *Chū* 柱 means a pillar, support, or a vital point. Ten-Chū is also effective in cases of occipital neuralgia, frozen shoulders, "a crick in the neck," high blood pressure, dizziness and car sickness. Aside from the above, interestingly enough, this tsubo behind the head is good for reducing swelling in the legs.

62. Dai-Jo 大杼 (UB-11)——*Tsubo for relieving pain in joints*

The location of Dai-Jo 大杼 (UB-11) according to the classical text *Su Wen* is, "below the back of the neck one and a half *cun* (two inches) to either side of the point under the first spine." Sit straight up and find the spine (spinous process) of the first thoracic vertebra (the second spine down). Then locate the tsubos four and a half centimeters to either side of the point just below that spine. Dai-Jo can be found on the sensitive points. This tsubo has traditionally been used for febrile diseases where there is no sweating, and for spasms in the muscles of the back and shoulder, as well as for convulsive fits in children.

The following is written concerning this tsubo in the classical text *Nan Jhing*; "Dai-Jo is the bone È 会 (meeting) point. All bones contain marrow. Marrow initially descends from the brain to pour through Dai-Jo. Then the marrow seeps down from Dai-Jo through the core of the spine and penetrates the coccyx to reach all the bones and joints of the body. This is the reason all the essence of bones meets at this point."

In this way, Dai-Jo is held to be an important tsubo for facilitating the flow of bone marrow. This tsubo is used for pain down the shoulders and back, headaches resulting from disfunctions in the five essential organs, as well as for pain in the joints such as rheumatism. The character *Dai* 大 is an honorific term, and *Jo* 杼 originally meant a loom, but it has come to mean scooping or drawing off water. Therefore, Dai-Jo together means an important tsubo which pumps out harmful energy collected in the bone marrow.

63. Fū-Mon 風門 (UB-12)——*Tsubo immediately effective for colds*

In Oriental medicine, diseases of the six *zang* and six *fu* are often referred to as *Fū* 風 (wind), and the causes of diseases from the environment are referred to as "pathogenic wind." There are said to be eight types of *Fū* coming from each direction including east, west, north and south, as well as the southeast, southwest, northeast and northwest. This "wind " becomes harmful energy to enter into the body and cause disease when the defenses of the body are weak, and this is called *Kyo-Fū* 虚風 (deficient wind). Otherwise, when there is strong reaction to "wind" as pain, fever and swelling, this is called *Jitsu-Fū* 実風 (excessive wind). This "pathogenic wind" is said to enter the body through Fū-Mon 風門 (UB-12), a tsubo located four and a half centimeters to either side of the point below the spinous process of the second thoracic vertebra.

If colds are not treated in their early stages at Fū-Mon, the "wind" supposedly goes to the tsubo Fū-Chi 風池 (GB-20) which lies to either side of Ten-Chū 天柱 (UB-10) on the hairline at the back of the head. This causes pain in the back of the head, the neck and down the back. When the cold progresses even further it is said to collect at the tsubo Fū-Fu 風府 (GV-16) right under the external occipital protuberance, and enter into the brain where it affects the "marrow." Since this "marrow" eventually reaches all the joints of the body including those of the legs, it was thought that pain spread to all joints of the body and caused a fever. The rule therefore, during the onset of a cold when the back of the head aches and there is tension in the back of the neck, is to first treat Fū-Mon; Fū-Chi and Fū-Fu are to be treated in the later stages of a cold. Symptoms such "a crick in the neck," occipital neuralgia, dizziness, car sickness and eye fatigue can also be remedied using this tsubo.

64. Hai-Yu 肺兪 (UB-13)——*Tsubo to check condition of lungs*

The *yu* points of various organs will be discussed for the tsubos which follow. *Yu* points begin at Hai-Yu 肺兪 (UB-13) and include Ketsu-In-Yu 厥陰兪 (UB-14) and Shin-Yu 心兪 (UB-15) which follow to total seventeen tsubos. These are all tsubos which lie in what is known as the greater yang area which is to both sides of the spine from the back of the head down the neck, shoulders, back, waist and hips. In Oriental medicine, all harmful influences from the environment are thought to enter into the body through these *yu* points and attack the associated organ to cause disease. The character *Yu* 兪 for *yu* point means a place where harmful energy pours in. Eventually this same harmful energy gathers at the *bo* points on the chest and stomach area. *Yu* points and *bo* points are thus very closely related, and by using the *yu* and *bo* points together, one can check for abnormalities in the associated organ systems.

Hai-Yu (lung *yu*) located about four and a half centimeters to either side of the point below the spinous process of the third thoracic vertebra is the *yu* point that is associated with the *bo* point Chū-Fu 中府 (LU-1), as explained earlier for the lung meridian. If there is some pain or tension when these points are lightly pinched, rubbed or pressed, this is a sign that there is some problem with the function of the lungs. In this case, there are usually accompanying symptoms such as discomfort in the chest, coughing, shortness of breath, mild fever, and tension in the back of the head, shoulders and down the back, Aside from the above symptoms, Hai-Yu is also used to treat symptoms like nettle rash (urticaria), colds, asthma, overexcitement and swelling in the legs.

65. Ketsu-In-Yu 厥陰俞 (UB-14)——*Tsubo for palpitation and enervation*

The tsubo Ketsu-In-Yu 厥陰俞 (UB-14) is located about four and a half centimeters to either side of the point right below the spinous process of the fourth thoracic vertebra. Ketsu-In-Yu, among all the *yu* points, should be remembered as a tsubo effective for people with poor circulation and those who tend to become chilled easily. Such people also seem to have no perseverance and tend to lack motivation at work. Applying gentle finger pressure and massaging Ketsu-In-Yu with a circular movement at the onset of palpitations or discomfort in the chest often proves very effective. *Yu* points have been discussed earlier, but more explanation regarding their significance is in order.

For man who stands upright on two legs, the spine is a crucial structure. The muscles which keep the spine in alignment and hold the body upright are referred to as the erector spinae or the sacrospinalis muscles. These muscles are like guy wires which support tall structures from four directions, and these muscles are only developed in man. When the functional condition of the organs in the chest and abdominal cavity are depressed or hyperactive, this creates tension and hypersensitivity in the supporting musculature. *Yu* points are an ingenious systematization of the reaction patterns of these muscles of the back in response to various organic disfunction. Ketsu-In-Yu is among the *yu* points used for “yin conditions,” or conditions of debility where an ailment is lodged deep in the body because of a decline in physiological functions.

66. Shin-Yu 心俞 (UB-15)——*Tsubo for weak heart*

Palpitations, pain and heaviness in the head, feverishness in the top half of the body and chills in the lower half of the body, a tendency for blood to rush to the head, and occasional piercing pain from the back to the chest, are all signs that there is some problem with the heart. In such cases, Shin-Yu 心俞 (UB-15), located four and a half centimeters to either side of the point below the spinous process of the fifth thoracic vertebra is often used.

Shin-Yu (heart *yu*) means the place where harmful energy pours into the heart. The corresponding *bo* point is Ko-Ketsu 巨闕 (CV-14) which lies right below the pit of the stomach. When there are mild heart attacks like angina pectoris, or symptoms like those mentioned above, and the area around Shin-Yu is sensitive, there is almost always a pain which runs down the inside of the left arm in line with the little finger. An effective treatment in this case would be to apply pressure slowly and firmly, not only on Shin-Yu, but also on Dan-Chū 膻中 (CV-17) right between the nipples, as well as on Ko-Ketsu, the *bo* point of the heart and Shō-Fu 少府 (HT-8) in the palm below the little finger. Shin-Yu may also be used effectively to relieve high blood pressure, headaches, and pain in the chest and side.

Shin-Yu is associated with the heart meridian discussed earlier which circulates through the heart. In Oriental medicine the heart houses one's "spirit." Supposedly the heart is filled with "essential fluids" in which the spirit resides. Thus it is considered a most important organ in the body which serves to coordinate the function of the mind and body. The fact that heart attacks are often associated with shock or mental distress, lends support to this Oriental concept.

67. Kaku-Yu 膈兪 (UB-17)——*Tsubo for food lodged in stomach*

There are many people who have poor digestion whose stomachs feel distended and uncomfortable after meals. This is a sure sign of a weak stomach, and Kaku-Yu 膈兪 (UB-17) is very effective in such cases. Kaku-Yu is located four and a half centimeters to either side of the point below the spinous process of the seventh thoracic vertebra.

In Oriental medicine the human body has three "heaters," or locations where heat is produced, and these are the upper, middle and lower heaters. The upper heater covers the area between the neck and the pit of the stomach, while the middle heater covers the area down to the navel and the lower heater covers the area from the navel down to the pubic hair. The upper heater is related to the respiratory and circulatory systems, the middle heater is related to the digestive system and the lower heater is related to the urogenital system which expels waste products from the body. These heaters, together, are called the triple heater, and they are the three sources of heat or energy in the body.

The tsubo Kaku-Yu happens to be located right on the border line of the upper and middle heaters. Kaku-Yu is therefore a very valuable tsubo effective for treating symptoms of both areas including that of the respiratory, circulatory and digestive systems. To list a few symptoms treated with this tsubo, for the middle heater there is food retention in the stomach, distention of the stomach and belching, and for the top heater there is coughing, shortness of breath, pain in the chest and side, as well as the sensation of feverishness in the upper half of the body.

68. Kan-Yu 肝兪 (UB-18)——*Tsubo to strengthen weak liver*

Kan-Yu 肝兪 (UB-18: liver *yu*) is an important tsubo for checking the condition of the liver. Since the condition of the liver affects all the rest of the body, Kan-Yu is used for almost all types of symptoms from stomach trouble to nettle rash. Kan-Yu is located four and a half centimeters to either side of the point below the spinous process of the ninth thoracic vertebra. The *bo* point corresponding to this tsubo is called Ki-Mon 期門 (LV-14). It is located at the tip of the ninth rib, or in the hypochondriac region right on the lower border of the rib cage straight down from the nipple. The two tsubos Kan-Yu and Ki-Mon are used to check the condition of the liver meridian. It is interesting to note that both these tsubos, on the right side, correspond to the actual location of the liver.

Aside from the symptoms already mentioned, Kan-Yu is used for pimples, asthma, car sickness, pain in the chest and side, insomnia and swelling of the legs. In Oriental medicine it is thought that a person's soul or courage resides in the liver, and that in addition to housing one's thoughts and emotions, it serves as a coordinating center for the muscles and tendons in the body. The tsubos Kin-Shuku 筋縮 (GV-8) located between the spinous processes of the ninth and tenth thoracic vertebra, Kan-Yu four centimeters to either side of this, and Kon-Mon 魂門 (UB-42) another four centimeters to the outside, are a row of five tsubos which lie on the same level as the liver. Therefore, these tsubos can used to regulate the function of the liver and to calm one's emotions.

69. Tan-Yu 胆兪 (UB-19)——*Tsubo for diseases of digestive organs*

Tan-Yu 胆兪 (UB-19) is located four and a half centimeters to either side of the point right below the spinous process of the tenth thoracic vertebra. It is effective for symptoms such as a bitter taste lingering in the mouth, a dry mouth, an oppressive pain extending from the pit of the stomach around to the side with hard spots under the ribs, and also difficulty in getting food down. In the Orient there is the expression "inseparable as the liver and gallbladder." Friends who always work together cheerfully are often referred to as "inseparable friends like the liver and gallbladder." This indicates how the *zang*, liver, and the *fu*, gallbladder, function in mutual cooperation and support to perform their respective roles.

It follows that symptoms Kan-Yu 肝兪 (UB-18: liver *yu*) is effective for are also treatable by Tan-Yu (gallbladder *yu*). Acupuncture and moxibustion treatments on these tsubo are quite effective against diseases of the liver and gallbladder, especially chronic cases of cholecystitis. Also, as just discussed before, the liver was considered as being the seat of thoughts and emotions. In the Orient, there are expressions like "pulverizing one's liver and gallbladder" which means to exhaust oneself completely, mentally and physically, after an all out effort. This expression is among many in the Orient which point out the close-knit relationship between the liver and gallbladder.

70. Hi-Yu 脾兪 (UB-20)——*Tsubo to strengthen weak "spleen"*

Hi-Yu 脾兪 (UB-20) is located about four and a half centimeters to either side of the point below the spinous process of the eleventh thoracic vertebra. Hi-Yu (spleen *yu*) is the *yu* point of the spleen meridian, and this is where harmful energy can enter the "spleen." Shō-Mon 章門 (LV-13), at the tip of the eleventh rib, is the *bo* point of the spleen meridian.

Even when we refer to the "spleen," it is not the same thing as understood by modern medicine. Instead, as explained earlier, it refers to the pancreas which is a leaf-shaped yellow and greyish organ lying sidewise behind the stomach. The pancreas secretes a hormone called insulin, and when its secretion becomes impaired, diabetes results. Diabetes has been called a "disease of affluence," and has been on the increase recently, not just among the middle-aged, but among young people as well. Hi-Yu is effective in treating jaundice, lassitude, drastic loss of weight and excessive thirst which occur in diabetics. Also, Hi-Yu is indispensable for treating chronic stomach problems, loss of appetite, acne and overexcitement. In Oriental medicine it is said, "one's will is housed in the spleen," so Hi-Yu acts to control the mind and is good for "quieting the nerves."

71. I-Yu 胃兪 (UB-21)——*Tsubo to improve stomach function*

When there seems to something wrong with the stomach, check either I-Yu 胃兪 (UB-21) located about four and a half centimeters to either side of the point below the spinous process of the twelfth thoracic vertebra, or Chū-Kan 中脘 (CV-12) at the midpoint between the pit of the stomach and the navel. I-Yu (stomach *yu*) is where harmful energy can enter into the stomach, so it is used often for various symptoms associated with stomach problems such as heartburn, feeling of pain or oppression in the stomach area, belching, feeling of distention in the stomach, and otherwise, when infants with digestive problems throw up milk. Tension and pain around the middle of the back and muscular tension from the shoulders down to the back are also typical signs of a weak stomach, for which I-Yu is used. This tsubo has been used in Japan since the olden days along with the "six moxa points for the stomach," Hi-Yu 脾兪 (UB-20) and Tan-Yu 胆兪 (UB-19). In addition, this tsubo is used together with other tsubos to treat hemorrhoids.

Chū-Kan, the *bo* point of the stomach meridian, is located over the area where blood vessels branch off from the abdominal aorta to supply the stomach, pancreas and liver, and also, this is where there is an important nerve cluster of the autonomic nervous system which controls the function of the internal organs in conjunction with the blood vessels. The basic rule for treating stomach problems in Oriental medicine is to first check for signs of stomach disfunctions at I-Yu and Chū-Kan, and then to select the appropriate tsubos along the stomach meridian.

72. San-Shō-Yu 三焦兪 (UB-22)——*Tsubo to improve overall condition*

The triple heater (San-Shō 三焦) is the source of energy for warming the human body, as was explained earlier. San-Shō-Yu 三焦兪 (UB-22: triple heater *yu*) is the point where harmful energy can enter the triple heater. This tsubo is located four and a half centimeters to either side of the point below the spinous process of the first lumbar vertebra. San-Shō-Yu is used for fevers caused by overwork, growling stomachs due to poor digestion, tension in the muscles down the back and pain in the lower back, as well as skin breaking out for no apparent reason, a decline in vitality, hemorrhoids or "slipped disks."

The *bo* point of the triple heater meridian is Seki-Mon 石門 (CV-5) which is approximately six centimeters below the navel. The four tsubos San-Shō-Yu, Seki-Mon, Dan-Chū 膻中 (CV-17) right between the nipples, and Chū-Kan 中脘 (CV-12) at the midpoint between the pit of the stomach and the navel, are most important tsubos for fully regulating the functions of the body. Whenever you feel that your physical condition is less than perfect and your work is suffering as a result, try massaging or giving finger pressure to these vital tsubos. If it is just a simple case of fatigue, taking a hot bath and getting a good night's sleep should take care of the problem. But if there is an unusual amount of pain or tension around these tsubos, giving a thorough treatment to the meridians associated with these points will provide welcome relief.

73. Jin-Yu 腎兪 (UB-23)——*Tsubo to increase stamina*

The kidney in Oriental medicine is said to house the congenital essence, or the basic life force present in each one of us at birth. This "kidney" in today's terms can be understood as the adrenal glands. The point where harmful energy can enter the "kidney" is Jin-Yu 腎兪 (UB-23: kidney *yu*). The overall condition of the body can be checked at this tsubo.

Jin-Yu is located about four and a half centimeters to either side of the point below the spinous process of the second lumbar vertebra, which is level with the bottom rib at the side. If there is no big hard spots or pressure sensitive areas in the muscles to either side of the spine at the waist, it means that the person is in satisfactory condition. On the other hand, if the muscles here are very tense and are sensitive to the slightest amount of finger pressure, and also, there are large lumps as hard as rocks, it is a sure sign that the person is generally overworked. In such cases the blood pressure tends to rise, vitality decreases, the feet swell up, and insomnia and acne become a problem. In the case of women, there are menstrual irregularity accompanied with low back pain and chilling of the feet.

Jin-Yu, in the same manner as Kan-Yu 肝兪 (UB-18), is used for a wide variety of symptoms throughout the body such as asthma, coughs, "slipped disks" and fatigue in the legs. Right between Jin-Yu on the right and left sides lies Mei-Mon 命門 (GV-4) which is directly under the spinous process of the second lumbar vertebra. Mei-Mon is very effective when used together with Kan-Gen 関元 (CV-4), about nine centimeters under the navel, for treating persons who are thin and have symptoms of anemia, poor digestion and susceptibility to colds.

74. Dai-Chō-Yu 大腸兪 (UB-25)——*Tsubo to improve condition of large intestine*

Often, when people have digestive problems, they complain of stomach trouble in general, but the symptoms of digestive problems differ according to whether the function of the stomach, large intestine, or small intestine is affected. When the problem lies in the large intestine to which Dai-Chō-Yu 大腸兪 (UB-25) is related, the intestines make noises and there is pain in the lower abdomen accompanied with diarrhea or constipation. In addition, there is tension down the back and pain in the lower back area. When the problem lies in the small intestine, the pain is centered around the navel, and this is accompanied with severe diarrhea. The stomach growls and people rush to the toilet to find in many cases that they are too late. On the other hand, when there is a sense of oppression in the pit of the stomach, this is a sign that the function of the stomach has weakened, and this is often accompanied with a feeling of distension in the stomach, nausea and repeated belching. If there is a dull or piercing pain about an hour after a meal, this could be the sign of an incipient peptic ulcer. Even though the complaints may be just stomach trouble in general, use the tsubos I-Yu 胃兪 (UB-21), Dai-Chō-Yu and Shō-Chō-Yu 小腸兪 (UB-27) selectively.

Dai-Chō-Yu is located four and a half centimeters to either side of the point below the spinous process of the fourth lumbar vertebra. As its name implies, Dai-Chō-Yu (large intestine *yu*) is used when the function of the large intestine deteriorates. Aside from improving the function of the large intestine, Dai-Chō-Yu is used for nettle rash, "slipped disks." and fatigue in the legs.

75. Shō-Chō-Yu 小腸兪 (UB-27)——*Tsubo to improve condition of small intestine*

Shō-Chō-Yu 小腸兪 (UB-27: small intestine *yu*) is the point where harmful energy enters the small intestine. Therefore, it is effective for such symptoms as tension and pain in the lower abdomen, swelling of the legs, or mucus mixed with the stools. For women, this tsubo is also used for excessive menstrual discharge. Massaging around this tsubo after applying hot compresses is especially effective in relieving low back pain which stems from organic disorders in the lower abdomen.

Shō-Chō-Yu is located about four and a half centimeters to either side of the point below the spinous process of the first sacral vertebra. This may be a little bit difficult to understand, so an explanation of skeletal anatomy is in order.

The spine in the neck are called cervical vertebra. The sternum is the breast bone in the middle of the chest to which the clavicles attach, and the ribs extend from both sides of the thoracic vertebrae to form the rib cage. The spine becomes lumbar vertebrae from around the level of the navel. The sacrum and coccyx (tailbone) form the lower end of the vertebral column. The sacrum is a bone shaped like an inverted isosceles triangle located in the middle of the hips, and it composes the back of the pelvis along with the coccyx at its tip. The sacrum is a bone comprised by the fusion of what were originally five separate sacral vertebrae, and individual spinous processes (spiny protrusions to back) stick out as a reminder of this. These section of the sacrum are identified from the top as the first, second, third, fourth and fifth sacral vertebrae. Shō-Chō-Yu happens to be on either side of the point below the first spinous process of the sacrum.

76. Bō-Kō-Yu 膀胱兪 (UB-28)——*Tsubo for enuresis*

In Japan, many people of the older generation remember receiving moxibustion on their lower back from their mothers when they wet their bed as little children. Moxibustion was not done on these children for punishment, but instead the mother was burning moxa on Bō-Kō-Yu 膀胱兪 (UB-28) to cure the habit of bed-wetting, even though she did not always know what she was doing.

Bō-Kō-Yu (urinary bladder *yu*) is the place where harmful energy enters the urinary bladder, so it is very effective against bed-wetting, otherwise known as nocturnal enuresis, and this tsubo has been used for this purpose in Japan from times past. Further, Bō-Kō-Yu is also effective for the women with poor circulation who tend to contract cystitis.

Bō-Kō-Yu is located about four and a half centimeters to either side of the point below the spinous process of the second sacral vertebra. Any symptoms of the urinary bladder such as chilling of the extremities, should be relieved simply by applying heat stimulation around this tsubo using moxa sticks, heat pads, or hot compresses. Generally speaking, thermal therapy is most appropriate for all the tsubos in the lower abdominal, pelvic and sacral regions. The reason for this is that from a functional and structural standpoint, the lower abdomen tends to get poor circulation and blood has a way of getting congested here. Therefore, warming this area improves circulation and alleviates chilling, numbness and pain.

77. Jō-Ryō 上髎 (UB-31)——*Tsubo for menstrual disorders*

There seems to be a great number of women who suffer from menstrual problems, especially people like waitresses in dining cars and tour bus guides who have to remain standing in unstable conditions. The menstrual problems occur especially in these women because they keep their center of gravity low and an excessive amount of blood remains in the lower half of the body, and this causes a congestion of blood in the pelvic area. Applying thorough heat stimulation around the tsubo Jō-Ryō 上髎 (UB-31) gives a considerable amount of relief.

In the classics, the location of Jō-Ryō is stated as being "in the first space of the sacrum on either side of the spine." This refers to the intervertebral foramen (opening for spinal nerve) of the sacrum next to the spinous processes of the sacral vertebrae, which are fused together as explained earlier. There are four pairs of sacral foramina, and they are numbered from the first posterior sacral foramen down to the fourth posterior sacral foramen, from top to bottom. Above each one of these foramen are tsubos respectively named Jō-Ryō 上髎 (top sacral), Ji-Ryō 次髎 (UB-32: second sacral), Chū-Ryō 中髎 (UB-33: middle sacral) and Ge-Ryō

下髎 (UB-34: bottom sacral), from top to bottom. Since these are a total of eight points, they are also called the "eight *ryō* points." These "eight *ryō* points" are very effective for diseases of organs in the pelvic cavity; especially symptoms associate with gynecological disorders including menstrual problems. Other symptoms which women suffer from and treatable by these tsubos are tension and pain in the lower abdomen, swelling in the legs, excessive discharge, blood rising to the head, feeling of heaviness in the head and constipation.

78. Fu-Bun 附分 (UB-36)——*Tsubo for stooped backs in the elderly*

Fu-Bun 附分 (UB-36) is located on the line running parallel to the spine and nine centimeters to either side. It is to either side of the point below the spinous process of the second thoracic vertebra. All the tsubos from Fū-Mon 風門 (UB-12) to Bō-Kō-Yu 膀胱兪 (UB-28) are located on lines which run down from the shoulders to the hips four and a half centimeters away and parallel to the spine. The tsubos from Fu-Bun to Hō-Kō 胞肓 (UB-48) are located on the lines also running from the shoulders down to the hip another four and a half centimeters to the outside of the first lines.

Fu-Bun (next to divide) got its name from being close to the area where the spinal nerves going to the arms branch off. It is a very effective tsubo for ankylosing spondylitis where the spine becomes inflexible with age. The spine has a tendency to become bent with age. On top of this, the spongelike disks between the vertebrae lose their moisture and harden, and gradually the vertebrae start to become fixed to each other from the top downward to eventually become like one long bone. This is what is referred to as ankylosing spondylitis, and it becomes hard for a person to lean back or to twist to the side. Thus, the back becomes stooped and the chest becomes compressed to cause discomfort in the chest, coughing, shortness of breath and palpitations. Fu-Bun is the tsubo used to relieve such symptoms.

79. Hak-Ko 魄戸 (UB-37)——*Tsubo for tension in the neck and shoulders*

In Oriental medicine the organs are each considered to have a mental and emotional aspect along with physiological functions. The lungs are said to house *kihaku*, or spiritedness. The name *Hak-Ko* 魄戸 (UB-37: spirit door) implies that this tsubo is an entrance to the lungs. Hak-Ko is located about nine centimeters to either side of the point below the third thoracic vertebra. It is very effective against stiffness in the neck and shoulders, frozen shoulders, blood rising to the head, coughing, discomfort in the chest, asthma, palpitations and shortness of breath. Hak-Ko is also used to treat the psychological symptoms of anxiety which often accompany lung diseases, especially the tendency to worry over the slightest thing, being continually depressed and unable to keep up one's motivation.

In the anciet text, *Su Wen*, there are five tsubos, or a total of ten points on both sides of the *yu* points of the five essential organs (liver, heart, spleen, lung, kidney), listed as being four and a half centimeters to the outside. These ten tsubos are supposed to be used when there is "heat" in the essential organs. These tsubos are, Hak-Ko next to Hai-Yu 肺兪 (UB-13) which is beside the point below the third thoracic vertebra, Shin-Dō 神堂 (UB-39) which is next to Shin-Yu 心兪 (UB-15) which is beside the point below the fifth thoracic vertebra, Kon-Mon 魂門 (UB-42) next to Kan-Yu 肝兪 (UB-18) which is beside the point below the ninth thoracic vertebra, I-Sha 意舎 (UB-44) next to Hi-Yu 脾兪 (UB-20) which is beside the point below the eleventh thoracic vertebra, and Shi-Shitsu 志室 (UB-47) next to Jin-Yu 腎兪 (UB-23) which is beside the point below the second lumbar vertebra.

80. Kō-Kō 膏肓 (UB-38)——*Tsubo for chilled condition*

Kōyaku in Japan today means ointment, but once it meant a medicine effective for hard to cure illnesses. The character *Kō* means an incurable disease, and the second *Kō* 肓 means a hole or tsubo. Thus Kō-Kō 膏肓 (UB-38) means a place to treat difficult and hard to cure illnesses. This tsubo is located about nine centimeters to the outside of the point below the fourth thoracic vertebra. It is used often for loss of stamina and general fatigue. There is an old saying which goes, "Burn five hundred pieces of moxa here and there is no disease which cannot be cured." Moxibustion at Kō-Kō is, in fact, effective for discomfort in the chest, palpitations, sharp pain in the pit of the stomach, and pain which extends from the shoulders down the back and to the arms.

Also, in acupuncture, this tsubo is used often for those with heart trouble such as angina pectoris from myocardiac infarctions, and those with various symptoms caused by hardening of the arteries. Often people are said to have poor circulation, but this is chiefly because of problems in the heart which is the central organ of the circulatory system. Once the function of the heart is improved, the chronic symptom of feeling chilled will disappear. For this reason, moxibustion at Kō-Kō is effective for those whose hands and feet are always abnormally cold.

81. I-Ki 譩譆 (UB-40)——*Tsubo for fevers with perspiration*

In one classic of Oriental medicine it is written, "When a big wind causes sweating and fever, burn moxa on this tsubo." Coming down with a fever and sweating copiously after exposure to a strong wind is therefore supposed to be treated by moxibustion at I-Ki 譩譆 (UB-40). Such symptoms can also be relieved by applying acupuncture or acupressure here instead of moxibustion. This tsubo is also effective for pains in the chest, the side or the back, as well as dizziness, shortness of breath, difficulty in breathing and coughs. I-Ki is located about nine centimeters to the outside of the point below the sixth thoracic vertebra.

When there are symptoms in the respiratory or circulatory systems, tension and hard spots appear between the shoulder blades on the shoulders and back. Hard spots like "lumps" tend to occur especially around I-Ki, and if this is successfully removed, surprisingly enough, this makes the whole chest area feel much better. Those with even slightly high blood pressure most often feel a sense of oppression in their back along this tsubo, and the stifling feeling in their chest never seems to go away. In such cases, try massaging this tsubo thoroughly with your fingers.

The character *I* 譩 of I-Ki means to belch, or otherwise to heave a big sigh and *Ki* 譆 means to cry out in pain. This tsubo is named this because the patient reacts strongly and begins belching in some cases when this tsubo is pressed, or when acupuncture and moxibustion are applied.

82. Kaku-Kan 膈関 (UB-41)——*Tsubo for trouble in getting food down*

The character *Kan* 関 of Kaku-Kan 膈関 (UB-41) means a border or check point, and *Kaku* 膈 means to separate or to distinguish. This tsubo is, in other words, a gateway between the chest and abdomen. The tsubo Kaku-Yu 膈兪 (UB-17) is located about four and a half centimeters to either side of the point below the seventh thoracic vertebra, and Kaku-Kan is located another four and a half centimeters to the outside of this tsubo. Kaku-Kan is used whenever a person feels nauseous and cannot stop belching, or otherwise when food gets stuck in the gullet and does not go down.

In the classical texts "ailments of *Kaku*" referred to food becoming lodged in the gullet and not reaching the stomach. In one sense, this is a condition which has similarities with cancer today, because cancer develops easily close to the entrance of the stomach (the cardia) which is right below the diaphragm. The reason for this is supposedly because this part of the gullet (esophagus) is crimped in and narrower than other parts, and is therefore more susceptible to irritation.

Cancer of the stomach, or of the esophagus is quite common in Japan. The esophagus passes right next to the place where the trachea (wind pipe) splits in two at the height of the fifth thoracic vertebra to reach either lung. This is the first narrow part the food has to get past. Further down the esophagus narrows again where it penetrates the diaphragm, so food must pass through another narrow part. From the standpoint of Oriental medicine, excessive constriction of these areas cause symptoms such as food becoming lodged in the chest or gullet.

83. I-Sha 意舎 (UB-44)——*Tsubo for strengthening one's will*

I-Sha 意舎 (UB-44) is effective in cases of diarrhea resulting from intestinal problems, a sensation of distention in the stomach, urine turning reddish in color, as well as occasional nausea and fever with yellowing of the eyes. *I-Sha* means the place where one's will is housed, and it was thought that this tsubo exerts control over one's will. It was explained earlier in the section for Hi-Yu 脾兪 (UB-20) how the will was housed in the spleen, so therefore these tsubos are intimately related, and I-Sha can be used for those symptoms Hi-Yu is used for.

The spleen and stomach meridians in Oriental medicine are a yin-yang pain pair in an interior-exterior relationship, and thus they mutually assist and cooperate in each other's functions. Because the spleen determines one's will power, those who have stomach trouble tend to be weak willed, and often are anxious and worry about every little thing people say. It is a fact that stomach problems are common among nervous types, and it has been demonstrated by modern medicine how there is a close relationship between the function of the stomach and mental stress. Pressing I-Sha, the tsubo for "strengthening one's will," under stressful situations will serve to improve the stomach condition. This tsubo, located nine centimeters to either side of the point below the eleventh thoracic vertebra, is indispensable for people with weak stomachs or weak wills.

84. Shi-Shitsu 志室 (UB-47)——*Tsubo to increase stamina*

In the classics of Chinese medicine it is written, "One's intentions are housed in the kidney." Shi-Shitsu 志室 (UB-47: intention room) is a tsubo where the quotient of energy a person has been endowed with from birth can be determined. If a person has kidney problems, this means his motivation and aspirations are weakened because intentions are housed in the kidney. This is often seen in the "kidney deficient condition" where one tires easily, sexual performance declines, the body becomes flaccid, one's motivation to work is lost and illnesses are the worst in the winter. Shi-Shitsu is used just for such a condition, and aside from this, it is used for lumbago or sudden low back pain.

This tsubo is located nine centimeters to either side of the point below the second lumbar vertebra. This is just to the outside of the tsubo Jin-Yu 腎俞 (UB-23) and is level with the tip of the lowest rib. Shi-Shitsu is used together with Jin-Yu to treat pain in the upper and lower back, as well as when there are symptoms like hardness and pressure sensitivity around the navel, a paucity of urine, impotence, a lack of sexual drive and total exhaustion.

Thermal therapy known as *on-ho* (warm and reinforce) method has been used in Japan since the early days, in addition to the standard moxibustion where moxa cones are burned directly on the skin. In this method a slice of garlic or ginger is placed on the skin and the moxa is burned on top of this for a milder form of heat stimulation. Another name for Shi-Shitsu is *Sei-Shitsu* 精室 (sperm room) so it is easily to understand how this tsubo is known as one which increases a person's sexual prowess.

85. Hō-Kō 胞肓 (UB-48)——*Tsubo for gynecological problems*

Hō-Kō 胞肓 (UB-48) is located about nine centimeters on either side of the point below the spinous process of the second sacral vertebra, along with the tsubo Shi-Shitsu 志室 (UB-47) on both sides of Jin-Yu 腎俞 (UB-23). Hō-Kō is an important tsubo for treating diseases of the sexual organs, especially gynecological disorders.

The character *Hō* 胞 of Hō-Kō can be interpreted to mean the uterus. The uterus is the organ in which the fetus grows, and this tsubo is therefore particularly important for women. Gynecological disorders are always accompanied with symptoms such as heaviness of the head, stiff shoulders, fatigue in the waist area, tension in the lower abdomen, uterine discharge and chilled feet. Many women past their prime complain of being cold in their waist area, tension in their lower abdomen and chilling of their feet. In these cases, it is best to warm up the body below the waist. In Japan people used to take what were called *koshi-yu* (waist bath) where only the lower half of the body was soaked in hot water. This method of warming up all the tsubos in the sacral region, which are very important for gynecological problems, to restore circulation in the lower half of the body is greatly recommended.

86. Shō-Fu 承扶 (UB-50)——*Tsubo to relieve sciatica*

Shō-Fu 承扶 (UB-50) is located in the center of the horizontal crease which forms under the hips when standing straight up. This tsubo is most effective for a sharp pain along the nerve which runs down the back of the leg to the feet, known as sciatica. In this case, a hard spot can be found by pressing inside the crease below the buttock using the thumbs. This hard spot results from a defensive reaction in that part of the body to the pain in the leg. When this hard spot is pressed slowly and gently, the pain in the leg will ease and the person will feel much better.

Shō-Fu is an important tsubo right over the place where the sciatic nerve first makes its way out of the pelvis. This is the reason sciatica can sometimes be relieved instantly just by treating this tsubo. Aside from sciatica, this tsubo has been proven effective for excruciating pain from the thighs down to the knees, pain from hemorrhoids, swelling of hips, constipation, nocturnal enuresis and menstrual cramps. Relief can be provided to people with such symptoms by having them lay on their stomach and pressing this tsubo with the thumbs straight toward the center of the limb, going lightly at first and gradually increasing the pressure.

87. I-Yō 委陽 (UB-53)——*Tsubo for knee pain from aging*

Recently there seems to be an increase in the number of middle-aged women who complain of pain in their thighs and knees when standing up, sitting down, or when climbing up and down stairs. This is caused by the gradual deformation of the knee joint with age, where the muscles and tendons around the knees either become too tight or loose to impair the circulation. This used to be treated as a simple case of rheumatism, but now it is known as gonarthritis deformans (degenerative joint disease of the knees) which is caused by aging. I-Yō 委陽 (UB-53) is the tsubo used most often for this condition.

This tsubo is located in the back of the knee, or the popliteal fossa. There is a skin fold in the back of the knee, and I-Yō is on the outer edge of this crease (toward the little toe). The character *I* 委 means bend, and *Yō* 陽 (yang) means the outside of the leg (the inside of the leg toward the big toe is yin). I-Yō, therefore, means a tsubo to the outside of the fold in the knee. Aside from knee pain and sciatica, I-Yō is used quite often for hemiplegia after a stroke where the arms and legs on one side are paralyzed.

88. I-Chū 委中 (UB-54)——*Tsubo for cramps in the calf muscle*

I-Chū 委中 (UB-54), along with the previously mentioned I-Yō 委陽 (UB-53), is used often to treat knee pain. As its name implies, I-Chū (bend middle) is in the middle of the skin fold behind the knee. Traditionally this tsubo has been used as a point for letting blood (venesection) to provide relief whenever febrile, acute or heavy illnesses caused the calf muscles to cramp.

Just as explained before, degenerative joint diseases of the knee is seen just as often in middle-aged women, as baldness is seen in middle-aged men. The majority of middle-aged women with this condition complain of fatigue and pain in their lower back, thighs, calves and ankles. All this pain comes about because, when the knee is in pain, the muscles of the thighs are kept in a constant state of tension instead of being used properly to move the knee joint, and this causes fatigue and pain. Also, a greater burden is placed on the ankle joint to protect the knees, and so the calf muscles get tired and the ankles become worn out. Eventually the fatigue progresses upward to the muscles of the hips, and low back pain is the end result. The knee pain ends up causing pain in the thighs, calves, ankles and finally, the lower back. In such situations, trying to treat each painful area is ineffective unless the source of the problem, the knee pain, is cured. I-Chū is the tsubo to use in such situations.

89. Shō-Kin 承筋 (UB-56)——*Tsubo for cramps in the calves*

Every summer articles about accidents in the ocean and mountains can be seen in the newspapers. Even though the seasides have become quite crowded these days, people still throng to the beaches and drowning and missing persons are the inevitable result. It is interesting to note that the majority of drowning victims are able to swim. Those who are confident in their swimming ability venture farther offshore, but the farther out one gets, the colder the water becomes. This can cause cramping in the calf muscles if they react and contract suddenly. This is what places a swimmer in danger.

In such situations the best thing to do is not to panic, but float face up in the water and stretch out the cramped leg and grab the highest point of the calf muscle to apply strong pressure. This is usually right around where the tsubo Shō-Kin 承筋 (UB-56) is located. Shō-Kin means to control the muscles, and this tsubo is also named *Zen-Chō* 喘脹. Aside from cramps in the calf muscle, this tsubo is effective for sciatica which is a neuralgia where a sharp pulling pain runs down the back of the thighs to the knees. Also, Shō-Kin is used often to treat swelling in the armpit and nosebleeds.

90. Shō-Zan 承山 (UB-57)——*Tsubo to reduce swelling in calves*

Shō-Zan 承山 (UB-57) also has the name *Gyo-Fuku* 魚腹 (fish belly). The reason it got this name is because the calf muscle on which this tsubo is located somewhat resembles the belly of a large fish. *Shō-Zan* means to "control the mountain," and this comes from comparing the rise of the calf muscle to a hill or a small mountain, and further because this tsubo is used to control and relieve symptoms in this area.

Shō-Zan is located below the previous tsubo Shō-Kin 承筋 (UB-56) where the calf muscle turns into a hard tendon. Shō-Zan can be located by tracing up the back of the leg from the heels with your little finger. Dragging the finger up the center of the back of the calf, there will be a point where the finger comes to a stop at the rise of the muscle. This tsubo Shō-Zan is used often for fatigue in the knees and legs, swelling in the calves, cramps and constipation. This tsubo is especially effective when a person has been seated for a long time, like after watching a movie or long drives, and when the legs or calves become slightly swollen, or otherwise, the legs feel extremely dull and heavy.

91. Hi-Yō 飛陽 (UB-58)——*Tsubo for nasal congestion*

"The greater yang meridian of the foot is also called *Hi-Yō* 飛陽 (UB-58). When there is excess energy here, the nose becomes stuffy, the head aches and the back hurts. When energy is deficient, the nose becomes obstructed or bleeds. Treat this at the point where the meridian branches off."

The above is the explanation offered for the tsubo Hi-Yō in the classic text *Jin Mo Bian* 経脈編. It may come as a surprise that symptoms of the head and nose can be treated at a tsubo on the leg, but there is an old rule in Oriental medicine which goes, "If the disease is in the upper part of the body, use the points on the lower part, and if the disease is in the lower part, use points on the upper part." This means that when the illness is above the navel, tsubo located below the navel should be used, and conversely, if the disease is below, tsubo located above should be used. The validity of this approach has been verified today through studies on pressure sensitivity reactions showing that the upper and lower halves of the body are in a reciprocating relationship where one half controls and coordinates the other half.

The character *Hi* 飛 of Hi-Yō means high, and *Yō* 陽 means yang or the sunny side, so together it means a tsubo located high above the outside (yang side) of the foot.

Hi-Yō is located about twenty-one centimeters above the outer ankle bone and about three centimeters to the back of the leg. Putting strength in the calf muscle will cause a line to form on the outside edge of where the muscle tapers down at the bottom. Hi-Yō is located on the bottom edge of the calf muscle where it tapers off. Aside from the symptoms already mentioned, this tsubo is effective for pain in the toes, hemorrhoids, dizziness upon standing up and epilepsy.

92. Kin-Mon 金門 (UB-63)——*Tsubo for epilectic seizures*

Kin-Mon 金門 (UB-63) is the *geki* point of the urinary bladder meridian. As mentioned before, *geki* points are effective for acute symptoms. Keep this tsubo in mind because it can be used to treat all acute symptoms associated with this meridian. Regardless of the nature of the symptoms, if they are sudden or traumatic, apply pressure on this tsubo along with other tsubos indicated. Kin-Mon is immediately effective for epileptic seizures, sudden cramping of the calf muscles, or the ankle giving out without warning. It will surprise you how much this tsubo can alleviate the seizure or pain.

Kin-Mon is located below and slightly to the front of the outer ankle bone. This is right behind the tsubo Kei-Kotsu 京骨 (UB-64) which comes next. The character *Kin* 金 of Kin-Mon means gold or something precious, and *Mon* 門 is a gate or entrance. In other words, this tsubo is one important gateway in the flow of this meridian.

93. Kei-Kotsu 京骨 (UB-64)——*Tsubo to check condition of urinary bladder*

Kei-Kotsu 京骨 (UB-64) has been used to relieve pain in the feet since the olden days. It is written as being "on the greater yang area of the foot, a place where the meridian flows past, and designated as the *gen* point." Therefore, it is a very important tsubo for checking whether there are any abnormalities along the entire length of the greater yang urinary bladder meridian. Feeling the outside of the foot from the ankle bone toward the little toe, you will run across a prominent bump on the outside. This is the head of the fifth metatarsal bone, and Kei-Kotsu is located right in back of this.

Just like the tsubo Kei-Kotsu, all the tsubos used to check the condition over the whole meridian are called the *gen* points, and each of the twelve meridians have a *gen* point. The meridians which run down from the chest to the arms have this point on the wrist, while the meridians which run from the head to the feet have this point on the ankles. Whenever there seems to be a problem in the organs in the chest or stomach, this can be checked at the *gen* points around the wrists and ankles. In other words, if there is pressure sensitivity, hard spots, a sensation of being cold or hot, or otherwise, a pimple or a mark at the associated *gen* point, it is a sign that there is indeed something wrong with that organ in the chest or stomach area. In this way, the tsubo Kei-Kotsu is used more for the purpose of diagnosing and correcting the overall condition of the urinary bladder meridian than for symptomatic treatments.

8. Kidney Meridian

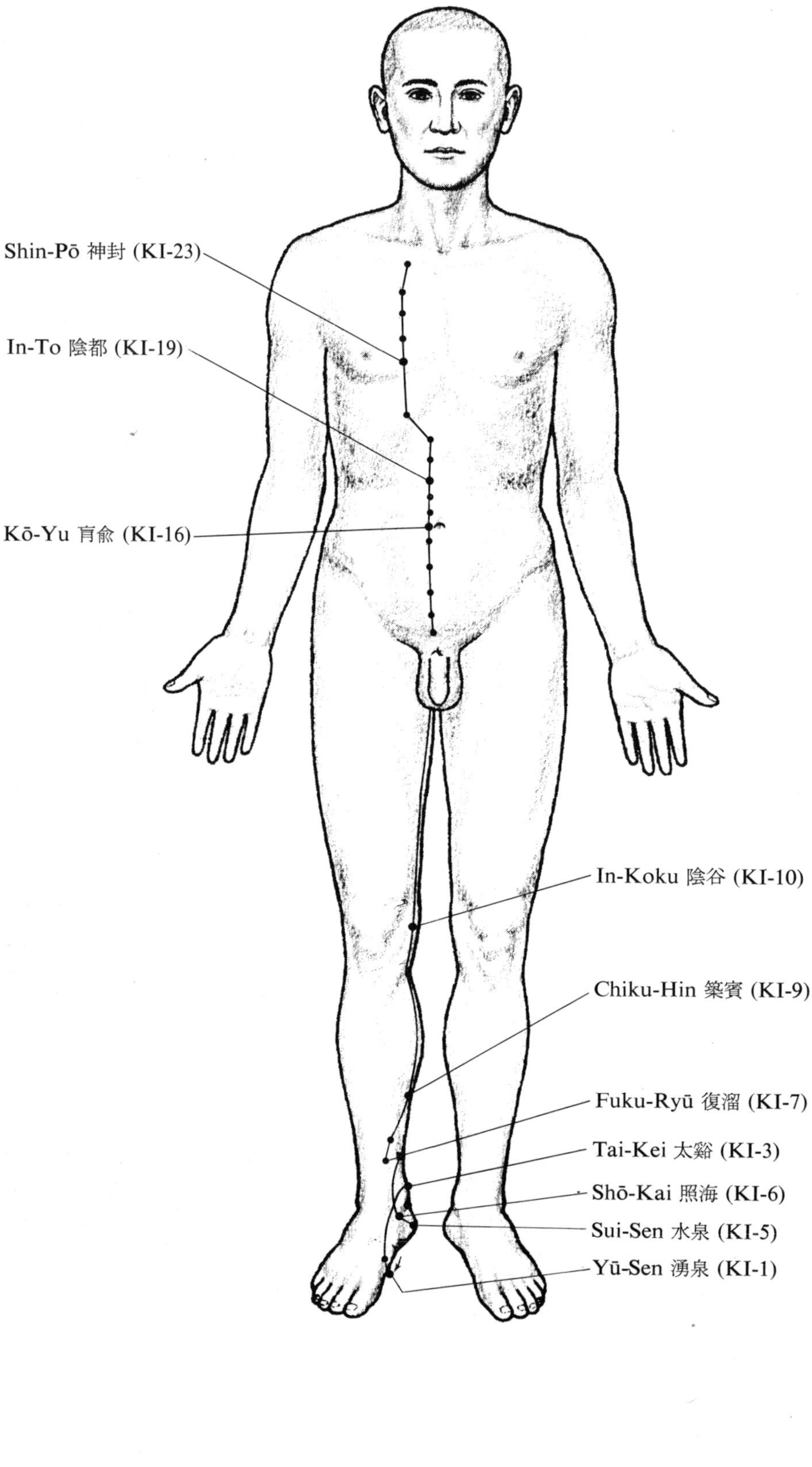

The kidney is among one of the five essential organs in Oriental medicine. The kidney was regarded as being the organ which contained the essential life force inherited from one's parents. As mentioned earlier, the "kidney" of Oriental medicine in its function more closely resembles the adrenal glands in modern medicine. The adrenal glands are yellowish small triangular endocrine glands on top of the kidneys which continuously regulate the metabolism in the whole body. They modulate the physical functions so that we may continue to live in health by adapting to changes in the weather and coping with daily stress such as troublesome human relationships. The "kidney" as described in Oriental medicine was intuitive knowledge of the adrenal glands derived from clinical experience.

The kidney meridian has a total of twenty-seven tsubos. It starts with the tsubo Yū-Sen 湧泉 (KI-1) on the soles of the feet. From here it passes behind the inner ankle bone and goes up the inside of the lower leg and reaches the tsubo In-Koku 陰谷 (KI-10) right beside the knee. The meridian continues up the inside of the thigh and goes up to the tip of the coccyx. From the tsubo Chō-Kyō 長強 (GV-1) it goes through to the lower abdomen where it travels up the lines one and a a half centimeters to either side of the anterior center line (the Conception Vessel). At the tsubo Kō-Yu 肓兪 (KI-16) just to either side of the navel, this meridian goes to the kidneys. The meridian divides in two after this, and one branch descends the Conception Vessel to go once around the urinary bladder, and the other branch goes straight up from the kidneys and reaches the lungs after going through the liver and diaphragm. The latter branch splits once more in the lungs, and one branch goes past the trachea to the root of the tongue, and the other branch circulates in the heart and connects with the heart constrictor meridian at the tsubo Dan-Chū 膻中 (CV-17) which is right between the nipples.

The following are some of the symptoms which tsubos of the kidney meridian are effective for; darkened face with no luster to the skin, dry tongue with sweaty palms, swelling of the throat, difficulty in breathing, dizziness upon standing, lack of appetite despite not having eaten, tendency toward diarrhea, getting tired easily, lack of muscle tone and loss of weight. Tsubos of the kidney meridian are also effective for those people whose physical condition deteriorates in the winter. The image of a person who is unable to stand up to things (keep a straight waist), or to put his weight (waist) behind something, particularly in the Orient, describes people who are indecisive and unsure of themselves. This is because in the Orient, the lower back or the area below the waist is considered to be of prime importance in centering the body. Along with the symptoms mentioned above, when the function of the kidneys are impaired, there is pain in the lower back and a loss of vitality.

Jin-Yu 腎兪 (UB-23) is one tsubo used to check the condition of the kidney meridian. One must keep a close watch on this meridian and check it periodically because it houses the basic source of vitality in human beings, and it is of primary importance as an indicator of our overall condition. Aside from Jin-Yu, the tsubos Kei-Mon 京門 (GB-25) at the tip of the twelfth rib, and Kō-Yu 肓兪 (KI-16) on either side of the navel, are used for the purpose of examining the condition of the kidney meridian. Eleven of the most often used tsubos of the kidney will be introduced below.

94. Yū-Sen 湧泉 (KI-1)——*Tsubo for gynecological disorders*

Tokujirō Namikoshi is the famous shiatsu instructor who said the words; "The essence of shiatsu is just like a mother's love, press and the spring of life wells up from within." These words were inspired when I introduced this tsubo during a lecture given in a seminar held by Mr. Namikoshi. *Yū-Sen* 湧泉 (KI-1: welling spring) means a tsubo where the life force present in a person from birth wells up. It is located to the front and in the middle of the soles. You can find this tsubo by pressing toward the center of the sole, behind the ball of the big toe, where there is a depression with a hard tendon underneath. The sole of the foot has been considered as being a very important place from ancient times because the energy of the earth is absorbed through the feet. At one time, it was even maintained that only experts could perform acupuncture or moxibustion here.

Perhaps for these reasons, there is something profound in the effects of this tsubo. Yū-Sen is especially effective for gynecological disorders, pain and chilling down the lower back and abdomen to the legs, as well as for blood rising to the head. Also, it is effective in preventing the general decrease in vitality which comes with age and for increasing stamina. In the "kidney decline condition" where a person's vitality declines greatly, this becomes quite apparent by the soreness and hard spots around this tsubo.

The best way to apply moxa on this tsubo is to place a slice of garlic or ginger between the skin and the moxa cone. This way no scar is left by the burning of the moxa, and no problem is created in walking. Shiatsu treatments to Yū-Sen are most effective when additional finger pressure is applied in succession up the kidney meridian to San-In-Kō 三陰交 (SP-6) and all the way up to the knee.

95. Tai-Kei 太谿 (KI-3)——*Tsubo to increase vigor*

The tsubo Tai-Kei 太谿 (KI-3) is located right in back of the inner ankle bone. This tsubo on the inside of the foot (side of big toe) is directly opposite of Kon-Ron 崑崙 (UB-60) which is on the outside of the foot (side of little toe). Tai-Kei is effective for overexcitement and an inability to calm down, pain in the calf muscle, the skin breaking out for no apparent reason, menstrual disorders and for making the legs more shapely.

Tai-Kei means a large ravine, and it is the *gen* point of the kidney meridian. This means that it is the place for checking and improving the condition of the kidney meridian. In the classics it is listed as being "the place where the lesser yin (kidney) meridian of the leg flows, designated as the *gen* (source)." It is thus clearly indicated as being the *gen* point of the kidney meridian where the energy in the meridian flows past. In other words, Tai-Kei is an important tsubo for determining whether the basic life force of a person endowed from birth is weak or strong. If this is found to be very weak, the treatment must concentrate on this tsubo.

The following symptoms are generalized under the "kidney deficient condition"; being weak and tiring quickly, decline in sexual drive, lack of muscle tone, chilling in the extremities, fatigue in the lower back and occasional feelings of heat in the soles of the feet accompanied with fatigue. In these cases, pain and hard spots appear around Tai-Kei. It goes without saying that this tsubo is used to treat all of the above symptoms.

96. Sui-Sen 水泉 (KI-5)——*Tsubo for acute symptoms of the kidney*

Among the five elements of wood, fire, earth, metal and water, the kidney corresponds to water. *Sui-Sen* 水泉 (KI-5: water spring) similar to Yū-Sen 湧泉 (KI-1), means a spring along the kidney meridian, or a spring from where the energy of this meridian flows. This tsubo, just as the three preceding tsubos of the kidney meridian, clearly shows the strength or weakness of one's inborn constitution since it is a spring along this meridian. Sui-Sen is also designated as the *geki* point of the lesser yin kidney meridian, so it is most effective in treating acute symptoms associated with the kidney. For example, it is used when one is fatigued and feeling dizzy, and when things appear hazy at a distance, menstruation is irregular, palpitations occur, one gets tired easily, or when the lower abdomen feels heavy and distended.

Sui-Sen is located to the back and below the inner ankle bone, about three centimeters below Tai-Kei 太谿 (KI-3). There are a great number of tsubos around the inner ankle bone, including that of the liver, kidney and spleen meridians. When man finally assumed the erect posture after having been a four legged creature, the ankles, knees, hips and waist came to play a crucial role. Therefore, if there was any weak point in his physical structure, it was these joints. This is the reason many important tsubos are located around the ankle, knee and waist. The secret to staying healthy is to keep the joints of the ankles, knees, hips and waist supple and free in movement.

97. Shō-Kai 照海 (KI-6)——*Tsubo for menstrual irregularities*

Menstrual irregularities are the source of a whole variety of other problems for women. It is not too unusual for women that irritability and becoming annoyed over minor things be connected with their period. Shō-Kai 照海 (KI-6) has been used from times past as a tsubo effective for menstrual irregularity and various other symptoms associated with this. These symptoms include psychological ones such as always being thirsty and unable to calm down, or for some reason feeling depressed and unable to enjoy oneself in the company of friends. Otherwise, this tsubo is very effective for troublesome symptoms such as low back pain, distention of the lower abdomen, fatigue and chilling of the arms and legs, and feeling slightly queasy or nauseous.

Shō-Kai is located right under the inner ankle bone. Touch the highest point of the inner ankle bone and then go down a little to where there is a small hollow area. This hollow place is Shō-Kai. The character *Shō* 照 means brightness, radiance or clarity. *Kai* 海 (sea) expresses a wide area where things collect. In other words, Shō-Kai denotes a place where harmful energy collects most clearly along the kidney meridian, and in this sense, Yū-Sen 湧泉 (KI-1) and Tai-Kei 太谿 (KI-3) together with this tsubo comprise three vital tsubos among those used to cure symptoms associated with the kidney meridian such as, chilling, heaviness, fatigue, or pain in the legs.

98. Fuku-Ryū 復溜 (KI-7)——*Tsubo for distention of abdomen*

The tsubo Fuku-Ryū 復溜 (KI-7) is located about six centimeters straight up from the inside ankle bone. Lightly pressing the inside of the leg upward from the inner ankle bone, there will be a slightly depressed area about six centimeters up. Pressing this point a little stronger, you may detect the pulsation of an artery deep down. The character *Fuku* 復 of Fuku-Ryū means to return, backtrack, or layer. *Ryū* 溜 means to collect or stagnate. So it means a place where the flow of the meridian energy is impeded and becomes backed up.

Fuku-Ryū, according to classical texts, is among the important tsubo of the kidney meridian along with those already mentioned. This tsubo has been used from times past for distention of the abdomen, swelling in the arms and legs, general fatigue, and lack of urine. This tsubo is also well-known as being able to relieve pain in the lower back and pelvic area, as well as toothaches. Personally, I use this tsubo with good results for the feeling of languor and dizziness, tinnitus caused by loss of vitality, as well as for night sweating and lack of appetite. Fuku-Ryū is well recognized as a tsubo effective in alleviating symptoms which are hard to cure from the standpoint of Western medicine using drugs and surgery. These symptoms include gynecological problems, general loss of vigor, low back pain and symptoms associated with high blood pressure (headaches, dizziness, shoulder tension, chilling of feet, insomnia, etc.).

99. Chiku-Hin 築賓 (KI-9)——*Tsubo for cramps in calf muscle*

The character *Chiku* 築 of Chiku-Hin 築賓 (KI-9) means to construct, and *Hin* 賓 is a character which has the meaning of beach. So, in a manner of speaking, it is a tsubo where the calf muscle (gastrocnemius muscle) gradually becomes smaller and the energy which flows through the meridian reaches a smooth shoreline where the energy forms waves. In more specialized language, these characters indicate a place between the soleus and gastrocnemius muscles. Find this tsubo by tracing a line up from the inner ankle bone to a point about eighteen centimeters above. The finger should come to a stop by itself. Chiku-Hin is located at this height and one finger width back from the shin bone.

The muscles around this tsubo often become cramped during long hikes, when swimming, or in athletic competitions, and otherwise, fatigue in the calf muscle creates lines of tension and stiffness. In order to relieve cramps in the calf muscle, first warm up the area and then massage the whole muscle slowly with large grasping movements.

Aside from the above applications, Chiku-Hin is used when there is a headache accompanied with a fever, and a person is nauseous or talks deliriously. In the past, Takeshi Sawada, a renowned Japanese acupuncturist, used this tsubo specially for its detoxification effect and he obtained good results in dispelling a wide variety of poisons from the body.

100. In-Koku 陰谷 (KI-10)——*Tsubo for impotence*

In-Koku 陰谷 (KI-10) is located on the back of the knee toward the inside, and is straight up from the inner ankle bone. A tsubo of the liver meridian, Kyoku-Sen 極泉 (LV-8), is located on the inside end of the crease in the leg when the knee is fully bent. In-Koku is separated from this tsubo by one muscle to the inside. In the classics of Oriental medicine the location of this tsubo is described as being "behind the medial condyle of the knee, behind and under the larger muscle and on top of the smaller muscle, a point responding to pressure, locate with the knee bent."

For women this tsubo is good for tension in the abdomen and discharge. For men, In-Koku is commonly used for impotence and disfunctions of the sexual organs. *In-Koku* (yin valley) means a valley along the course of the lesser yin kidney meridian. It is the sea point of the kidney meridian where the meridian energy flow converges to become one main channel. For this reason, this tsubo is also effective for neuralgia in the abdominal and lumbar region which produces severe pain in the lower abdomen and genital area, as well as down the inner thighs. Also, In-Koku of the kidney meridian and Kyoku-Sen of the liver meridian mentioned above are both vital tsubo for helping a person who has become weak in the knees from general fatigue or loss of vitality. Sometimes when people are extremely surprised or frightened, they feel faint and slump to the ground. This is called *koshi-ga-nukeru* in Japanese which means not being able to stand up to a situation. This is actually caused by becoming weak in the knees all of a sudden. In-Koku is a vital tsubo effective in such situations.

101. Kō-Yu 肓兪 (KI-16)——*Tsubo to increase vitality*

Kō-Yu 肓兪 (KI-16) has traditionally been said to "cure men unable to have children," and this means that it is a tsubo very effective for situations where a couple cannot have children because of some problem in the man. Kō-Yu has this effect because it corrects the energy balance in the body of those who have "kidney deficient condition." To treat such cases, moxibustion is applied on this tsubo one and a half centimeters to either side of the navel and slightly below. The character *Kō* 肓 of Kō-Yu is the same as that used for the tsubos Kō-Kō 膏肓 (UB-38) and Hō-Kō 胞肓 (UB-48), and it means a tsubo. Kō-Yu simply means a tsubo where the harmful energy of the kidney meridian flows.

This tsubo is also used often for such symptoms as palpitations, pain in the pit of the stomach and the tendency to have diarrhea because of a weak stomach. In addition to this, Kō-Yu is used to check the overall physical condition, especially the amount of fatigue, as well as to determine whether symptoms such as loss of stamina, blood rising to the head and chilling of the feet are present.

Lie on your back with your legs stretched out and bare your abdomen. Next, lightly touch the tsubo Kō-Yu on both sides of the navel with your middle finger, and then press the kidney points down toward the legs. If there is a disturbing sensation which extends down your legs when you do this, it means you are in a "kidney deficient condition." It is common that such people have mild low back pain or hard areas around the tsubo Yū-Sen 湧泉 (KI-1) in the sole of the foot.

102. In-To 陰都 (KI-19)——*Tsubo for gastroptosis*

The character *In* 陰 (yin) of In-To 陰都 (KI-19) comes from being on the lesser yin meridian of the legs, and *To* 都 (capital) means a place where people gather. Thus, this name indicates a place where harmful energy of the lesser yin kidney meridian gathers. This tsubo is located about thirteen centimeters above Kō-Yu 肓兪 (KI-16) which is one and a half centimeters to either side of the navel. In-To is just level with the midpoint between the navel and the pit of the stomach.

This tsubo is used most often for a persistent stifling sensation in the pit of the stomach, tension in the side, discomfort in the chest, palpitations, poor digestion, a heavy sensation in the stomach, and difficulty in getting to sleep. In-To is considered as being one of the more important tsubo in the kidney meridian. In-To, especially, is one tsubo which those suffering from gastroptosis should learn. Applying thermal therapy on this tsubo along with Kan-Yu 肝兪 (UB-18), Hi-Yu 脾兪 (UB-20) and I-Yu 胃兪 (UB-21) all on the back should provide amazing results. The most important thing, however, is to continue such treatments patiently over a period of time. Generally one complete treatment is given at least once a week in acupuncture, and this must be continued at least three times in a row to be really effective. It is rather hasty to conclude that it does not work after applying moxa or other treatments on a couple of occasions.

103. Shin-Pō 神封 (KI-23)——*Tsubo to stop acute chest pains*

In Oriental medicine one's spirit is said to be housed in the essential organ, the heart, so *Shin-Pō* 神封 (KI-23: spirit seal) means a tsubo where the subtle energy of the heart is sealed in. It is located about seven centimeters to either side of a line drawn straight down the center of the chest from the base of the throat to the pit of the stomach. It is just level with the nipples for men.

Shin-Pō has been noted from old times as being effective for heart disease, especially for various symptoms associated with angina pectoris. Aside from this, Shin-Pō is used often for blood rising to the head, discomfort in the chest, shortness of breath, coughing, distension from the chest around to the side, nausea and palpitations accompanied with pains which shoot through the chest to the back.

The following tsubos are intersected when a line is drawn around the torso from the back below the fourth thoracic vertebra to the side and on to the chest level with the nipples (below the fourth rib); Ketsu-In-Yu 厥陰兪 (UB-14) and Kō-Kō 膏肓 (UB-38) both on the back, En-Eki 淵液 (GB-22) under the armpit, Ten-Kei 天谿 (SP-18) and Ten-Chi 天池 (HC-1) just to the outside of the nipple, Nyū-Chū 乳中 (ST-17) right on the nipple, and Shin-Pō and Dan-Chū 膻中 (CV-17) to the inside of the nipple. These tsubos are all closely associated with the heart and the circulation of blood throughout the entire body. Even in Western medicine these tsubos all belong in the skin segment of the fourth thoracic nerve which manifests symptoms of the circulatory system. Therefore, even better results can be obtained by using these other tsubos together with Shin-Pō.

9. Heart Constrictor Meridian

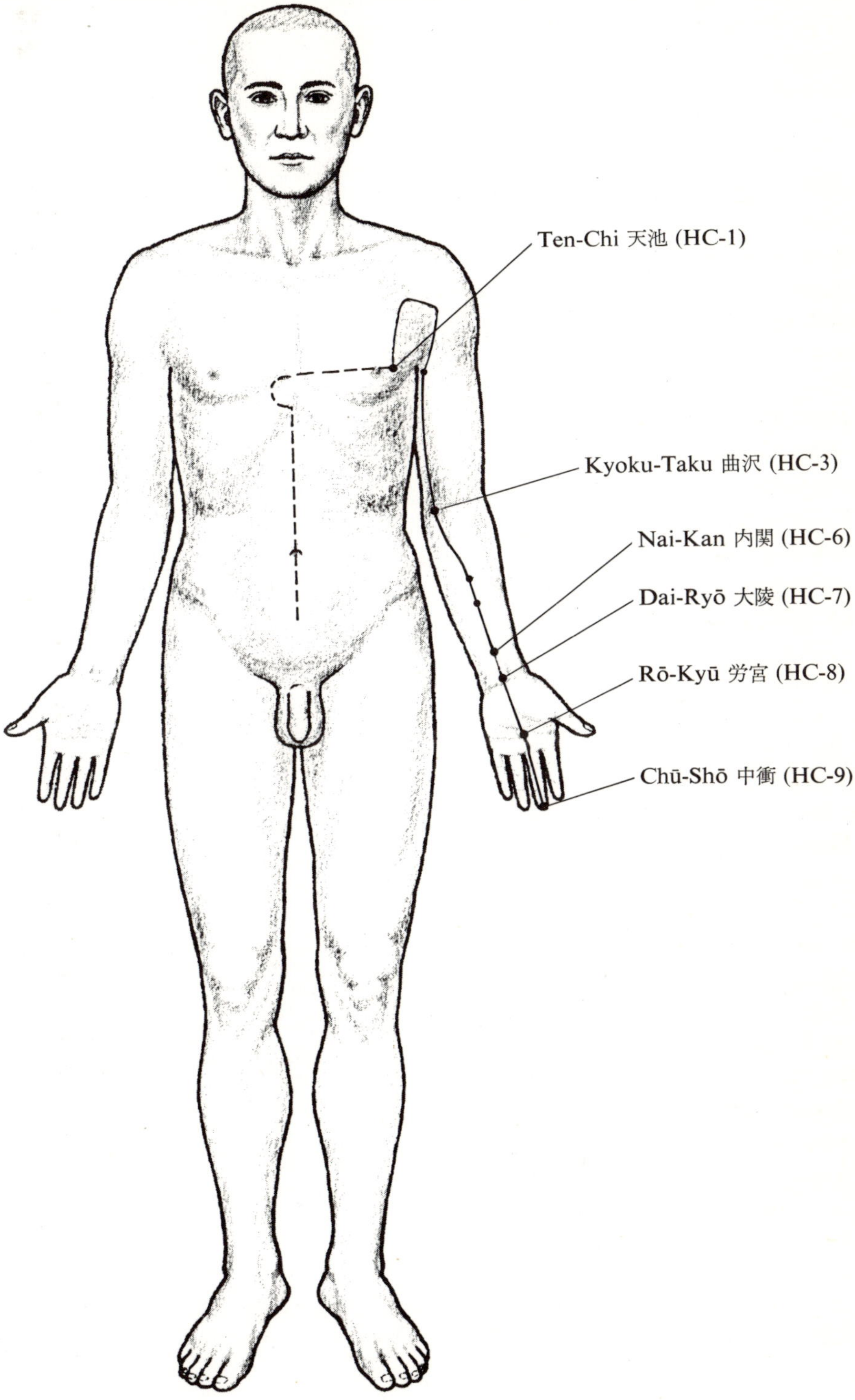

In Oriental medicine the heart is regarded as one of the most important organs among all of the organs, and the heart constrictor is the membrane (pericardium) which covers the heart. The heart constrictor meridian circulates through the pericardium and controls it. Traditionally, the heart was likened to the emperor of a state, and the heart constrictor was compared to a prime minister who governed a state by decree of the emperor.

In Oriental medicine, generally, the heart constrictor is not counted among the five *zang* and six *fu*. When the heart constrictor is included, it makes six *zang* and six *fu*. The reason the heart constrictor is not counted as a separate organ is because it does not have its own form or function. Its role is to cover and protect the heart—the central organ of the human body—and it serves to carry out the orders of the heart. For this reason, the symptoms treated with the tsubos of the absolute yin heart constrictor meridian and the lesser yin heart meridian are just about the same. This is one reason the heart constrictor is not counted among the five *zang* (essential yin organs).

For this same reason, the heart constrictor meridian is not an independent meridian, but is instead regarded as being a branch meridian. The heart constrictor meridian branches off from the previous kidney meridian and first goes through the diaphragm to go to three tsubos—Jō-Kan 上脘 (CV-13), Chū-Kan 中脘 (CV-12) and In-Kō 陰交 (CV-7)—and thereby connects with the triple heater meridian which comes next. Another branch from the kidney meridian goes through the chest and comes out to a point just to the outside of the nipple. From here it runs down the inside center of the arm. This is the surface branch of the heart constrictor meridian which has nine tsubos. This external branch begins at the tsubo just to the outside of the nipple and flows in front of the armpit and down the arm between the course of the lung and heart meridians. It travels down the inside of the elbow and the forearm to reach the palm. Here it divides into two, and one branch comes to an end at the base of the nail of the middle finger on the side of the thumb. The other branch goes to the base of the nail of the ring finger on the side of the little finger. This is the tsubo Kan-Shō 関衝 (TH-1) where the heart constrictor meridian connects to the first tsubo of the triple heater meridian of the arm.

As mentioned already, the heart constrictor covers the heart, and its meridian circulates around the heart, so almost all of the important tsubos used for heart conditions are located on this meridian. The following symptoms are said to be common when the function of the heart is impaired; flushed face, palpitations, yellowing of eyes, pain from the chest around to the side, pain, tension and numbness extending down the inside of the upper arm and forearm, and hotness in the palm of the hands. The nine tsubos of the heart constrictor meridian are used when these symptoms are present. Six tsubos among these which are most often used will be discussed below.

104. Ten-Chi 天池 (HC-1)——*Tsubo to relieve pain in underarm area*

Ten-Chi 天池 (HC-1) is located about three centimeters to the outside of the nipple. This tsubo is also called *Ten-E* 天会 (heaven meeting). It is the place where the absolute yin meridian of the arm and the lesser yang meridian of the leg, which is the same thing as saying, the heart constrictor and gallbladder meridians, meet each other. The character *Ten* 天 meaning heaven, generally refers to the Kingdom of God, but in terms of the body, it refers to the top half. *Chi* 池 is a pond where harmful energy collects. Thus, *Ten-Chi* means a place in the upper half of the body where harmful energy collects. Ten-Chi also refers to the place where all the harmful energy in the heart constrictor meridian collects, and the flow of energy backs up to become like a pond.

Ten-Chi is very effective when there is a sense of oppression and discomfort extending from the chest down to the pit of the stomach and lower abdomen, or when one does not perspire even with a high temperature, and otherwise for headaches, sore throats, swelling below the armpits, blood rising to the head and feelings of being chilled. When these symptoms are present, it is sometimes called "a voice in the chest" in Oriental medicine, and this describes a rushing sound in the chest or a sound from the throast.

There is a tsubo by the name Ten-Sen 天泉 (HC-2) about six centimeters down from the armpit on the inside of the arm. It lies right next to Ten-Chi when the arm is held down to the side. It is convenient to keep this tsubo in mind along with Ten-Kei 天谿 (SP-18) because both these tsubos have effects similar to that of Ten-Chi.

105. Kyoku-Taku 曲沢 (HC-3)——*Tsubo for brachial neuralgia*

The name *Kyoku-Taku* 曲沢 (HC-3) indicates the location of this tsubo. The character *Kyoku* 曲 means bend and this tsubo is at the bend in the arm, or inside the elbow. *Taku* 沢 means a place where the water of a river meets the grassy bank, and it refers to a hollow place. To find this hollow place inside the elbow, bend the arm and look at the hard tendon which appears below the biceps brachii muscle. Kyoku-Taku is in the hollow area to the inside of this tendon. More precisely, it is located on the skin fold of the elbow on the side of the little finger next to the big tendon. It is easiest to remember the location of this tsubo as being simply in the hollow part inside the elbow.

This tsubo has been used from times past as being very effective for neuralgia of the arms and hands. Aside from this, it is used for symptoms of pain in the pit of the stomach, fever, and a tendency for blood to rise to the head. Kyoku-Taku is the "sea point" of the heart constrictor meridian, and this is where the meridian grows in size and the flow of energy joins the main channel. The elbow is encircled with the "sea points" of the large intestine, lung, heart, small intestine and triple heater meridians. Actually, all the joints have many important tsubos around them, and since this is also the place where various problems occur, it is good to keep the tsubos around the joints in mind.

106. Nai-Kan 内関 (HC-6)——*Tsubo to stop heart attacks*

Flex your wrist with the palm facing upward, and two big tendons will appear in the middle of the forearm. Nai-Kan 内関 (HC-6) is located six centimeters up from the wrist between these tendons. This tsubo is located on the direct opposite side of the arm from Gai-Kan 外関 (TH-5) a tsubo of the triple heater meridian which goes up the center of the forearm on the outside.

Nai-Kan is known to be effective for paralysis of the arm from the elbow down, or when a person faints because of a heart attack like angina pectoris. Aside from this, Nai-Kan is effective for pain around the pit of the stomach, bloodshot eyes. headaches, and pain and numbness of the arm from the elbow down. It is written in a classical text as follows; "The heart meridian causes pain in the heart when energy is excessive, and causes headaches when energy is deficient; treat this at the point between the tendons (Nai-Kan)."

Besides Nai-Kan, there is another tsubo of the heart constrictor meridian located on the inside of the forearm which is on the midpoint between the elbow and the wrist, and it is called *Geki-Mon* 郄門 (HC-4). This is the *geki* point of the absolute yin heart constrictor meridian, and it too is a tsubo effective in relieving acute symptoms of mild heart attacks. As emphasized earlier, the *geki* point of any meridian is the tsubo which relieves acute symptoms.

107. Dai-Ryō 大陵 (HC-7)——*Tsubo to relieve pain and numbness in arms*

The tsubo Dai-Ryō 大陵 (HC-7) is also located between the two big tendons which start at the wrist. The character *Dai* 大 means a mound or hill, so just the name *Dai-Ryō* (large mound) indicates that this tsubo is next to a large tendon. Tsubos circled with the "sea points" of the large intestine, lung, heart, small intestine with the character *Dai* or *Tai* 太 are usually the most important tsubos along that meridian. Dai-Ryō is the *gen* point of the heart constrictor meridian. In classical text it is written, "The sun within the yang is the heart and its *gen* (source) is Dai-Ryō." Perhaps for this reason all symptoms associated with the heart constrictor meridian produce pain or hard spots around this tsubo. Thus, it is very important as the tsubo for checking the overall condition of this meridian. Otherwise, Dai-Ryō is used to treat pain and numbness in the arms.

Symptoms such as having a fever but not perspiring, hotness in the palm of the hands, swelling under the arms, pain in the pit of the stomach, swelling in the throat and dryness in the mouth are all associated with the heart. When these symptoms are present, pain or hardness can be felt just by lightly touching Dai-Ryō. Applying continued pressure on this tsubo in this case will relieve these symptoms naturally. Checking the *gen* points of each of the meridians in this way, one can learn whether there is any problem in the associated organ. An electro-acupuncture method called *Ryō-Dō-Raku* has become popular in Japan in the last few years, and it uses this principle to electrically diagnose the condition of each meridian at the *gen* points.

108. Rō-Kyū 労宮 (HC-8)——*Tsubo for relieving fatigue*

Many people experience a sensation of heat in the palm of their hands after staying up late a couple of nights in a row for work, or otherwise when a housewife has no time to relax between housework and caring for the children. This is a sign that one has become overworked. Pressing the middle of the palm between the points where the middle and ring fingers touch the palm will produce a sharp pain for such people. This is the tsubo Rō-Kyū 労宮 (HC-8).

The character *Rō* 労 means to work, and *Kyū* 宮 means palace. Whenever the body becomes exhausted, a reaction always appears here. Often, after an all night poker game, people massage this part of their hand without even knowing it. This is actually a very effective way to relieve fatigue. Aside from fatigue, Rō-Kyū is said to be very effective for rheumatoid arthritis. Arthritis has been called *Reki-Setsu-Fū* 歴節風 (moving joint affliction) in Oriental medicine, and supposedly this was a condition where pain raced through the joints because of exposure to the wind. Interestingly enough, this pain was said to vary according to the weather condition. Even though you may not have arthritis per se, if there is some pain in the joints, pressing the tsubo Rō-Kyū should ease the pain. Rō-Kyū is also used often for sensations of heat in the mouth as well as numbness in the arms.

109. Chū-Shō 中衝 (HC-9)——*Tsubo for oppressive feeling in chest*

When you go to bed at night, before going to sleep, lie on your back with your legs straight and open your mouth slightly to relax and press around the pit of your stomach using the palm of your hands. Then press slowly along the bottom of the rib cage on both sides. If this area feels soft and resilient, it is proof that you are in good health. Continue pressing between the pit of your stomach and the navel. If there are no hard areas or pain, it is almost certain that your stomach, pancreas and liver are functioning normally. In this manner, Oriental medicine attaches great importance to the tone and texture of the abdomen around the pit of the stomach. When a person becomes overworked, or is missing sleep, most often there is a stifling sensation in this area, and otherwise, there are hard places and tender areas.

Chū-Shō 中衝 (HC-9) is a very important tsubo for relieving such symptoms. When the pit of the stomach feels very distended and heavy, applying strong pressure on the base of the nail of the middle finger toward the thumb should provide relief from this stifling sensation, and also the feeling of lassitude and fatigue will begin to decrease. The name *Chū-Shō* (middle thrust) indicates that this is a tsubo at the tip of the middle finger where the meridian thrusts up against the end. Chū-Shō has traditionally been designated as being the well point from where the meridian wells up, and it is the end point of the heart constrictor meridian.

10. Triple Heater Meridian

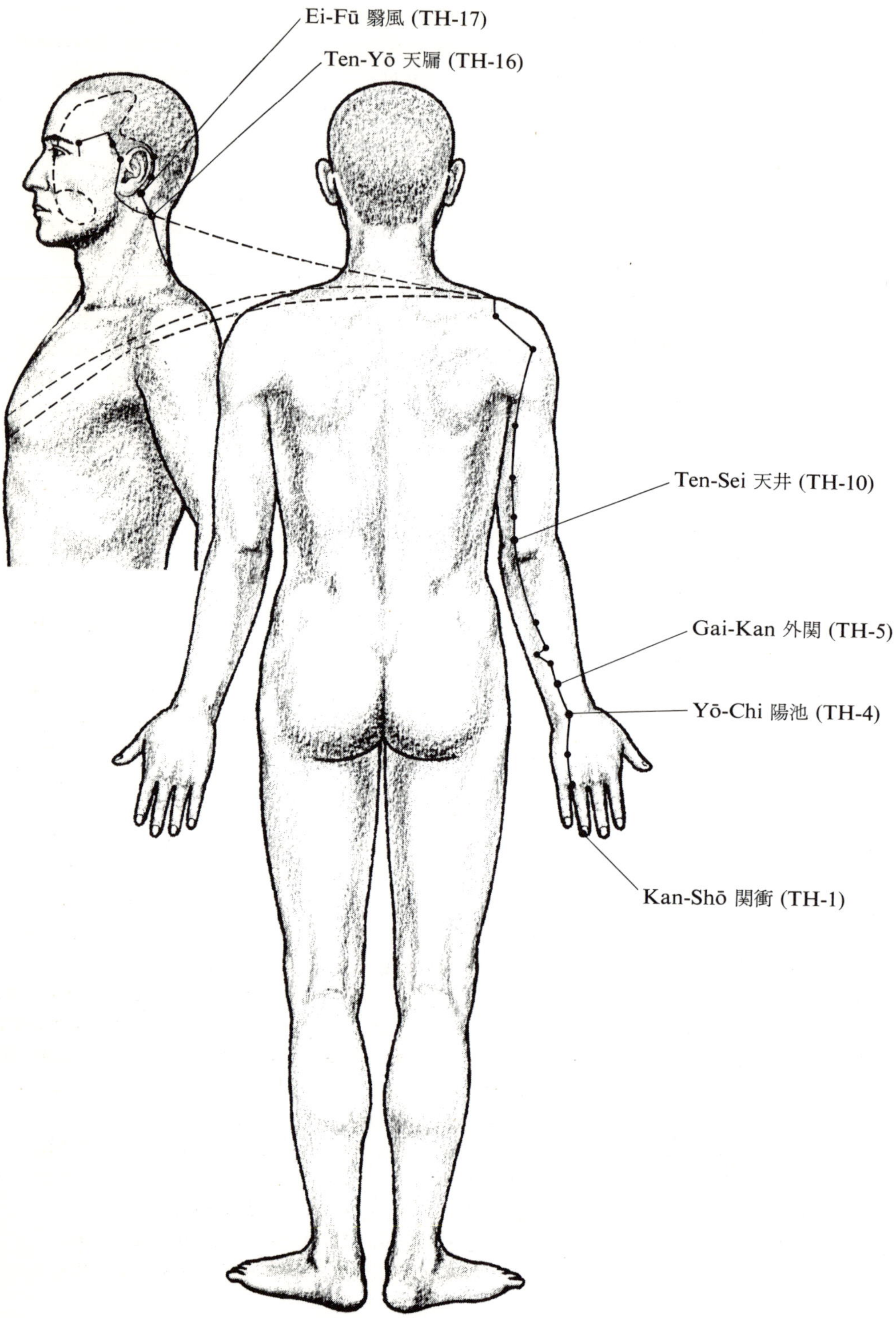

In Oriental medicine the triple heater is known as "the place where energy acquired after birth is absorbed." Thus, it is understood as a system whereby the congenital essence or energy quotient inherited from one's parents is activated and reinforced by the active absorption of the "energy of heaven (air)" and the "energy of earth (food)" through respiration and digestion which serve to circulate the essential life components through the six *zang* and six *fu*. Triple heater (San-Shō 三焦) also means three sources of heat. Even so, the triple heater which is described as "having a name, but no form," does not refer to an independent organ system. The upper heater is said to cover the area from the base of the neck to the pit of the stomach, the middle heater, from the pit of the stomach to the navel, and the lower heater, from the navel down to the pubic hair. The upper heater is associated with the circulatory and respiratory systems, the middle heater, with the digestive system, and the lower heater with the urogenital system.

The triple heater begins with the tsubo Kan-Shō 関衝 (TH-1) at the base of the nail in the ring finger. It travels past the wrist and up the back of the forearm and upper arm to reach the tsubo Ten-Ryō 天髎 (TH-15) on top of the shoulder, which is commonly used for "frozen shoulders." From here, it goes into the tsubo Ketsu-Bon 欠盆 (ST-12) in the supraclavicular fossa. This meridian then travels down the front of the body and circulates through the heart constrictor at the tsubo Dan-Chū 膻中 (CV-17). The meridian branches here and one branch descends to connect with the upper heater at the entrance to the stomach, or Jō-Kan 上脘 (CV-13), and with the middle heater at Chū-Kan 中脘 (CV-12), and finally with the lower heater at In-Kō 陰交 (CV-7) about three centimeters below the navel. The tsubo most important in treating the three heaters are therefore, Dan-Chū for the upper heater, Chū-Kan for the middle heater, and In-Kō for the lower heater.

The other branch from Dan-Chū goes up the chest and over to the back of the neck to the tsubo Dai-Tsui 大椎 (GV-14) of the Governor Vessel. This meridian then goes around behind the ear and crosses the temples to go to the tsubo Yō-Haku 陽白 (GB-14), and then to Sei-Mei 睛明 (UB-1) at the inner corner of the eye, and ends up at Ken-Ryō 顴髎 (SI-18) below the front of the cheek bone. Yet another branch of this meridian starts from the tsubo Ei-Fū 翳風 (TH-17) right below the ear, and goes in front of the ear to end up at the tsubo Dō-Shi-Ryō 瞳子髎 (GB-1). The path of this meridian is very complex, but it is equal in importance to that of the essential kidney meridian.

The symptoms for which the tsubos of the triple heater meridian are most effective include hearing problems, pain in the outer corner of the eyes, pain in the cheeks, pain and swelling in the throat, facial pain, pain in the lower jaw and down the side of the neck, as well as from the shoulder down the upper arm, and from the elbow down the back of the forearm to the thumb.

Also, even when there is no complaint of pain, a person's overall physical condition can be checked by inspecting the triple heater. For example, if the big muscles of the abdomen which extends down from the pit of the stomach down past the navel is very hard, this is a sign that the function of the stomach, pancreas, or liver is impaired. If this same muscles feels rigid below the navel especially, it is a sign of gynecological problems, or otherwise, of a weak constitution in general. Pressing the large abdominal muscle above and below the navel to compare the hardness of this muscle above and below is very important for diagnosis in Oriental medicine.

The triple heater meridian has a total of twenty-three tsubos. Six of the most used tsubos among these are discussed below.

110. Kan-Shō 関衝 (TH-1)——*Tsubo for chilling, numbness and pain in fingers*

There has recently been an increase of cases among elderly women where the cervical spine become deformed, or where the intervertebral disks of the cervical vertebrae lose moisture and result in what is known as degenerative cervical disease. This condition is more commonly referred to as the cervical syndrome. In this condition, the fingertips of the ring finger and little finger become chilled and feel numb, and otherwise there is a dull and heavy pain in the arm on the side of the little finger. Kan-Shō 関衝 (TH-1) is the tsubo used in such situations. It is located at the base of the nail of the ring finger toward the little finger. Kan-Shō is the "well point" as indicated in one text, "The place where the lesser yang meridian of the arm comes out; designated as the *sen* 泉 (well)."

This tsubo, aside from being effective for the above mentioned cervical syndrome with chilling, numbness and pain in the fingertips, is very effective in relieving swollen and hoarse throats. When such symptoms are present, even better results can be obtained by massaging and giving finger pressure along the triple heater meridian on the neck and shoulder while also treating Kan-Shō, or applying heat in this same area with a hair dryer.

The character *Kan* 関 of Kan-Shō originally came from the cross bar which is used to bar doors from inside, and it means to close or to seal off, but in addition its pronunciation is identical with another name for ring finger in Japanese. Since the character *Shō* 衝 means the tip or end, Kan-Shō means a tsubo at the tip of the ring finger.

111. Yō-Chi 陽池 (TH-4)——*Tsubo for pain in arms and greater stamina*

Bend your wrist forward as hard as you can and this will cause a thick tendon to appear on the back of your arm just above the wrist. The tsubo Yō-Chi 陽池 (TH-4) is on the wrist just to the side of this tendon toward the little finger, or slightly to the outside.

It is said that this tsubo is especially effective when there is an excruciating pain in the arm, or otherwise, when one's vitality has suddenly begun to wane. The most important feature of this tsubo is that it is the *gen* point of the triple heater meridian. It is written, "Whether the triple heater be deficient, or excessive in energy, (this tsubo) will show it." Therefore, one can check whether the function of the triple heater is underactive or overactive here.

One of the main schools of acupuncture in Japan is the Sawada style. In this approach the tsubo Yō-Chi, especially that on the left side, is held to be of primary importance. The rule in Oriental medicine has always been, "when a person faces southward the left side is yang." There are sayings like "the emperor faces south." Also, the Hall for State Ceremonies in the Imperial Palace of Kyoto faces south. This is because the south has always been considered the direction where yang is the most active. Naturally, when a person faces southward, the left arm points to the east which is the direction from which the sun rises. This is why the left arm came to be considered as being more important. In actual practice, however, there, is no need to be too concerned about this distinction.

112. Gai-Kan 外関 (TH-5)——*Tsubo for deafness and aural discharge*

The heart constrictor meridian has a tsubo named Nai-Kan 内関 (HC-6), and Gai-Kan 外関 (TH-5) is said to have a reciprocal relationship in its effects with this tsubo. Gai-Kan is especially effective for symptoms of deafness and aural discharge which are traditionally regarded as problems with the triple heater. Aural discharge is also known as otorrhea, and it is a disease where puss oozes out of the external auditory canal. Aside from this, Gai-Kan is effective for paralysis in the arms and legs, and for pain after a stroke. In one classic this tsubo is listed as, "Curing conditions where all five fingers are in pain and a person is unable to grasp anything."

The location of Gai-Kan is recorded as being "in the hollow place two *cun* (about two inches) up from the wrist." This is about seven centimeters above the wrist on the back of the forearm between two big tendons. When symptoms such as those just mentioned are present, the curative effect is increased considerably by also using the tsubos Shi-Kō 支溝 (TH-6) three centimeters above Gai-Kan, E-Sō 会宗 (TH-7) three centimeters to the outside of Shi-Kō, San-Yō-Raku 三陽絡 (TH-8) about five centimeters above Gai-Kan, and Shi-Toku 四瀆 (TH-9) about nine centimeters above Gai-Kan. There is no need to be too concerned with the exact location of these tsubos. Just lightly pinch or press the back of the arm from the shoulders down to the hand on the thick hard muscle in line with the finger. Find those points which are especially sensitive or tender, and these can be treated as tsubos.

113. Ten-Sei 天井 (TH-10)——*Tsubo for blood rising to the head*

Ten-Sei 天井 (TH-10) is referred to in the classics as "the place where the lesser yang meridian of the arm enters, designated as the *gō* (sea)." Thus, it is the tsubo where the triple heater meridian converges to form its main channel, or the place where all the small tributaries come together to join the main flow, just as rivers pour into the sea. The character *Ten* 天 of Ten-Sei means heaven, and *Sei* 井 means spring. Therefore, Ten-Sei is a spring from which water wells up, or the place where meridian energy passing up to the "heaven section" comes out. This tsubo is located on the back of the arm in a hollow area approximately three centimeters above the point of the elbow.

This tsubo is used often for pain in the corner of the eyes, hearing problems, sore throats, coughs, palpitations, and pain along the triple heater meridian from the shoulder down the arm. Above Ten-Sei are some of the best tsubos for relieving pain, numbness and chilling which extend along the triple heater meridian from the base of the neck down the shoulder and arm. These include, Sei-Rei-En 清冷淵 (TH-11) on the back of the arm seven centimeters above the elbow, Shō-Reki 消濼 (TH-12) on the middle of the backside of the upper arm, Ju-E 臑会 (TH-13) on the back of the arm about ten centimeters down from the back end of the shoulder, Ken-Ryō 肩髎 (TH-14) toward the back of the shoulder, and Ten-Ryō 天髎 (TH-15) just to the back of the midpoint between the base of the neck and the tip of the shoulder. These tsubos are also very important for treating cervico-brachialgia.

114. Ten-Yō 天牖 (TH-16)——*Tsubo for wryneck and nausea*

Ten Yō 天牖 (TH-16) is located to the bottom and back of the mastoid process which is a bony protrusion behind the ear where the sternocleidomastoid muscle attaches to the skull. Since it is on the side of the neck, Ten-Yō is used to treat wryneck and neck pain in general. It is also used for tinnitus, pain in the eyes, swelling in the face, tension in the back of the neck, and toothaches. There are the tsubos Ten-Chū 天柱 (UB-10), Fū-Chi 風池 (GB-20), Kan-Kotsu 完骨 (GB-12), Ten-Sō 天窓 (SI-16) and Ten-Tei 天鼎 (LI-17) located right around this tsubo. Treatments are most effective when these tsubos are used together with Ten-Yō to relieve pain in the head, eyes, ears and teeth, as well as pain and tension down the neck and shoulders.

The character *Yō* 牖 of Ten-Yō means window, or a place where light and fresh air are admitted. Thus, it is the tsubo where good energy is drawn into the "heaven section" to cure various symptoms associated with the triple heater meridian.

As already mentioned, there is a very important muscle called the sternocleido-mastoid which joins the trunk and the "heaven section" above the neck. Behind this muscle are important nerves and blood vessels which connect the head and the trunk. The area around the sternocleidomastoid muscle is therefore, a very vital place in the body. The sensations in the organs of the chest and abdominal cavity are controlled by the vagus nerve which is a parasympathetic nerve running behind the sternocleidomastoid muscle down to the chest and abdomen. So it is understandable how the tsubos in this area with the character of *Ten* 天 are effective in curing problems in the chest and abdomen.

115. Ei-Fū 翳風 (TH-17)——*Tsubo for dizziness and facial pain*

With the condition called trigeminal neuralgia, a strong pain is felt around the forehead and eyes, as well as from the cheeks down to the chin. The most effective tsubo for treating this condition is Ei-Fū 翳風 (TH-17). Some acupuncturists insert a needle diagonally in this tsubo aiming the tip toward the tsubo Hyaku-E 百会 (GV-20) on the top of the head. A strong sensation may be felt in the eardrums that can make a person temporarily deaf, but inserting the needle a little deeper and leaving it there for a while will make the pain from neuralgia disappear. Also, finger pressure on this point is quite effective against dizziness or car sickness. There is another tsubo effective for trigeminal neuralgia called Yō-Haku 陽白 (GB-14) that is located slightly above the center of each eyebrow, which is also used for beauty massage.

Ei-Fū is located in the hollow place right under the earlobe and to the front of the mastoid process. A penetrating pain can be felt when this tsubo is lightly pressed or massaged with the tips of the thumb or index finger. This tsubo is effective for a wide variety of symptoms in the head and facial area. The triple heater meridian has a number of tsubos beginning at Ei-Fū which encircle the ear from behind. They are, Kei-Myaku 瘈脈 (TH-18), Ro-Soku 顱息 (TH-19), Kaku-Son 角孫 (TH-20), Ji-Mon 耳門 (TH-21) and Wa-Ryō 和髎 (TH-22). These are all tsubos used to treat deafness and tinnitus. Recently it was reported in China that the hearing of numerous deaf children had been restored almost completely by giving them acupuncture treatments using these tsubos.

11. Gallbladder Meridian

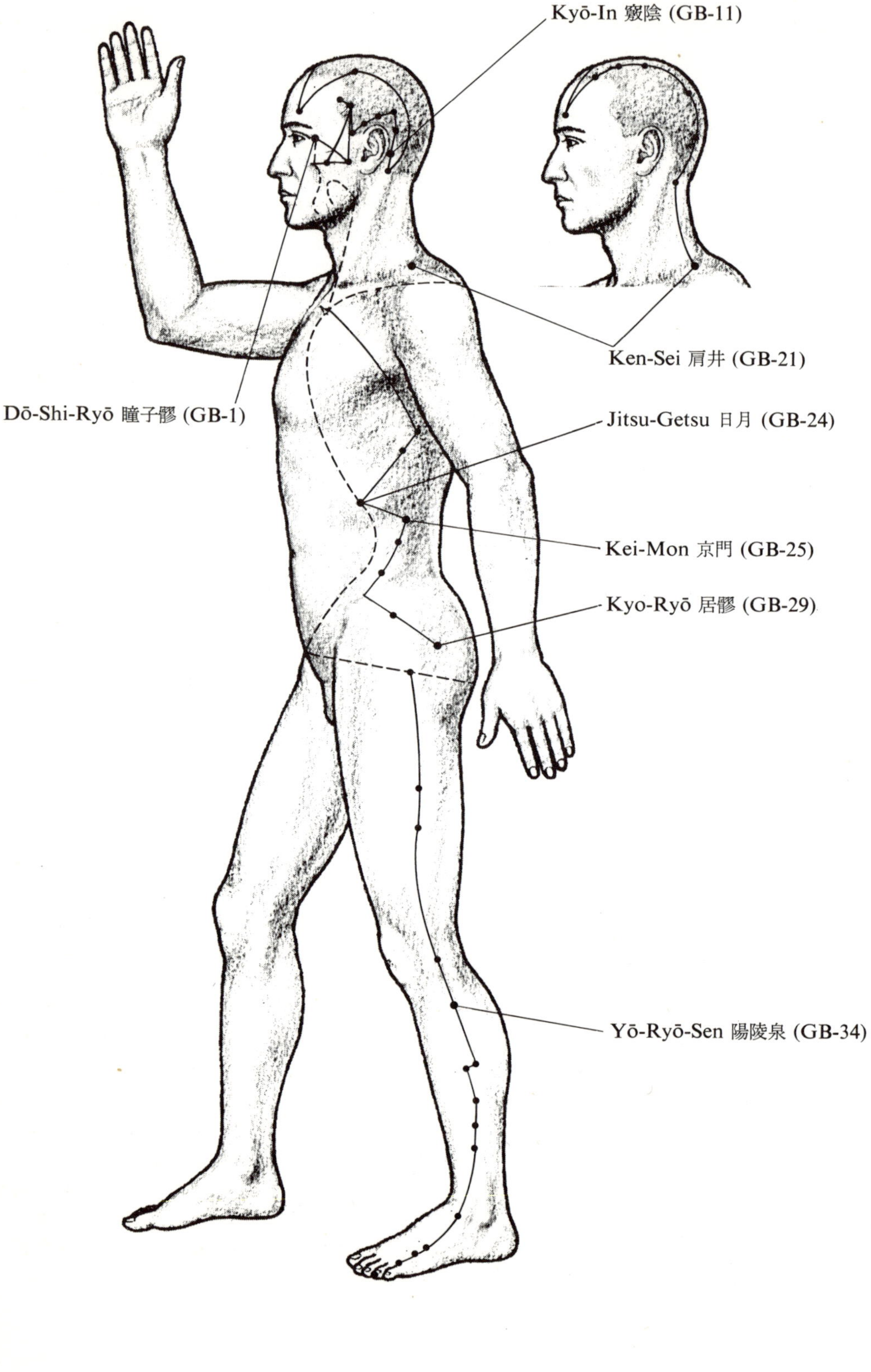

After the triple heater meridian comes the gallbladder meridian which circulates through the gallbladder, a *fu* (yang organ). This gallbladder is the same one referred to in Western medicine. In the classics of Oriental medicine the gallbladder is recorded as follows: "The *fu* of the gallbladder is shaped like a gourd. It lies hidden beneath the folds of the liver. It attaches to the tenth spine. It contains three *gō* (slightly more than a U.S. pint) of clear fluid which is bitter in taste."

The gallbladder is the *fu* connected with the liver and associated with the element wood. As described in the Japanese expression "inseparable friends like the liver and gallbladder," the gallbladder forms an interior-exterior relationship with the liver to assist in its functions.

The gallbladder meridian is quite a long meridian with as many as forty-four tsubos which go all the way from the head down to the toes. As can be seen in the figure, this meridian begins at the tsubo Dō-Shi-Ryō 瞳子髎 (GB-1) at the outer corner of the eye and goes to the tsubo Kan-Kotsu 完骨 (GB-12) behind the ear. From here it goes back to the forehead and down between the eyes and then straight back over the head to reach the tsubo Fū-Chi 風池 (GB-20) behind the skull. Here the meridian branches in two, and one branch goes down the shoulders and the other goes up to the ear and then travels around the lower jaw and cheek, before going down into the supraclavicular fossa. The former branch goes down the side of the trunk and splits once more at the tsubo Jitsu-Getsu 日月 (GB-24) at the tip of the ninth rib where one branch goes inside to circulate through the liver and gallbladder, and then rejoins the main channel at the outside of the hip joint. The main channel goes down from Jitsu-Getsu and goes past the tsubo Kei-Mon 京門 (GB-25) on the side and joins up with the other branch down at the hip joint. Here this meridian converges to form a large channel and descends on the outside of the thigh and calf to come to an end at the base of the nail of the fourth toe.

Tsubos of the gallbladder meridian are used to treat a wide variety of problems because the meridian covers such a large area. These tsubos are effective for such things as pain down the side of the body which includes headaches, pain in the side of the neck to its base whenever the neck is turned, pain in the underarm or flank region, and pain in the outside of the knees or legs. These tsubos are also effective for people who seem to lack vitality and have dark and dingy looking complexions, swelling of lymph nodes below the ear and on the jaw, sensation of heat on the outside of the legs, or pain in the fourth toe.

The following traits can be listed for discriminating those people with problems in their liver and gallbladder. Their eyes appear bluish in color and vacant, and their tone of voice is high pitched. Also, such people tend to get sick in the springtime when plants are budding. They usually prefer foods with a sour taste and oily foods like tempura or Chinese dishes. In order to confirm the diagnosis, lightly press the tsubo Jitsu-Getsu which is located at the tip of the ninth rib where the finger comes to a stop when tracing down the rib cage from the pit of the stomach. Also, press Tan-Yu 胆兪 (UB-19) which is to either side of the point below the tenth thoracic vertebra. If there is pain or stiffness here, it is a sure sign that the person has problems in these organs. The tsubos discussed next are the best points for curing the symptoms listed above.

116. Dō-Shi-Ryō 瞳子髎 (GB-1)——*Tsubo to remove "crow's feet"*

It is said that once women reach the age of twenty-five, they suddenly begin to age. It may be rather extreme to say that all women begin to age in their mid-twenties, but this is said because once a woman reaches this age there is a tendency for small wrinkles to form on the face more easily, especially the variety known as "crow's feet" on the outside corner of the eyes. Just these wrinkles make a woman's face appear quite a bit older. Dō-Shi-Ryō 瞳子髎 (GB-1) which is located in the hollow place at the outer corner of the eye is the tsubo most effective in removing small wrinkles like "crow's feet."

Dō-Shi-Ryō has also been used together with the tsubo Chō-E 聴会 (GB-2) in the depression just to the front of the ear when pressed, Kyaku-Shu-Jin 客主人 (GB-3) above the cheek bone just in front of the ear, Gan-En 頷厭 (GB-4) at the top of the temples, Ken-Ro 懸顱 (GB-5) right below Gan-En, and Ken-Ri 懸釐 (GB-6) just below this, as a tsubo indispensable for migraine headaches, dizziness, blurring of vision, tinnitus, facial paralysis and neuralgia, especially trigeminal neuralgia or spasms and numbness going from the temples down to the jaws.

The interesting name of *Kyaku-Shu-Jin* (guest and host) comes from likening the cheek bone to a gateway where two tsubos on either side face each other just as a visiting guest comes up to face his host at the gate. Kyaku-Shu-Jin is right above the tsubo Ge-Kan 下関 (ST-7) of the stomach meridian, and it displays equal effectiveness when the upper teeth are in pain due to trigeminal neuralgia.

117. Kyō-In 竅陰 (GB-11)——*Tsubo for dizziness and tinnitus*

The character *Kyō* 竅 means a hole in the skull, or the ear, while *Yin* 陰 means in the shadow, or behind the ear. The *Kyō-In* 竅陰 (GB-11) means a tsubo just behind the flap of the ear (the auricle). There are many tsubos around the ear, but Kyō-In among them is famous from the olden days as being especially effective for ear problems. It performs wonders when a person is hard of hearing, dizzy, or has tinnitus. This is among the tsubos used in China to restore the hearing of deaf children.

When elderly persons complain of getting tired easily, feeling poorly, or becoming hard of hearing, applying finger pressure on this tsubo can improve their physical condition and hearing. Also, similar effects can be obtained by just taping on a tiny wad of tinfoil or a steel grain (e.g., a small ball bearing) to this tsubo. Those who hear a loud ringing in their ears and are hard of hearing quite often have high blood pressure. The overall deterioration in their physical condition is manifesting as hearing problems.

Kyō-In is also a place where the gallbladder and the urinary bladder meridians cross each other. As explained before, the urinary bladder meridian is in an interior-exterior relationship with the kidney meridian so this tsubo has a deep relationship with the "kidney deficient condition," or the loss of vitality. It is said that the kidney deficient condition" shows up most clearly in the ears and the "two orifices" (the sex organs and anus). It is sound reasoning, therefore, to use this tsubo in conjunction with other important tsubos associated with the kidney meridian such as Jin-Yu 腎兪 (UB-23), Kō-Yu 肓兪 (KI-16), Kei-Mon 京門 (GB-25) and Tai-Kei 太谿 (KI-3).

118. Ken-Sei 肩井 (GB-21)——*Tsubo for shoulder tension*

Ken-Sei 肩井 (GB-21) is located on top of the shoulder at about the midpoint between the base of the neck and the tip of the shoulder. Ken-Sei is indispensable for all of the following symptoms; a sense of oppression in the back of the head, tension from the neck down to the shoulders, eye fatigue, tinnitus, toothaches, pain from the shoulder down to the arm, poor digestion and pain in the joints from a cold. This tsubo is particularly effective for "cricks in the neck," shoulder tension, frozen shoulders, a pain like neuralgia in the back of the head, over-excitation and high blood pressure.

Ken-Sei (shoulder well) is sometimes referred to as the "well of the shoulder." This denotes a "spring" on the shoulder where meridian energy flows out. Those who suffer from chronic stiffness in their shoulder area should lie on their stomachs and have either their spouse or children give them strong thumb pressure here. The tension will in most cases be relieved just by pressing this tsubo for a while. In Oriental medicine there is even a massage technique called the "Ken-Sei Technique," where the treatment concentrates on this tsubo. It is not too advisable, however, to press or pound this area too much. It is important to exercise caution specially with those who have high blood pressure. It has been said from the old days that novices should be careful about using this tsubo. Even experienced acupuncturists treat this point with due caution. This is because inserting a needle too deeply here or overdoing the amount of stimulation can cause a person to faint with cerebral anemia. This just goes to show what a powerful effect this tsubo can have.

119. Jitsu-Getsu 日月 (GB-24)——*Tsubo for pain in the gallbladder*

Jitsu-Getsu 日月 (GB-24) is located just below the tip of the ninth rib. It is said to be a place where the energy of the gallbladder meridian penetrates into the abdomen, and this tsubo is used often for excruciating pain from the chest down to the stomach, or else, when one is unable to breathe deeply. Jitsu-Getsu (sun moon) was called the light of God in ancient times, and being the *bo* point of the gallbladder meridian, it has been used extensively. This tsubo, coupled with Tan-Yu 胆兪 (UB-19) of the urinary bladder meridian, has a deep significance as a tsubo for inspecting the functional condition of the gallbladder. Thus, this point is used to check for abnormalities in the gallbladder, an organ that temporarily stores bile which assists the digestion of fats.

To examine this tsubo, first lay down on a bed in the supine position and open your mouth slightly and relax. Then use both thumbs to slowly press just below the rib cage from the side of the stomach and work toward the chest. If there is any pain in the area that the right thumb is pressing as you inhale slowly and deeply, it is a sign that there is some problem in the gallbladder. This simple examination can be done at home in private after you go to bed at night.

120. Kei-Mon 京門 (GB-25)——*Tsubo to strengthen the digestive organs*

Symptoms such as a heavy oppressive pain going from the chest around to the side, rumbling in the stomach with diarrhea, poor digestion with belching, nausea, heartburn, and stiffness of the shoulders going down between the shoulder blades with occasional oppressive pain, all indicate a "kidney deficient condition." In Oriental medicine this is regarded as a decline in the function of the kidneys. Kei-Mon 京門 (GB-25) is the tsubo used often to treat this condition. This tsubo is the *bo* point of the kidney meridian and it is used to check the condition of the kidney meridian. Therefore, Kei-Mon is a very important tsubo which provides warning signals for the kidney that houses the "basic life force" acquired at birth.

Since Kei-Mon is located at the tip of the twelfth rib, it becomes hard to find when people lie on their back. It is better for a person to sit up or to lie on the stomach to locate this tsubo. Feeling the ribs on both sides of the back, there will be a short rib at the level of the waist which does not attach at the end. This is the twelfth rib.

The name *Kei-Mon* (city gate) means a gate to the capital where the emperor lives. This name, in other words, comes from this tsubo being the gate where harmful energy can enter the place where the "basic life force" from birth resides. After Kei-Mon comes the tsubos Tai-Myaku 帯脈 (GB-26) and I-Dō 維道 (GB-28) which are also located on the side and used in the same way as Kei-Mon.

121. Kyo-Ryō 居髎 (GB-29)——*Tsubo to relieve fatigue in knees and legs*

Kyo-Ryō 居髎 (GB-29) is located about fifty-five centimeters below the tip of the eleventh rib, which can be slightly difficult to find. This tsubo is level to the public area just below the front of the hip bone. In more specialized terms, it is below to the anterior superior iliac spine.

This tsubo is especially effective for such symptoms as a heavy sensation or fatigue in the knees, as well as the legs being tired and heavy with a pulling sensation in the muscles. Kyo-Ryō is also used for tension and pain in the lower abdomen, and pain extending down the legs from the waist, or going up to the shoulders, as well as the condition known as sciatica where there is a sharp wrenching pain which extends from the back of the thighs to the outside of the calves. This pain can be relieved by pressing Kyo-Ryō toward the center of the pelvis using both thumbs.

When neuralgia occurs along the sciatic nerve, the ankle, knee and hip joints become less movable and low back pain in the hip muscles is the inevitable consequence. This is when the tsubo Kyo-Ryō becomes important. Low back pain results from a wide variety of causes, and it is often referred to as the "lumbagosciatica syndrome." The deformation of the lumbar vertebrae, in pariticular, is often the cause of severe low back pain extending down the thighs.

122. Yō-Ryō-Sen 陽陵泉 (GB-34)——*Tsubo for "top hot bottom cold" condition*

Yō-Ryō-Sen 陽陵泉 (GB-34) is recorded in the classics as, "the place where the lesser yang meridian enters; designated as the *gō* (sea)." Thus, Yō-Ryō-Sen is a very important tsubo. In the *Ling Shu*, the original classic of Oriental medicine, the use of this tsubo is outlined as follows; "For symptoms of the interior up high, use the Ryō-Sen on the yin side, for symptoms of the exterior up high, use the Ryō-Sen on the yang side."

This, in other words, is saying that In-Ryō-Sen 陰陵泉 (SP-9) should be used for yin symptoms primarily involving chilling in the area above the navel, and that Yō-Ryō-Sen should be used for symptoms such as fever, swelling, or pain which appear on the exterior. The "yang Ryō-Sen" is located on the side of the little toe and the "yin Ryō-Sen" (spleen meridian) is located on the opposite side, or the inside. Yō-Ryō-Sen is located about three centimeters below the knees at the bottom and just to the front of the apex of the head of the fibula (the prominent bump below the outside of the knee).

In Oriental medicine the term "ailments above and below" is used. This is because there are times when the symptoms on the upper half of the body differ completely from those on the lower half. This is the so-called "top hot bottom cold" condition or conversely, the "top cold bottom hot" condition. The rule for treatment in these cases is to treat ailments affecting the upper half of the body by using points on the lower half. Great importance is attached to Yō-Ryō-Sen as the tsubo for restoring the balance when there is disharmony in the upper and lower halves of the body, or when there are differences in the manifested symptoms. Even more dramatic results can be achieved by using both the yin and yang Ryō-Sens together.

12. Liver Meridian

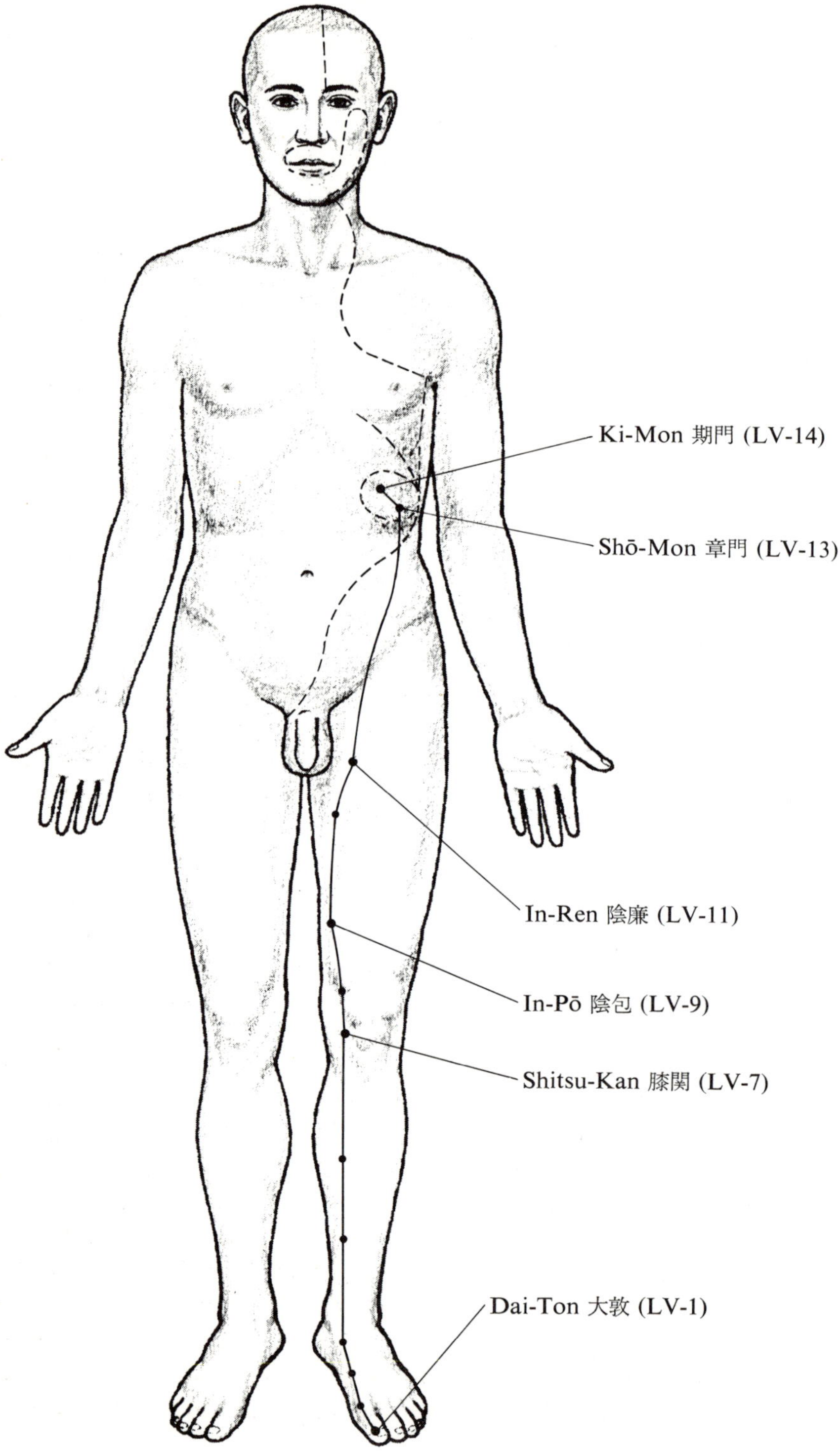

The liver meridian is the last meridian among the twelve meridians. Traditionally, it is referred to as the absolute yin liver meridian of the leg. The liver as understood in Oriental medicine is somewhat different than that of Western medicine. In the classical texts the liver is described as follows;

"The essential organ, the liver, attaches to the ninth spine. It is bluish in color and shaped like cedar leaves. Three leaves hang to the left and four leaves hang to the right. The gallbladder is the *fu* associated with the liver and these organs belong to the element of wood. This is the organ where decisions are made."

In Japan, the liver has been called *kimo* 肝 from ancient times, and it is used as an allusion to one's innermost feelings or "gut intentions." The common phrases like "bearing it in the *kimo*," or "having a strong *kimo*," in the Japanese language are examples of this. The character for liver 肝 (*kan*) is also used to denote something important as evident in phrases like "vital as the liver," or "inseparable friends like the liver and gallbladder." In addition, the liver was regarded to perform a vital function in maintaining the basic life functions in the body along with the kidney.

The liver, because it is so important, is associated with a wide variety of symptoms both physical and psychological. The main symptoms associated with the liver include, a dark and dingy complexion, dry throat, oppressive feeling in the chest, nausea, tendency to have diarrhea, pain in the toes around the third toe, chilling of the extremities, feverishness, low back pain in women, difficulty in urinating at night, pain in the inguinal region and genital area, as well as continual tension in the lower abdomen. Since the liver is also deeply connected with one's thoughts and emotions, a disfunction can cause irritability or an inability to make decisions. Among all the symptoms mentioned, those related to the reproductive organs are most notable because the liver meridian circulates through the sex organs in both men and women, and for this reason many tsubos of the liver meridian are effective in relieving such symptoms.

The course of the liver meridian follows an ascending path as seen in the figure. It begins at the tip of the big toe and passes in front of the inner ankle bone and climbs upward after mingling with the kidney and spleen meridians. It then travels up the inside of the knees and the thighs to go on to the lower abdomen from the place the leg attaches to the trunk. Here it circulates through the reproductive organs, and then goes up to the point nine centimeters below the navel. The meridian branches to the right and left here and goes up to the tip of the eleventh rib and then to the tip of the ninth rib where it encircles the stomach area and circulates through the liver and gallbladder. The tsubos of the liver meridian all appear below this point, but the meridian continues to go farther on up to the throat and below the eyes where it splits into two. One branch goes to the very top of the head to connect with the kidney meridian, and the other branch circles once around the mouth. Yet another branch splits off from the tip of the ninth rib and connects with the lung meridian which is the first meridian among the twelve meridians. In this way all twelve of the ordinary meridians are connected in sequence to each other in the *zang-fu*-and-meridian theory of Oriental medicine, and vital energy is thought to circulate through the body unceasingly. The liver meridian has a total of fourteen tsubos, and six of the most used tsubos among these will be discussed below.

123. Dai-Ton 大敦 (LV-1)——*Tsubo for nocturnal enuresis*

The liver meridian begins with the tsubo Dai-Ton 大敦 (LV-1). The character *Ton* 敦 means to stagnate, so *Dai-Ton* (large stop) is the place where the energy flowing through this meridian is stopped up in a big way and the flow is impeded. This tsubo which corresponds with Dai-To 大都 (SP-2) of the spleen meridian, is also called *Sui-Sen* 水泉 (water spring). Dai-Ton is recorded as "the place where the flow of the absolute yin meridian of the leg begins; designated as the *sei* (well)." Therefore, this tsubo has been regarded as being a very important one from the early days.

Dai-Ton is located at the base of the big toenail toward the little toe, and if there are any symptoms of the liver, this point is often sensitive to the slightest amount of pressure. This tsubo is well known as being good for pain which goes from the flank to the lower abdominal region, and for pain down the inside of the legs known as lumbo-abdominal neuralgia, femoral neuralgia, or saphenous neuralgia. This tsubo is also used often for treating gynecological disorders.

Another tsubo effective for the same symptoms is Kō-Kan 行間 (LV-2) located right between the big toe and the second toe. Also, tracing up the back of the foot between the big toe and the second toe with a finger, it will come to a stop where the back of the foot rises. You can detect a pulse by lightly touching this point with your finger. This is the *gen* point of the liver meridian, the tsubo Tai-Shō 太衝 (LV-3). Keep Kō-Kan and Tai-Shō in mind along with Dai-Ton as being important tsubos for treating most all symptoms associated with the liver meridian.

124. Shitsu-Kan 膝関 (LV-7)——*Tsubo for knee pain and increasing stamina*

The name *Shitsu-Kan* 膝関 (LV-7: knee gate) means that this tsubo is like a gateway where the energy of the liver meridian enters the knees. The liver meridian travels upward past Chū-Hō 中封 (LV-4) in the hollow place above the inner ankle bone, and Rei-Kō 蠡溝 (LV-5) about fifteen centimeters above the ankle bone, to reach Shitsu-Kan. This tsubo is located on the inside of the knee about five centimeters below the bend in the knee. Shitsu-Kan is used primarily for knee pain or sore throats, but it is also used for the loss of sexual drive in both men and women, as well as for menstrual irregularities in women.

Right above this tsubo is Kyoku-Sen 曲泉 (LV-8) which is located in the hollow place to the inside of the fold in the knee when it is flexed. The name means a spring at the bend in the knee where meridian energy wells up. In traditional terms, it is said that when harmful energy becomes stopped up in the knees, Kyoku-Sen is treated to make pure meridian energy pour out and wash away the harmful energy. When this tsubo is used together with Shitsu-Kan, even better results can be obtained for the symptoms listed above. Just a little pressure on these tsubos will be extremely painful especially when there is knee pain from aging, also known as degenerative joint disease of the knees. Burning small pieces of moxa on these two tsubos is remarkably effective in alleviating pain in such cases.

125. In-Pō 陰包 (LV-9)——*Tsubo for loss of stamina and menstrual irregularities*

The tsubo In-Pō 陰包 (LV-9) is located on the inside of the thighs and is about forty centimeters up from Kyoku-Sen 曲泉 (LV-8). In more specific terms, tracing up the thigh with a finger on the sartorius and gracilis muscles (inside back of thigh), a point will be reached where these two muscles separate. In-Pō is above place where these two muscles divide, and it is often tender when pressed.

In Japanese, impotence is called *inpo*, so sometimes when I teach students, they begin to snicker when they hear the name of this tsubo. Once a student caused an outburst of laughter in the class when he asked outright, " Is that tsubo really effective for impotence?" In any case, In-Pō, just the same as the other tsubos of the liver meridian, is effective for various symptoms related with the reproductive organs. It is especially effective for menstrual irregularities, infrequent urination or incontinence of urine. It is also effective for low back pain, pain or dull and heavy sensations in the lower abdomen, as well as for pain, numbness and chilling of the feet associated with the "liver deficient condition" of Oriental medicine. When the muscles on the inside of the thighs become as stiff as a board and the feet are cold, and also there is low back pain, this is a sign that one's stamina has declined greatly. It does one little good just to worry about this. It is best to take a hot bath and massage along the liver meridian in such cases, and to give thorough finger pressure, concentrating around the tsubo In-Pō.

126. In-Ren 陰廉 (LV-11)——*Tsubo for menstrual disorders*

The tsubo In-Ren 陰廉 (LV-11) is located on the inside of the upper thighs, and is listed as being "two *cun* (about two inches) under the tsubo Ki-Shō 気衝 (ST-30)." This means that it is about six centimeters below the place where the leg connects to the trunk. In-Ren is among the tsubos effective for gynecological disorders, and it is often used together with other tsubos of the liver meridian.

This tsubo is recorded in the classics as "curing infertility, pain in the lower abdomen, and chilling of feet for women; burn three pieces of moxa here and a child will come." This tsubo has therefore been known from the olden days as being effective for infertility. Three pieces of moxa means that three small cones of moxa are burned on each point. However, this is very difficult in practical terms because of the extreme sensitivity of this location. Therefore, I have yet to confirm the validity of this practice. In *Wakan Sansai Zu E*, a Japanese classic, it is written as follows; "(In-Ren) controls infertility and menstrual problems for women."

The character *Ren* 廉 of In-Ren refers to a corner or edge, and *In* 陰 (yin) refers to the reproductive organs. Thus, In-Ren is a tsubo on the outer edge of the sex organs. When there are menstrual problems, the best results can be obtained by using other effective tsubos along with In-Ren including, Jin-Yu 腎兪 (UB-23), Jyō-Ryō 上髎 (UB-31), Ji-Ryō 次髎 (UB-32), Chū-Ryō 中髎 (UB-33), Ko-Ketsu

巨闕 (CV-14) and Tai-Kei 太谿 (KI-3). In-Ren, in addition to menstrual problems, is effective for distention of the lower abdomen and chilling below the waist.

127. Shō-Mon 章門 (LV-13)——*Tsubo for pain in the chest and side*

Shō-Mon 章門 (LV-13) is located at the tip of the eleventh rib. Lie on your back and start counting down your ribs from the top, beginning from the first one below the clavicle. The ribs will begin to get shorter from around the fifth and sixth ribs. Feel along the tip of the ribs as they join and curve around to the side until you reach the eleventh rib. Shō-Mon is almost on the side of the abdomen at the tip of the first floating rib. The character *Shō* 章 of Shō-Mon means clear, and *Mon* 門 means a gate where harmful energy enters and exits. Thus, Shō-Mon is a tsubo where the coming and going of harmful energy can be most clearly seen. Interestingly enough, although this tsubo is on the liver meridian, it is the *bo* point of the spleen meridian, and this is where the function of the pancreas can be checked.

The symptoms for which Shō-Mon is effective include; firstly, pain from the chest going around to the side, rumbling in the intestines with poor digestion, nausea, occasional stiffening of the joints and the arms and legs becoming very tired. For infants, this tsubo is used when they vomit milk or get diarrhea. Since this tsubo is the *bo* point of the spleen meridian, it is also used to treat diabetes.

It is written in *Sen Kin Pō*, a classical text, "When there is blood in the urine, burning one hundred pieces of moxa here is effective." Thus, Shō-Mon can be effective when there is blood mixed in with one's urine.

128. Ki-Mon 期門 (LV-14)——*Tsubo to relieve pain in chest and side*

The tsubo Ki-Mon 期門 (LV-14) is located at the tip of the ninth rib. Tracing the bottom of the rib cage from the pit of the stomach, this tsubo is just about at the midpoint between the front center and the side. This tsubo is of particular importance among the fourteen points of the liver meridian as the *bo* point of the liver meridian. When a person stays up late for a poker game or some other reason, or has had one too many to drinks the night before, blood becomes congested in the liver and a person is unable to keep up one's vitality and stamina. In these cases, there is usually a strong pain when Ki-Mon is pressed lightly upward from below while drawing a deep breath. This proves that blood has become stagnated in the liver, so massage or apply finger pressure to this point and relieve the tension in this area. Breathing is sure to become easier, and one's vitality will be restored.

Ki-Mon is used particularly for symptoms such as insomnia, pain in the chest and side, lack of appetite, post pregnancy disorders, and when food becomes lodged in the gullet and one has a hard time getting food down. This tsubo is considered as a point where the yin energy of the body collects because the greater yin spleen meridian, the absolute yin liver meridian, and the In-I Vessel 陰維脈 of the extra meridians all cross here. Yin energy refers to cold energy, so this tsubo is indispensable for acute febrile and infectious diseases. There are actually records of how such diseases were cured by administering acupuncture to Ki-Mon.

13. Governor Vessel

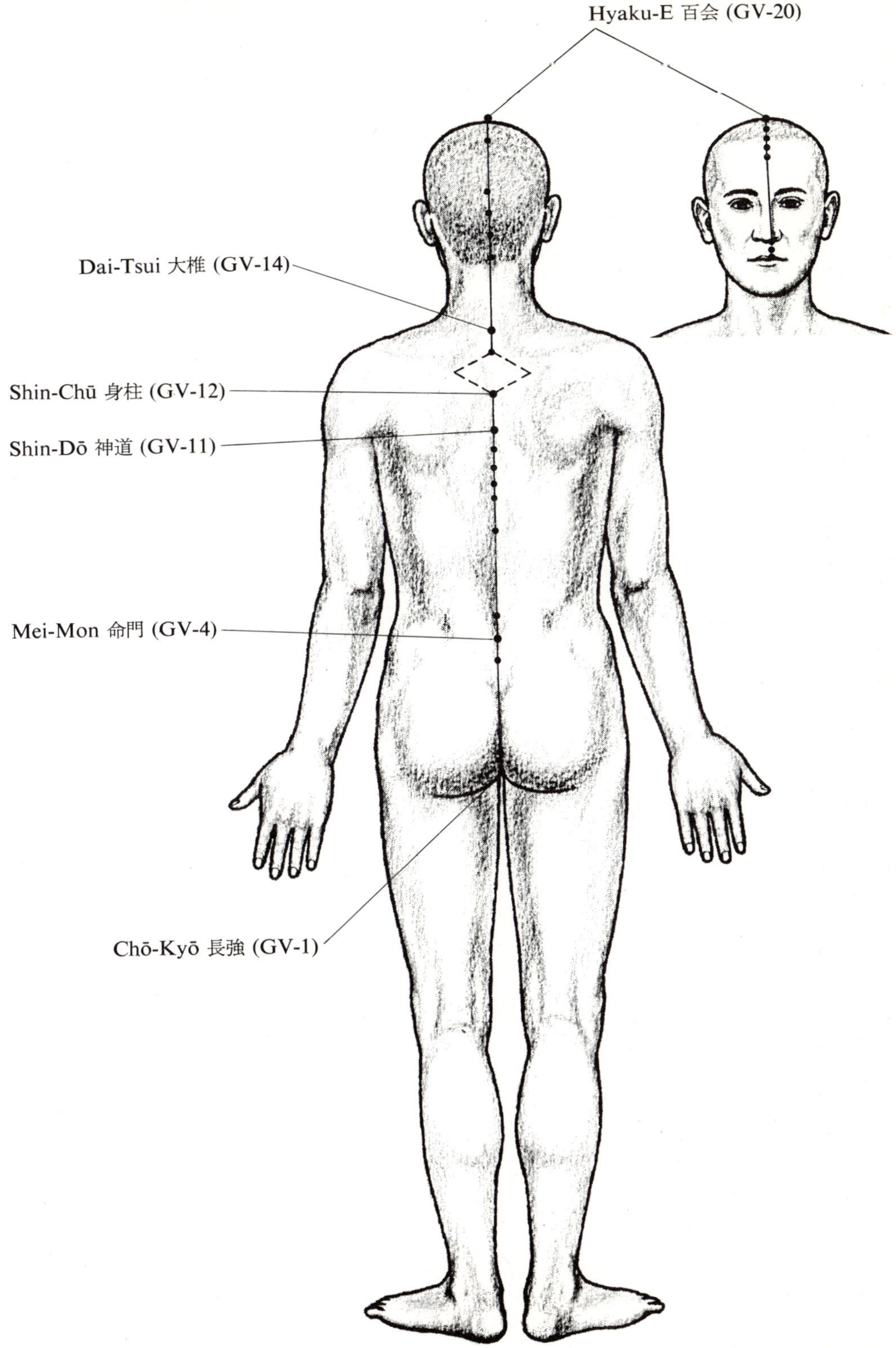

The twelve meridians and their respective tsubos have been discussed thus far, and these meridians are known as the twelve ordinary meridians. In addition to these, according to Oriental medicine, there are eight extra meridians in the human body. These extra meridians are thought to constantly adjust the amount of energy flowing through the twelve meridians so that just the right amount of energy circulates in the six *zang* and six *fu*. The eight extra meridians are, the Governor Vessel (Toku-Myaku 督脈), Conception Vessel (Nin-Myaku 任脈), Yō-Kyō Vessel (Yō-Kyō-Myaku 陽蹻脈), In-Kyō Vessel (In-Kyō-Myaku 陰蹻脈), Yō-I Vessel (Yō-I-Myaku 陽維脈), In-I Vessel (In-I-Myaku 陰維脈), Tai Vessel (Tai-Myaku 帯脈) and Shō-Vessel (Shō-Myaku 衝脈). These extra meridians connect the twelve ordinary meridians in the body vertically, horizontally, and diagonally, and perform the vital role of regulating the flow of energy. The Conception and Governor Vessels which lie on the very center line of the body on the front and the back from the head down to the buttocks are especially important in regulating the energy circulation system known as the triple heater meridian which affects the functions of the organs in the thoracic, abdominal and pelvic cavities. The two extra meridians above, and their tsubos will be discussed in the two sections which follow.

Discussion will begin with the Governor Vessel which is spoken of as "controlling (the body) from the back." In other words, it oversees, takes charge or supervises from the back. The Governor Vessel is on the vertical midline to the front of the body from the top of the head down the back, waist and hips. It covers a wide area including the anus, the sexual organs, the spine, the head, the nose and the upper teeth. It can be said to cover the entire back. Therefore, when the Governor Vessel becomes obstructed, a large number of symptoms result. The tsubos along this meridian are used to alleviate these symptoms. These tsubos are used especially to treat symptoms in the head area, or those caused by diseases in the reproductive organs, as well as for a wide variety of symptoms associated with the digestive and respiratory systems.

A few examples of the symptoms for which tsubos of the Governor Vessel are used include pain which thrusts upward from the lower abdomen to the pit of the stomach, an increase of pain whenever the body is bent forward, feeling giddy and the sudden occurrence of sharp pain, as well as a dry and sore throat. In addition to this, tsubos of the Governor Vessel are used for hemorrhoids and nocturnal enuresis, as well as a paucity or retention of urine in women.

The Governor and Conception Vessels respectively have twenty-seven and twenty-four tsubos. The rule in Oriental medicine is that symptoms at the front of the body are treated by using tsubos of the Conception Vessel, and symptoms of the backside are treated with tsubos of the Governor Vessel. There is a condition in Oriental medicine called *Hai-Kyō* (back hardening) where the back becomes very rigid. This is a disease resulting from aging which is called ankylosing spondylitis or spondylitis deformans today. The classics say to use points "where they separate." This is saying, in other words, to treat mainly those places around the points where the Governor and Conception Vessels branch off or intersect other meridians. Six of the most commonly used tsubos among the tsubos of the Governor Vessel will be discussed next.

129. Chō-Kyō 長強 (GV-1)——*Tsubo for hemorrhoids and gonorrhea*

The Governor Vessel begins at the tsubo Chō-Kyō 長強 (GV-1) which is located at the tip of the coccyx (tailbone). *Chō-Kyō* (long strong) got the name because it is a tsubo which makes one's life long and makes the body strong. This tsubo is used to treat rigidity and inflexibility of the back, constipation and hemorrhoids, convulsive fits in children, difficulty in urination and gonorrhea (called *Go-Rin* 五淋 in Oriental medicine). Excellent results can be obtained for headaches and hemorrhoids when the tsubo Hyaku-E 百会 (GV-20) located on the top of the head is used together with this tsubo.

In Oriental medicine the type of headache where there is pain along the Governor Vessel from the front of the head to the back is called "Governor Vessel headache." In this case, the tsubos of the Governor Vessel are inspected from Hyaku-E down to Chō-Kyō to find the one indicated for treatment. Once you learn the course this meridian follows, it becomes very clear why both Hyaku-E and Chō-Kyō can be effective for hemorroids. In Oriental medicine there is a therapeutic principle where symptoms on the top half of the body are treated at the bottom half, and those of the bottom half are treated at the top. In other words, for symptoms which are clearly in the upper half of the body, or otherwise the lower half, the symptoms are treated on the opposite end of the body above or below. There is another principle in Oriental medicine where symptoms on the left side are treated on the right, and those on the right side are treated on the left. Also, there is a principle for *yu* points and *bo* points where symptoms on the front of the body are treated on the back and vice versa.

130. Mei-Mon 命門 (GV-4)——*Tsubo for building stamina*

Mei-Mon 命門 (GV-4: life gate) is also known as the "gate of life," and it is said to be the place where the life force inherited from one's parents resides. This tsubo got this name because it is located close to the center of a person's life force. Jin-Yu 腎兪 (UB-23) is located adjacent to the spinous process of the second lumbar vertebra, which is just between the kidneys. Therefore, Jin-Yu also goes by names like "energy between kidneys," or "the seat of inherited life force."

As is evident from its name, Mei-Mon is a tsubo for strengthening one's inborn constitution and physical capacity. Thus, it has been used from times past for treating people with weak and sickly constitutions or with low back pain. It is also very effective for tinnitus, headaches, menstrual disorders and discharge generally accompanied by a decline in vitality. Even more substantial effects can be obtained by using this tsubo together with Jin-Yu, also said to be the seat of inborn energy, as well as San-Shō-Yu 三焦兪 (UB-22), known as the seat of acquired energy, and Kan-Gen 関元 (CV-4), the tsubo for increasing vitality.

Straight above Mei-Mon, under the spinous process of the ninth thoracic vertebra lies Kin-Shuku 筋縮 (GV-8). This tsubo is also used when a person's back becomes rigid and bending forward and backward is difficult. In Oriental medicine it is stated that "the liver controls the tendons." Kin-Shuku lies right between Kan-Yu 肝兪 (UB-18), which are the liver *yu* point. This tsubo is another one well worth remembering.

131. Shin-Dō 神道 (GV-11)——*Tsubo for a weak heart and angina pectoris*

As stated many times already, a person's spirit is thought to reside in the heart in Oriental medicine. In other words, one's personality, capabilities and level of health are all determined by the heart. *Shin-Dō* 神道 (GV-11: spirit path) means that this tsubo is on the path which leads to one's spirit. It is located below the spinous process of the fifth thoracic vertebra, and to both sides of this lie the tsubo Shin-Yu 心兪 (UB-15). This point is noted in the classics as "the heart attaches to the fifth spine." Therefore Shin-Dō is located just below the spine of the fifth thoracic vertebra.

Shin-Dō is often used together with Shin-Yu to treat disorders of the circulatory system. The symptoms for which these tsubos are effective include feverishness in the upper half of the body, tension in the neck and shoulders, palpitations and shortness of breath. Shin-Dō is also a remarkably effective tsubo for relieving pain from a mild attack of angina pectoris.

Right below Shin-Dō, under the spinous process of the sixth thoracic vertebra, there is a tsubo called Rei-Dai 霊台 (GV-10). The name *Rei-Dai* (spirit pedestal) is also related to the spirit being housed in the heart, and presumably it serves as the pedestal on which the spirit sits. As mentioned before, all the tsubos with the character *Shin* 神 or *Rei* 霊 are tsubos used to treat the heart which houses the spirit. In addition to bolstering the physiological function of the heart, these tsubos are used to restore a person's emotional and psychological balance. People with health problems stemming from disturbances of the autonomic nervous system, who tend to be emotionally unstable, anxious, introspective and afraid of people, can derive great benefits from acupuncture and moxibustion treatments over a long period. The reason for the effectiveness of these treatments can be explained by the principles of Oriental medicine, yet seeing the results can be quite amazing.

132. Shin-Chū 身柱 (GV-12)——*Tsubo for convulsive fits in children*

In Japan people used to burn moxa on the backs of children who were weak or given to convulsive fits. This is not done any more, but acupuncturists still use this same method to cure convulsive fits in children. This tendency is most often seen in children who are hypersensitive, and especially in children with parasitic worms that cause them to become irritable. This is the origin of the word *kan-no-mushi* (mad bug) and the best way to cure this condition is to burn moxa on the tsubo named *Shin-Chū* 身柱 (GV-12) located right below the third thoracic spine. This was the reason moxibustion was applied on children's backs in times past.

Another name for Shin-Chū is *chiriki* 散り気 which means a tsubo where the harmful energy which has collected in the body is dispelled. This tsubo is especially noted as one which strengthens and improves the general condition of infants. In Japan, "moxa at *chiriki*" is still well known as being the most important tsubo for moxibustion of children.

Aside from treating children, Shin-Chū is used to relieve pain and tension from the head down the back of the neck and shoulders and back. It is written in one classic that, "The point below the third spine (Shin-Chū) controls heat in the chest." Shin-Chū is level with Hai-Yu 肺兪 (UB-13) located on either side, and these tsubos have been used since the olden days to reduce fevers caused by diseases in the respiratory organs.

133. Dai-Tsui 大椎 (GV-14)——*Tsubo for nettle rash*

Dai-Tsui 大椎 (GV-14) is located at the base of the neck on the back between the spinous process of the seventh cervical and first thoracic vertebrae. This may be difficult to locate, so bend the head slightly forward and then turn it from side to side, keeping the shoulders still. Looking at the top of the spine when a person does this, there is one spine which moves with the head, and another below it which does not. The spine that moves is the cervical vertebra, so Dai-Tsui is just below the lowest spine that moves.

When a person has an allergic condition, this point will be extremely sensitive when pressed or hit lightly. This tsubo is used when there is a considerable amount of tension from the neck down to the shoulders. Also, amazing results can be obtained in relieving migraine headaches, nettle rash, hemorrhoids, nose colds, and digestive problems by applying moxibustion on this tsubo. This is especially effective for people who tend to get nettle rash, migraine headaches and sore eyes, and otherwise those who catch colds easily, and have digestive problems with occasional diarrhea, or those with a constant feeling of oppression like asthma in their chest, as well as those with pimples or rough skin in the triangular area on their back below Dai-Tsui and between the shoulder blades. When this is the case, burning small pieces of moxa around Dai-Tsui, above and below, and to either side, usually gives remarkable results. The tsubo Fū-Fu 風府 (GV-16) is also a very important tsubo, but it will not be covered here because it was already mentioned with Fū-Mon 風門 (UB-12).

134. Hyaku-E 百会 (GV-20)——*Tsubo for headaches and hemorrhoids*

There is a point at the very top of the head which feels tender when pressed, and this is where the imaginary line drawn from the top of each ear and the centerline running back from between the eyebrows intersect each other. This is the tsubo Hyaku-E 百会 (GV-20). It is said to be the point where all the meridians meet, and thus, a tsubo effective for all symptoms in any part of the body. Hayaku-E is especially effective for hemorrhoids which is classified among the "ailments above and below" in Oriental medicine.

Just three centimeters to the front of Hyaku-E is the tsubo Zen-Chō 前頂 (GV-21) and three centimeters to the back is the tsubo Go-Chō 後頂 (GV-19). These tsubos are very effective for headaches when used together with Hyaku-E. Pain and heaviness in the head can be roughly divided into two types. In one type there are various other symptoms on the face such as with the eyes or nose, and in the other type there is a heavy sensation like something is covering the head, and this is accompanied with occipital neuralgia, tension down the neck and fatigue in the shoulders and back. The rule in treatment, therefore, is to use Hyaku-E and Zen-Chō when there are symptoms in the facial area along with a headache such as eye fatigue, blurring of vision, nasal obstruction, or tinnitus. Hyaku-E and Go-Chō are used when there are symptoms of tension and stiffness down the neck and shoulders along with a headache.

In addition to this, Hyaku-E gives good results for high blood pressure, hemorrhoids and car sickness.

14. Conception Vessel

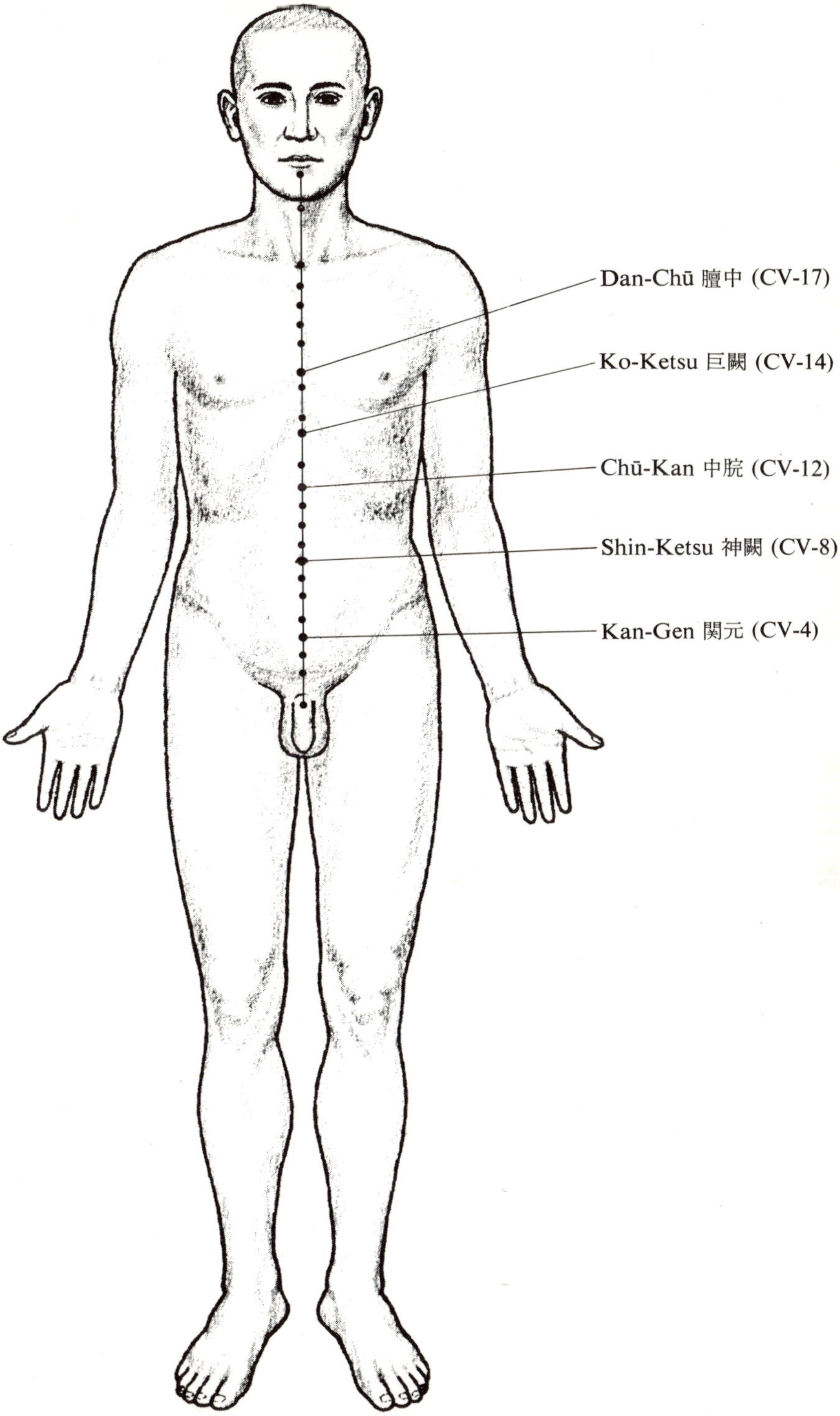

The Conception Vessel lies on the median line which runs down the front of the body from the center of the face to the neck, the center of the abdomen and the pubis, and is spoken of as "controlling (the body) from the front." This means that this meridian controls things in the front of the body. The Conception Vessel has twenty-four tsubos starting with E-In 会陰 (CV-1) which is located on the perineum (a point just to the front of the anus). From E-In, this meridian travels up the front of the body going over the lower abdomen and chest to end at the tsubo Shō-Shō 承漿 (CV-24) in the middle of the lower jaw.

As may be expected, the Conception Vessel has a very close relationship with pregnancy in women, and this meridian is characterized by having many tsubos that are very effective for gynecological problems. In a classical text it is written, "The Conception Vessel relates to pregnancy; it flows along the midline of the abdomen to facilitate conception and the growth of the fetus in women."

The tsubos E-In, Kyok-Kotsu 曲骨 (CV-2), and Chū-Kyoku 中極 (CV-3) which form a row on the line going up from the perineum to the navel, are noted especially as being tsubos indispensable for treating symptoms of the urogenital organs. There is a condition called *naiketsu* commonly seen in men where a hard lump forms in the lower abdomen. In more current terms, it is a hard growth under the white line (linea alba), the vertical groove in the center of the abdomen between the muscles, and it is a condition where a large amount of gas collects in the intestines. Aside from the symptoms of infertility and menstrual problems in women, the tsubos of the Conception Vessel are very important for stimulating the self regulating mechanism of the body.

The most important tsubos Kan-Gen 関元 (CV-4), Shin-Ketsu 神闕 (CV-8), Chū-Kan 中脘 (CV-12), Ko-Ketsu 巨闕 (CV-14) and Dan-Chū 膻中 (CV-17), among the twenty-four of the Conception Vessel, will be discussed in detail. There are other tsubos on the Conception Vessel such as E-In, Seki-Mon 石門 (CV-5), In-Kō 陰交 (CV-7) and Kyū-Bi 鳩尾 (CV-15) which are equally important, but it is really difficult to rank them in order of importance. Kyū-Bi is located below the sternum at the tip of the xiphoid process. This is above the tsubo Chū-Kan which will be discussed in detail later. E-In is the first tsubo of the Conception Vessel and lies between the anus and the genitals. For men, this is between the anus and the scrotum, and for women, this is between the anus and the labium majus. The tsubo In-Kō is located about three centimeters below the navel and is the source point for the lower heater of the triple heater as discussed previously. Seki-Mon is about three centimeters down from In-Kō and is an important tsubo as the *bo* point for checking the condition of the triple heater meridian. Kan-Gen will be explained in detail next, but it is just three centimeters below Seki-Mon. The three tsubos, In-Kō, Seki-Mon and Kan-Gen are each vitally important points located directly under the navel evenly spaced on a line going down toward the genital region.

135. Kan-Gen 関元 (CV-4)——*Tsubo for increasing vitality*

As just explained above, this tsubo is located about nine centimeters directly under the navel in line with Seki-Mon 石門 (CV-5) and In-Kō 陰交 (CV-7). Kan-Gen 関元 (CV-4) is a very important tsubo governing one's basic energy level determined by birth, and is also the *bo* point of the small intestine meridian. For this reason, Kan-Gen is used to treat a great variety of symptoms. Among these, it is especially effective for loss of vitality, loss of weight, high blood pressure, insomnia, and chilling of the extremities, as well as pimples and nettle rash. The Conception Vessel has a deep connection with the reproductive organs in both men and women. In particular, Kan-Gen, located on the lower abdomen between the navel and the genitals, is the perfect tsubo for treating diseases having to do with the sex organs.

Another tsubo, Kyok-Kotsu 曲骨 (CV-2), lies on the center line of the lower abdomen right above the symphysis pubis, and this point also shows a reaction when there are gynecological disorders, and is very effective in treating them. Also, Chū-Kyoku 中極 (CV-3) which is located about twelve centimeters below the navel on the center line going down toward the pubis, is another tsubo that is, just like Kyok-Kotsu, very effective for disfunctions in the urogenital organs, especially gynecological disorders.

As for Kan-Gen, it is a tsubo well worth remembering as being effective not only for stopping the loss of weight, but also for middle-aged and obese women, as well as young ladies worried about the shape of their legs.

136. Shin-Ketsu 神闕 (CV-8)——*Tsubo for warming the stomach*

Shin-Ketsu 神闕 (CV-8) also goes by other names such as *Sai-Chū* 臍中 (navel middle) or *Mei-Tai* 命帯 (life cord), and it is located right on the navel. This tsubo should not be pressed very strongly. In Japan, practices such as heating up a piece of *konnyaku* (devil's tongue jelly) and placing this on the navel, or otherwise, packing the navel with salt and burning moxa on top of this, have been common from the old days.

The navel is obviously a depression in the skin, but there is no fatty tissue, fascia or muscle under the navel, and here the skin attaches directly to the peritoneum. This is why methods like those mentioned above are used instead of pressing the navel. There is an old wives' tale in Japan about how lint must not be removed from the navel. This is not because taking lint out of the navel causes stomach pains as the tale goes, but because poking the navel stimulates the peritoneum directly to sometimes cause discomfort.

For this reason, Shin-Ketsu is never used directly for acupuncture, moxibustion or shiatsu treatments. Nevertheless, this tsubo is the best place for warming up the inside of the abdomen from the outside, so it is used to warm up the body whenever a person feels chilly and has stomach pains. There are many important tsubos right around the navel. The area immediately around Shin-Ketsu is used in Oriental medicine to diagnose the condition of the abdomen overall.

137. Chū-Kan 中脘 (CV-12)——*Tsubo for improving digestion*

Chū-Kan 中脘 (CV-12) is located about twelve centimeters above the navel on the center line of the upper abdomen. This is around the midpoint between the navel and the pit of the stomach. The character *Kan* 脘 of Chū-Kan denotes the opening of the stomach. Thus, the tsubo over the top opening of the stomach is called Jō-Kan 上脘 (CV-13), and the tsubo located over the bottom opening of the stomach, about three centimeters above the navel, is called Ge-Kan 下脘 (CV-10). *Chū-Kan* 中脘 (middle opening) is located right between Jō-Kan and Ge-Kan, or between the top and bottom openings of the stomach.

As for the symptoms for which Chū-Kan is effective, there are of course, those related with stomach problems, as well as diarrhea, constipation, nettle rash, dizziness, tinnitus and pimples. In addition to this, Chū-Kan is used to increase one's stamina.

When the stomach feels distended and heavy after an evening meal, give light massage and finger pressure on Chū-Kan. One will begin to feel amazingly better as the tension and sensitivity in this area diminishes, and the hard areas in the back are also relieved. This will naturally cause one to sleep better, and one will wake up bright and fresh the next morning with a healthy appetite. This same tsubo is also effective for calming a person down, and is very much related to weight problems of either being too fat or too thin.

Chū-Kan is of great importance as the source point of the middle heater of the triple heater which covers the area from the pit of the stomach to the navel and associates with the digestive system.

138. Ko-Ketsu 巨闕 (CV-14)——*Tsubo to relieve palpitations*

As written in the classics, Ko-Ketsu 巨闕 (CV-14) is the *bo* point of the heart meridian and is a very important tsubo as the principal point for treating heart conditions. This tsubo is located above Chū-Kan 中脘 (CV-12), right below the pit of the stomach. In Oriental medicine, any hardness or stifling sensation here is referred to as "obstruction and hardness in the epigastrium," and the tone and resiliency of skin around this area is regarded as being an important barometer of a person's health. If this area seems to be hard, it is a good idea for that person to get some rest because even though there may not be any symptoms as such, it is a sign that the heart is overworked.

Ko-Ketsu is an invaluable tsubo for those people with high blood pressure who constantly seem to have palpitations. Aside from this, it is effective for chronic stomach problems and menstrual disorders. Also, Ko-Ketsu is used to treat asthma which was once regarded as being a disease of the elderly, but now has become more widespread among the youth as the air has become more polluted by such things as auto emissions.

Aside from Ko-Ketsu, there is a tsubo called Kyū-Bi 鳩尾 (CV-15) in the pit of the stomach. It is located just above Ko-Ketsu and below the tip of the sternum.

The name *Kyū-Bi* (dove tail) came from the shape of the xiphoid process being likened to the tail of a dove.

139. Dan-Chū 膻中 (CV-17)——*Tsubo for coughs and shortness of breath*

The tsubo Dan-Chū 膻中 (CV-17) is located in the front center of the sternum right between the nipples. Symptoms related to the heart such as palpitations, coughing, shortness of breath, and pains going from the pit of the stomach around to the side can be treated with this tsubo. In addition, conditions of being under weight and lacking in stamina can be improved along with poor lactation in nursing mothers.

Angina pectoris may be suspected whenever a piercing pain is felt from this tsubo to the area below the spinous process of the fourth thoracic vertebra. When this occurs, finger pressure on Dan-Chū should help relieve the pain. Dan-Chū also happens to be the source point for the upper heater of the triple heater which covers the area from the top of the chest to the pit of the stomach. This is the reason this tsubo can be used to quiet pains in the chest and flank region.

The area around Dan-Chū is known to be very important in Western medicine also, and it is of significance as a "Head's zone," named after a British physiologist, Sir Henry Head. Directly above Dan-Chū is Gyoku-Dō 玉堂 (CV-18) which is level with the third intercostal space, and Shi-Kyū 紫宮 (CV-19) which is level with the second intercostal space. Another important tsubo above Dan-Chū is Ten-Totsu 天突 (CV-22) in the center of the notch above the sternum. This is at the front of the neck at the base. All of the tsubos mentioned are effective for respiratory problems, but Ten-Totsu is especially effective for asthma when used in conjunction with the other effective tsubos.

Part Two:

Tsubo Treatments for Symptoms Caused by Fatigue

The health products industry has enjoyed a great boom in recent years. All kinds of devices, from adhesive tape with small magnets to electric massage chairs, have been marketed in Japan with the claim of providing relief from symptoms of fatigue, and many of these have become very popular. This points to how fatigued people have become in this day and age. Perhaps fatigue and overwork can be counted among modern afflictions. As segments of our society become more and more specialized and compartmentalized, personal relationships seem to have become that much more complicated. While at work, a person has to deal with superiors and co-workers, and after returning home, one has to face involved relationships with one's spouse and children. Often a person is left with very little time to really relax, and stress just keeps piling up.

Stress can trigger mental fatigue which often makes a person's head feel clouded and causes one's thoughts to become disorganized, and a person becomes unable to concentrate at work. Moreover, mental fatigue is often accompanied with physical symptoms such as a dull and tired sensation all over the body, tension in the neck and shoulders, an oppressive feeling in the chest, and insomnia, as well as headaches and heavy sensations in the head. What condition do symptoms of fatigue indicate in terms of modern medicine? There are many theories regarding this, and although it is difficult to say which is the most correct, the following five theories are representative of the current medical understanding regarding fatigue.

1) The chemical components of fatigue build up in the muscles and tissues as well as the internal organs to cause fatigue. These are waste products resulting from the oxidation of sugars obtained from food, and these include lactic acid, pyruvic acid and ammonia.
2) All activities in life involve the contraction and relaxation of muscles. Fatigue results when there is a shortage of biochemical components necessary for this activity (e.g., glycogen, adenosine triphosphoric acid, various vitamins, minerals and hormones).
3) Fatigue is caused by a deterioration in the physiological function of expelling waste products produced by the oxidation or combustion of organic compounds and nutrients transported to the cells by blood circulation.
4) The autonomic nervous system automatically regulates the metabolic rate of the body so that it is able to adapt to the external environment whether it be warm or cold. Imbalances in this control mechanism could be the cause of fatigue.
5) Fatigue is a condition where the body is subjected to conditions exceeding its capacity to adapt, and normal functioning is thereby impaired as in cases of overexertion or mental fatigue.

It is no simple matter to define fatigue precisely in medical terms, but generally speaking, fatigue is manifested in the form of muscular tension or stiffness. This is not to imply that all muscular tension is a sign of fatigue. Nevertheless, tension in the muscles of the head, neck, back, arms, pelvic region, thighs and calves can cause sensations of dullness and fatigue over the entire body. This tension is caused by the lack of sufficient circulation of blood through the muscles and connective tissues of the area. Furthermore, this tension causes blood to become congested in the affected area to aggravate the symptoms, and this begins a vicious circle which only compounds the fatigue.

All of our bodies have certain physiological limits that vary with each individual, whether it be for mental activity, or muscular and organic functions. This may be called the margin of safety we have in which no problems or illnesses will result so long as we work within these limits. However, if a person places too great a burden on the mind at work, or gets overworked to become "stressed out" and full of anxiety, or otherwise overworks certain muscles in sports or physical labor, obviously these limits are exceeded and the body begins to manifest symptoms of fatigue.

The first sign of fatigue to appear is the dulling of mental acuity, and eventually muscular strength begins to decrease and the whole body is overtaken with tiredness and one does not feel like moving at all. This condition is accompanied with various symptoms of fatigue such as tension down the back of the neck and shoulders, pain in the back, chilling of the extremities, headaches and a heavy sensation in the head. Once these symptoms of fatigue become fixed as a chronic condition, one's physiological functions can no longer be kept up at a normal level and eventually a particular function or organ becomes abnormal and the body contracts a disease.

In this sense, fatigue can be regarded as a phenomenon where the body has come a step closer to disease and that much farther from health. At the same time, fatigue serves as a warning light which tells a person that the body is approaching an abnormal state. In this context, feeling tired and listless is a natural defense mechanism of the body which is not really a bad thing in itself. The important point is to quickly relieve the fatigue whenever the warning light begins to flash on and off. It goes without saying that fatigue is most easily removed when the amount is small. This may seem like an obvious point, but the greatest key to staying healthy and for avoiding illness is to take immediate steps to counter the effects of fatigue at the appearance of the first signs of fatigue.

The best way to stay free of fatigue is to live an ordered life, and to take a hot bath and get plenty of sleep whenever one becomes tired, and in general, to get an ample amount of rest and relaxation in one's life. Be that as it may, people living in this busy world today seem to have a hard time living up to this simple ideal. This is why the maintenance of one's own health through tsubo therapy is recommended wholeheartedly.

There is much mention in Oriental medicine about "curing illnesses before they occur." The basic principle followed is to take steps to retain health well before disease sets in. The maintenance of health and the prevention of disease by providing relief from fatigue can be called the most prominent feature of Oriental physiotherapy including massage and acupuncture. With these therapeutic principles of prevention in mind, ninty-one examples of tsubos specially effective in relieving fatigue and restoring vitality are presented in this section according to symptoms. One thing must be said about these symptom specific tsubos, and this is that there is usually more than one tsubo effective for any given symptom. Fatigue causes a wide variety of symptoms, and in many cases, using a combination of tsubos gives best results. These specially effective tsubos should be regarded as a group of tsubos, selected from among the numerous tsubos on the body, that are most effective in relieving one particular manifestation of fatigue.

1. Treating Symptoms in the Head and Facial Area

A. Heaviness over the whole head——Hyaku-E 百会 (GV-20)

Perhaps you have had the experience of waking up in the morning to discover that your head feels dull and heavy. Often this feels as if something heavy is covering the head like a hat, particularly for middle-aged people, and at times a person has to go through the whole day with this dull headache. This type of headache appears most often when one is behind in sleep or when the blood pressure is fluctuating because of a decline in one's physical condition. In any case, this symptom is obviously a sign of overworking the mind and body.

The specially effective tsubo in this case is Hyaku-E 百会 (GV-20) at the very top of the head. This is located by drawing an imaginary line over the head connecting the top of the ears (the ears can be folded forward to find the right point) and locating the point where the center line drawn straight back from between the eyebrows intersects this. Hyaku-E is easy to locate because it usually feels tender when pressed. This is the tsubo where all the channels of energy in the body meet. The name *Hyaku-E* (hundred meeting) presumably comes from one hundred channels meeting at this point. It is known as a tsubo effective for all diseases, but it is especially effective for symptoms accompanied with a headache.

Whenever there is a sensation of heaviness over the head, place the index and middle fingers of both hands together on Hyaku-E and press straight down forcefully as if trying to make it penetrate to the stomach. Pressing and moving the fingers back and forth slightly on this tsubo is amazingly effective in relieving the heavy feeling over one's head.

Just the above treatment should provide relief, but even better results may be obtained by applying pressure on Ten-Chū 天柱 (UB-10) at the edge of the hairline on the outside of the big muscle at the back of the neck, and on Fū-Chi 風池 (GB-20) which is located just one finger width to the front of Ten-Chū. To apply pressure on Ten-Chū, hold your head from behind with the four fingers to the side of the head and

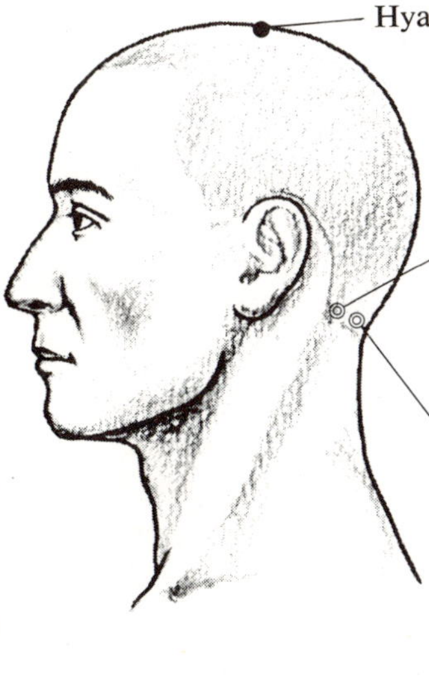

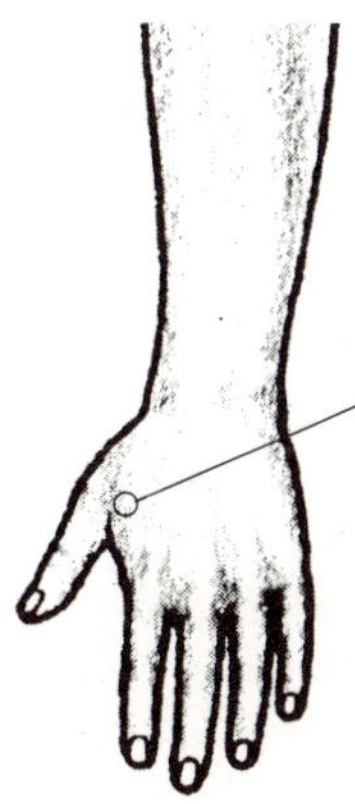

press the tsubos upward toward Hyaku-E with your thumbs. One can move the thumbs back and forth slightly, the main point being to press strongly enough so that these points feel slightly sore.

If these treatments are not totally effective, supplement this with pressure on the tsubo Gō-Koku 合谷 (LI-4). This tsubo on the back of the web between the thumb and the index finger is pressed strongly with the other thumb. Gō-Koku is another tsubo used often to relieve headaches and fatigue.

B. Pain on one side of the head——Ken-Ro 懸顱 (GB-5)

There are many people who suffer from what is called a migraine headache. This is a throbbing pain on one side of the head that occurs most often during the change of seasons. At times, this headache occurs so suddenly and strongly that it makes tears come to one's eyes. This headache occurs on either side, but generally there seems to be more people who suffer from migraine headaches on the left side. This condition is also referred to as "cerebral allergy" in Japan, and it appears most commonly among people with allergic constitutions. However, similar symptoms also appear quite commonly among healthy people when they become fatigued. People with stubborn migraine headaches associated with allergic conditions should consult a specialist and try to improve their basic physical condition, but migraine headaches caused by fatigue can be cured easily through tsubo therapy.

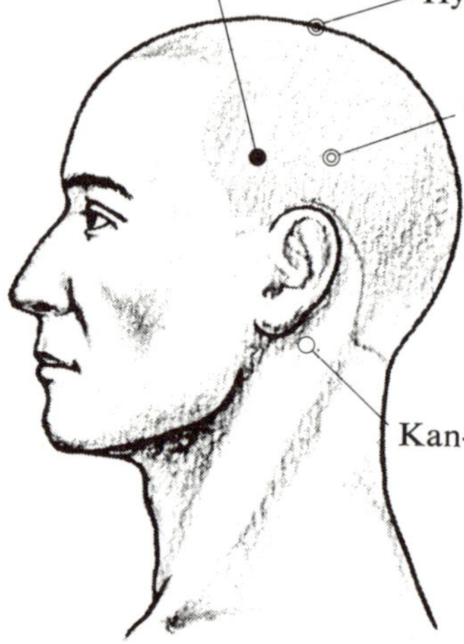

The tsubo specially effective for migraine headaches is Ken-Ro 懸顱 (GB-5) which is at the top of what is called the temples. This tsubo is located at about the midpoint between the corner of the hairline on the forehead and the earlobe. A hard muscle can be felt by feeling this area with the fingertips while biting hard with the back teeth. This is the temporal muscle which is used in chewing and this area is generally known as the temples. The hardest point in this muscle is a tsubo which can be remarkably effective in alleviating migraine headaches. When you have severe migraine headaches, press this tsubo firmly from both sides with the middle fingers so that the right and left hands are pushing against one another, and then add small circular movements while pressing. This will cause a penetrating sensation which will reach the very center of one's head, and after this the pain will go away mysteriously.

Adding the tsubos Hyaku-E 百会 (GV-20), Ten-Shō 天衝 (GB-9) and Kan-Kotsu 完骨 (GB-12) in this treatment should be thoroughly effective. The location of Hyaku-E has already been covered in the preceding section. Ten-Shō is located two finger widths just above the top of the ear. which happens to be just to the back of Ken-Ro. Kan-Kotsu is located to the back of the bony protrusion in the skull behind the ear. Pressing these tsubos firmly with the thumbs toward the front from the back should ease the pain and provide prompt relief.

All the tsubos just mentioned are on both sides of the head, but when migraine headaches occur just on the left side, then treating only those tsubos on the left is usually quite effective in providing relief.

C. Heaviness in forehead——Zen-Chō 前頂 (GV-21)

A sensation of heaviness in the head is generally a symptom resulting from overworking the mind and body. Heaviness mainly in and around the forehead is usually due to psychological fatigue. Therefore, this is a symptom which appears often among people who work at desks all day long. Stress tends to accumulate easily when one does too much desk work, and even though there may not be a severe headache, there is discomfort in the head. The tendency is for the forehead area to feel heavy and uncomfortable when one is looking downward. This symptom can sometimes be very stubborn and persist throughout the day. Under these circumstances it is best to get plenty of rest and to relieve the basic cause of stress. Otherwise, in tsubo therapy, the tsubo Zen-Chō 前頂 (GV-21) is used to relieve such symptoms.

The location of Zen-Chō is just two finger widths (using index and middle fingers) in front of Hyaku-E mentioned previously, which is easy to find. Zen-Chō is also used when there is swelling in the forehead and facial area, or when one's head feels hazy. The sensation of heaviness in the forehead will go away and you will feel much better after applying pressure on Zen-Chō. This is done in the same way as for Hyaku-E 百会 (GV-20), where the index and middle fingers of both hands are placed on the tsubo to apply firm pressure toward the center of the head.

Another tsubo which should not be overlooked for relieving heaviness in the forehead is Zu-I 頭維 (ST-8), which is one finger width behind the corner of the hair-

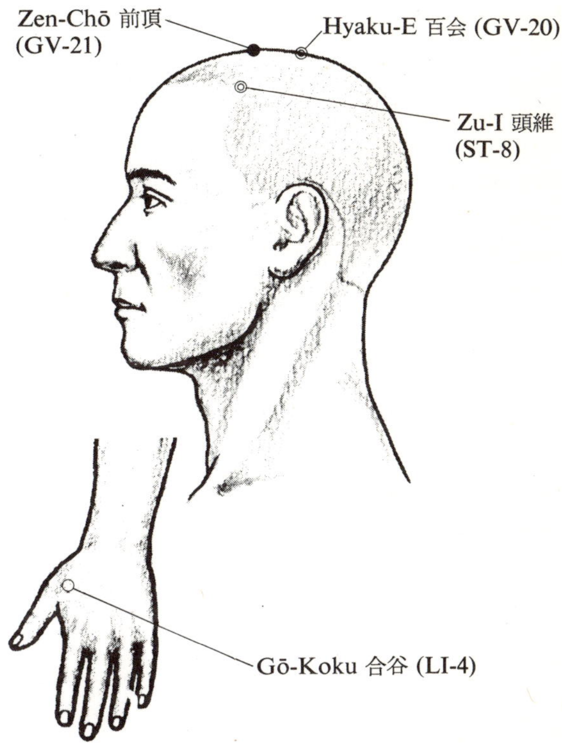

line on the forehead. The character *I* 維 of Zu-I means a big event, so the name *Zu-I* (head event) indicates an important tsubo used for headaches, eye fatigue, nasal obstruction, or any substantial symptom in the forehead or facial area.

When the forehead area feels heavy, the effect of treatments are heightened by also using Hyaku-E. The important point is to use the tsubos Zu-I and Hyaku-E together with Zen-Chō for the best results. If this does not seem to provide relief, press the tsubo Go-Koku 合谷 (LI-4) on the back of the hand. This is one of the easiest tsubos to press, and it also happens to be one of the most effective.

D. Heaviness in back of head——Go-Chō 後頂 (GV-19)

A healthy blood supply is vital for supplying the brain cells with the necessary oxygen and nutrients, and for removing cellular waste products. The blood vessels which supply the brain go up either side of the neck and join inside the head. On the other hand, in the human body the weight of the head is only supported by the cervical vertebrae and the muscles going down from the back of the head to the shoulders. Therefore, when these muscles become very tense, the blood vessels going to the brain are compressed and circulation to the head decreases. This then causes a heavy sensation in the back of the head. The second most common location where the sensation of heaviness occurs is in the back of the head, the most common sensation is one of the whole head being covered. The tsubo most effective for the former symptom is Go-Chō 後頂 (GV-19), two finger widths to the back of Hyaku-E 百会 (GV-20). This is on just the opposite side of Hyaku-E from the tsubo Zen-Chō 前頂 (GV-21) mentioned previously. Just keep in mind that for heaviness in the front of the head the tsubos Zen-Chō, Hyaku-E and Zu-I 頭維 (ST-8) are used, and for that in the back, Go-Chō and Hyaku-E are used.

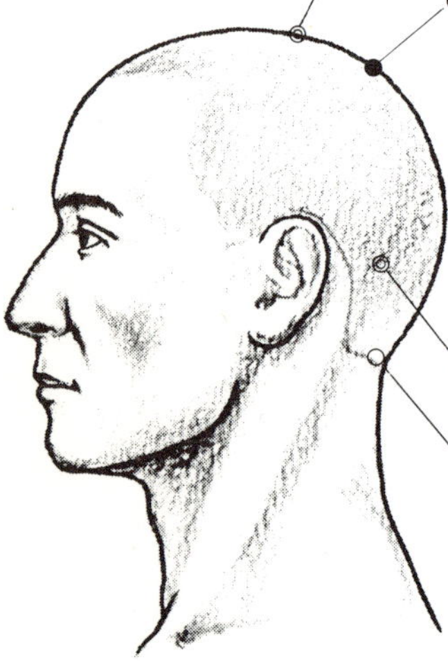

In addition to this there is the tsubo Nō-Kū 脳空 (GB-19) located two finger widths to either side of the external occipital protuberance. Nō-Kū (brain empty) just as the name implies, is used in situations where the whole head is in a daze as if it were actually empty. Chiefly, Go-Chō is the tsubo used to relieve sensations of heaviness in the back of the head, and Nō-Kū and Hyaku-E are used as supplementary tsubos. The method of pressing Go-Chō is just the same as that for pressing Hyaku-E and Zen-Chō. Applying pressure on Nō-Kū, however, differs from this; it is pressed firmly from behind with both thumbs. The key point here is to make small circles with the thumbs so as not to pull the hair, and to provide strong stimulation which penetrates to the center of the head.

As stated in the beginning of this section, the cause of heaviness in the back of the head is usually muscular tension down the back of the neck and the shoulders, so this condition is most often accompanied with stiffness and discomfort in the neck and shoulders. For this reason, even better results can be obtained by also applying pressure on Ten-Chū 天柱 (UB-10) along with Go-Chō, Hyaku-E and Nō-Kū. Ten-Chū is also known as a tsubo remarkably effective for headaches, so it proves most useful for this purpose also.

E. Lack of luster in hair——Shō-Kō 承光 (UB-6)

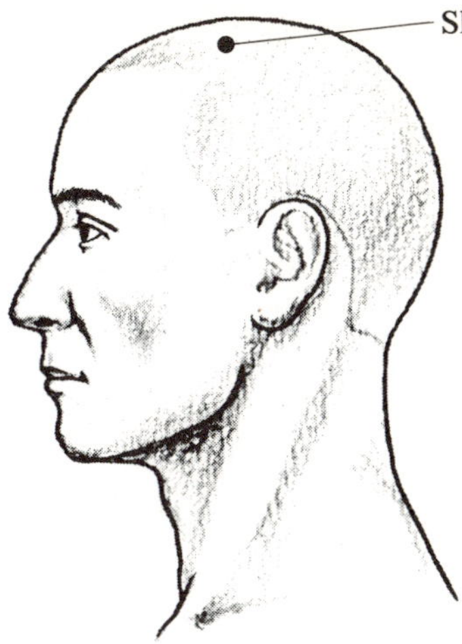

Most everyone loses hair with age and also for older people hair loses the luster it once had. Even young people, when they are overworked or become worried about something, get white hairs overnights, or otherwise their hair loses its shine and body. This is evidence that the autonomic nervous system, which aside from controlling the functions of the internal organs, regulates the excretion of sweat and body oils, has been impaired in its function by mental and physical fatigue. Therefore, in order to maintain shiny and healthy hair, it is first necessary to restore the function of the autonomic nervous system. The tsubo to be used for this purpose is Shō-Kō 承光 (UB-6), located on the top of the head.

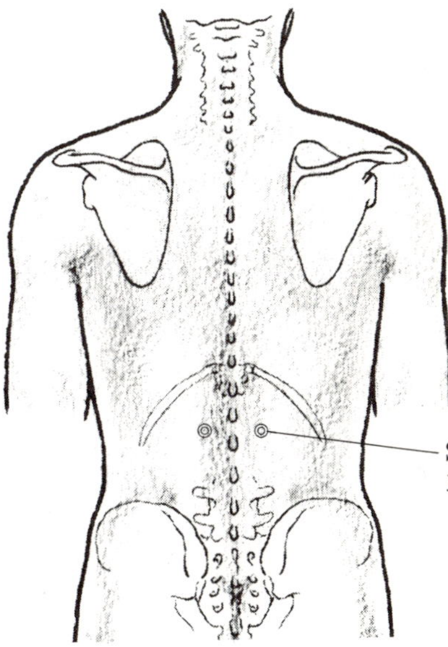

Generally, the tsubos on the head are difficult to find because no one method for locating tsubos on the head works in every case. Find Shō-Kō by placing the index, middle and ring fingers to the front of the top of the head and then locate the points in front of the ring finger four centimeters to either side of the center line. Two places can be found where the pain reaches the eyes when these points are pressed strongly. This is Shō-Kō, the tsubo specially effective for keeping one's hair shiny and full of body.

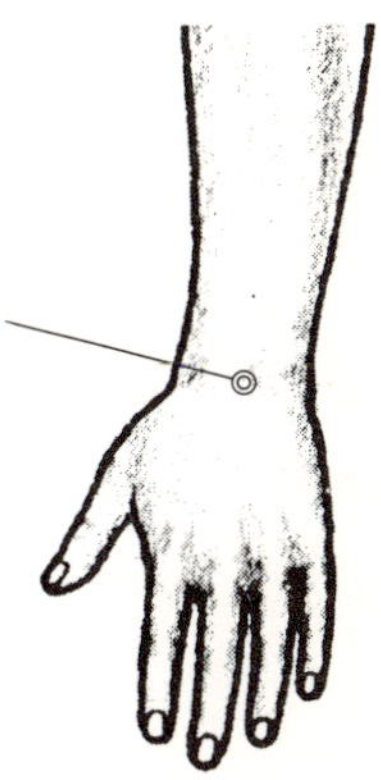

Hair tends to lose its luster when one's vitality is waning. In order to restore luster to hair which has lost its shine, one must revitalize the energy through the whole body. The tsubos effective for revitalizing body energy is San-Shō-Yu 三焦兪 (UB-22), to either side of the first lumbar vertebra, and Yō-Chi 陽池 (TH-4) in the middle of the back of the wrist. San-Shō-Yu, especially, is a vital tsubo directly linked with the triple heater which is regarded as being the source of body heat in Oriental medicine. San-Shō-Yu has long

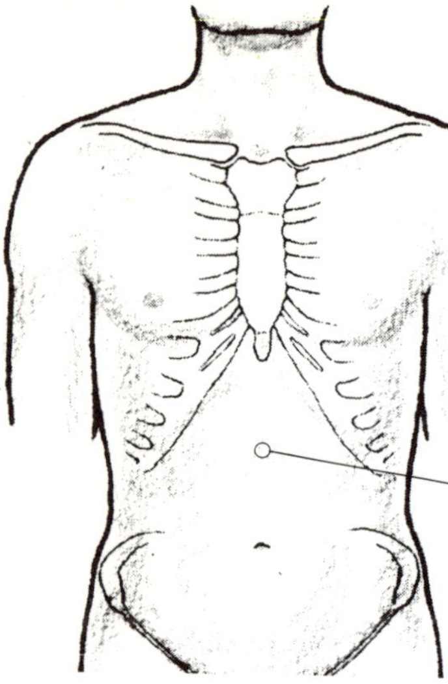

been known as a tsubo for improving the overall physical condition and thereby adding a healthy shine to one's skin and hair. When hair has lost its shine by the cumulative effect of overwork and anxiety, apply firm finger pressure on San-Shō-Yu and Yō-Chi along with Shō-Kō.

Furthermore, when the digestive organs are not in very good condition, one's nutritional state deteriorates in proportion, and hair also loses its luster. In this case, giving finger pressure to Chū-Kan 中脘 (CV-12), located right between the navel and the pit of the stomach, will further improve the effect.

F. Vertigo and dizziness in general——Ten-Yō 天牖 (TH-16)

After becoming middle-aged, people often begin to experience vertigo or dizziness when standing up from a chair, or when going up and down a flight of stairs. Dizzy spells are often accompanied with tinnitus, and these symptoms appear frequently when one is overworked and lacking in sleep. When dizzy spells occur repeatedly, some disorder in the cerebrum or cerebellum may be suspected, so one should consult a specialist. If it is a simple case of dizziness caused by nothing more than fatigue, however, tsubo therapy is usually enough to cure the problem.

There are some people who mistakenly think that dizziness is a condition having to do with poor eyes, but in fact, this is a symptom which is caused by disfunctions in the semicircular canals of the inner ear. In Oriental medicine, therefore, dizziness is treated by using the tsubo Ten-Yō 天牖 (TH-16) located on the neck behind the ear. There is a hard bone behind the ear, and the bottom end of it is called the mas-

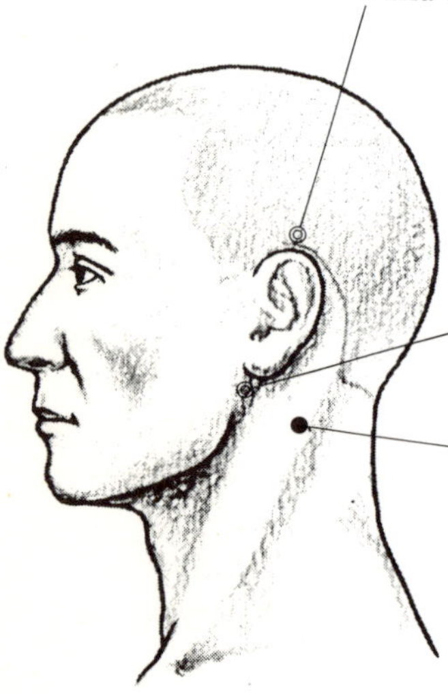

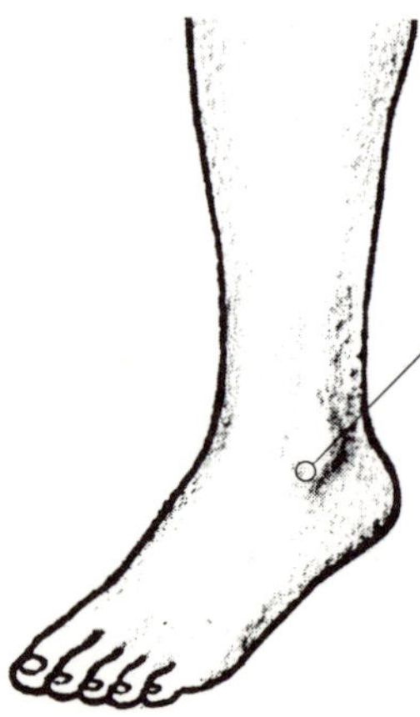

toid process. Ten-Yō is located just to the back of the large muscle (sternocleidomastoid) which attaches to this bony protrusion.

The character *Yō* 牖 of Ten-Yō means a window, so the name means a place where light is admitted into the "heaven section" as spoken of in Oriental medicine. When the area around this "window" for the upper part of the body becomes blocked with tension, dizziness results, and this same point can be stimulated to relieve the problem.

The best way to press Ten-Yō is to place each middle finger on the tsubo to either side and press firmly toward the throat until the large muscle on the side of the neck is reached. The tsubo is stimulated by kneading this point back and forth, and this should cause the dizziness to go away. Also pressing the tsubos Kaku-Son 角孫 (TH-20), on the head just above the ear, and Ei-Fū 翳風 (TH-17), just behind the earlobe, should provide prompt relief.

If you become dizzy while at work, take your shoes and socks off and use your thumbs to press the hollow spot just one finger width in front of the outer ankle bone until it hurts. This is the tsubo called Kyū-Kyo 丘墟 (GB-40), and it often gives quick relief from dizzy spells. It may be hard to comprehend why a tsubo on the leg is used to dispell dizziness, but points on the leg (earth section) are often used in Oriental medicine to relieve symptoms in the "heaven section."

G. Dizziness upon standing——Kyō-In 竅陰 (GB-11)

When the condition of being mentally and physically overworked continues over a period of time, symptoms of vertigo, tinnitus, and dizziness upon standing begin to appear one after another. Vertigo is an abnormality in the balancing mechanism of the body where one's surroundings seem to be whirling. Dizziness upon standing is where a person becomes dizzy and unsteady when trying to stand up. Both these symptoms occur when fatigue causes the blood pressure to fluctuate, and further, when there is a tendency for blood to rise to the head. In addition, since it is said that "the kidneys open to the ears" in Oriental medicine, the above symptoms appear more often when a person's vitality has waned (kidney deficient condition).

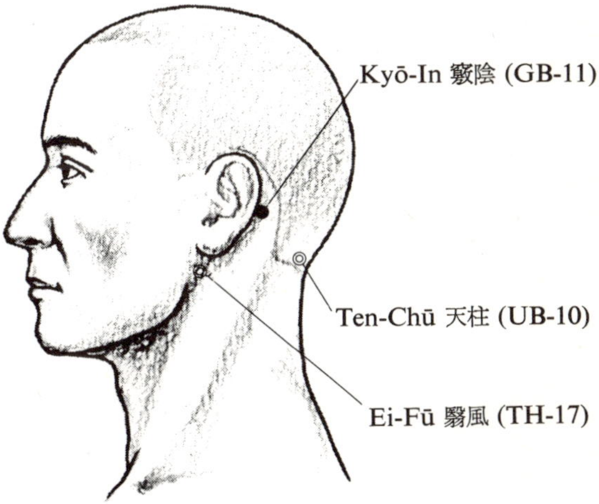

Since dizziness upon standing is an abnormality in the inner ear just like vertigo, a tsubo just behind the ear named Kyō-In 竅陰 (GB-11) is the main point used for effective treatments. The character *Kyō* 竅 of Kyō-In denotes an orifice in the skull, which refers to the ears, and the character *In* 陰 means yin, or a part in the shadow. This point is not very difficult to locate, and simply stated, it is in the hollow place between the hard bone behind the ear and the base of the ear. There are many tsubos around the ear, but among them, Kyō-In has been well known since the olden days as being particularly effective for symptoms related to the ears such as vertigo, tinnitus and dizziness upon standing. In addition to this, the tsubos Ei-Fū 翳風 (TH-17) and Ten-Chū 天柱 (UB-10) are used when a person has been working too hard on the job with accumulated fatigue, and feels dizzy just after standing up.

The best way to press Kyō-In is to use the middle fingers to press as hard as one is able. This will cause the ears to ring, and as soon as this happens, knead this point as if drawing three small circles. Place your thumbs on Ei-Fū next and press so that it can be felt inside the ears. Ten-Chū should be pressed after this. The key point here is to place the thumbs on the tsubos and the four fingers on the side of the head to press firmly so that the force come to bear on only the thumbs. Inexperienced people often put strength in the four fingers instead of the thumbs, but this is not very effective.

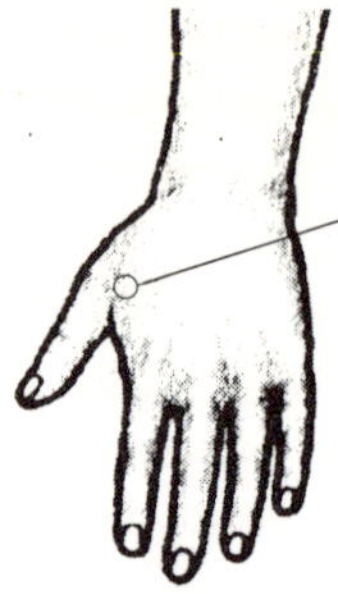

When the treatment is done correctly, dizziness upon standing should cease to occur. Finger pressure to Gō-Koku 合谷 (LI-4) may be added in the treatment for good measure.

H. Dazed feeling in head——Tsū-Ten 通天 (UB-7)

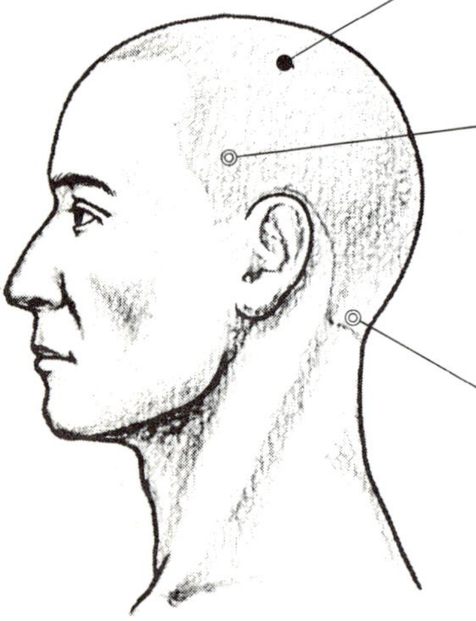

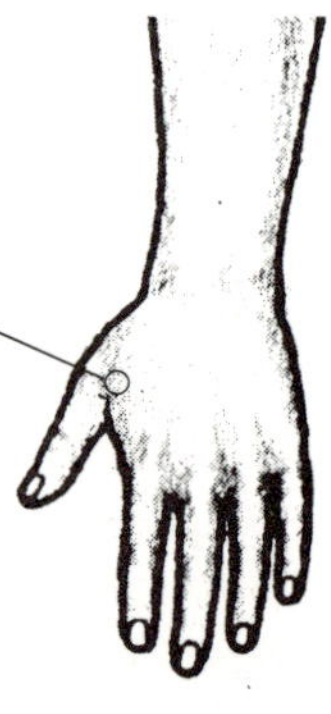

When a person goes without sleep for a while, the head begins to feel dazed and one begins to yawn uncontrollably. There may be no headache or sensation of heaviness in the head, but one does not want to think about anything, or to do anything. This is a state where one is sapped of motivation. Such a lack of drive may be caused by a variety of reasons, but quite often, it stems from overwork and exhaustion. In such cases, the best thing to do, of course, is to get plenty of sleep to rest one's body and mind. This, however, is not always possible when some important job needs to be done. For this reason, it is very convenient to keep in mind the specially effective tsubos which give a surprising amount of relief from symptoms of fatigue.

There is a tsubo called Tsū-Ten 通天 (UB-7) close to Hyaku-E 百会 (GV-20), which has already been mentioned repeatedly. The name *Tsū-Ten* (passing heaven) comes from the meridians, or channels of energy in the body, passing to the top of the head and circulating in the brain from this tsubo. In other words, Tsū-Ten is an exceptionally effective tsubo for all symptoms in the "heaven section." Locating tsubos like Hyaku-E and Tsū-Ten can be difficult because of the hair. When the head feels hazy, first locate Hyaku-E at the very top of the head, and then find the points two finger widths to either side of this. This is Tsū-Ten, and it is able to clear up the head to a surprising extent. In my experience, pressing tsubos like Hyaku-E and Tsū-Ten for people who complain of their head always feeling hazy and unclear, sometimes causes their scalp to dent in somewhat. In this way, Tsū-Ten can be quite dramatic in its effects for symptoms of the head.

When one's head is unclear, this is often accompanied with migraine headaches, and in this case, the tsubo Ken-Ro 懸顱 (GB-5) introduced earlier should also be pressed. When there is a sensation of heaviness in the head also, apply additional finger pressure on Ten-Chū 天柱 (UB-10). Also pressing Gō-Koku 合谷 (LI-4) just for good measure should provide even better results.

l. Lack of color in face——In-Dō 印堂 (extra tsubo)

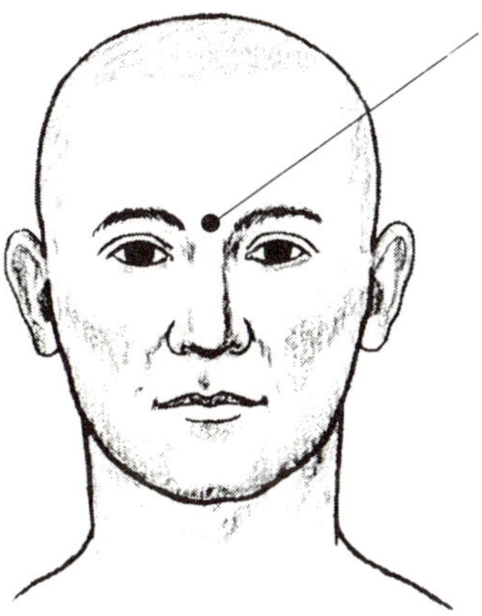

Sometimes even when we do not feel especially fatigued, people still say to us, "You look rather pale; is something the matter?" It is only obvious that for humans, the clearest sign of fatigue appears on the face. When fatigue builds up and a person is unaware of it, often when waking up in the morning, one will find that his body does not feel fully rested. When this is the case, the face lacks color and wrinkles and sags appear on the face. Fatigue causes the facial skin of women to become rough and their makeup does not go on as good as usual.

In this way, one's complexion can be called an indicator of one's physical and mental condition. It goes without saying that when one's face is lacking in color, restoring one's vitality by ample rest and relaxation should be the first priority. Finger pressure on the tsubo In-Dō 印堂 (extra tsubo), nevertheless, is very effective as a temporary measure. In-Dō is located right between both eyebrows. Figures of Buddha often have a mark on the forehead between the eyebrows. This can be thought of as the location of the tsubo In-Dō. The character *In* 印 means mark, and *Dō* 堂 means a house. In other words, In-Dō is a very important tsubo, just like the name plate on one's residence.

This tsubo is very easy to press. All you need to do is use your middle finger to firmly press this tsubo straight toward the center of your head. This will improve circulation and color will return to your face. Another tsubo which should not be

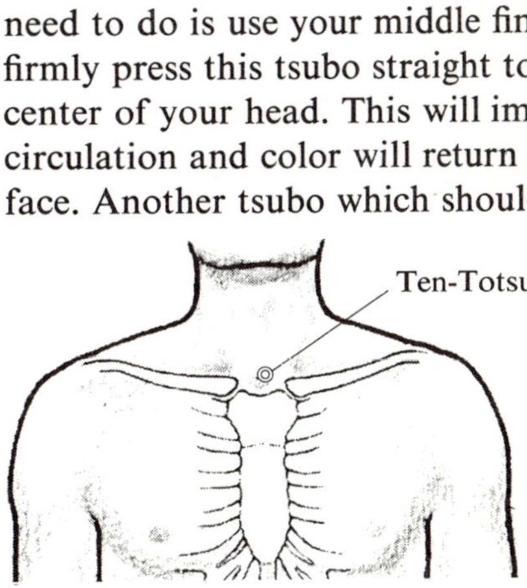

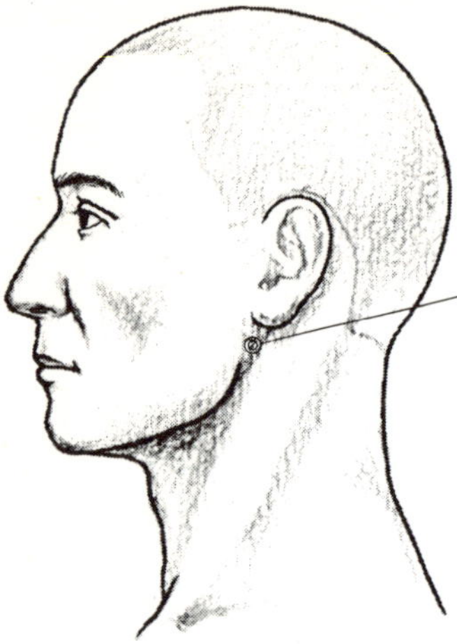

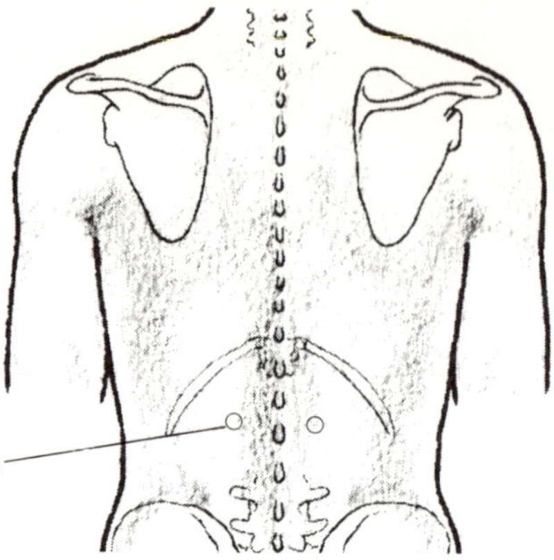

overlooked for improving your complexion is Ten-Totsu 天突 (CV-22) which is located directly below the Adam's apple on top of the sternum. To press Ten-Totsu, hook your index finger around the top of the sternum and press downward. Pressing the tsubo Ei-Fū 翳風 (TH-17) in addition to this should enhance the effect.

It is obvious that lack of color in the face is not just a problem in the face. This means that one's physical condition has deteriorated and that the skin over the entire body is lacking in color and luster. It is necessary that the proper functioning of the internal organs be restored so that nutrients are able to reach all parts of the body. For this purpose, applying finger pressure on the tsubo San-Shō-Yu 三焦俞 (UB-22), located to either side of the first lumbar vertebra is recommended.

J. Dry facial skin——Kan-Yu 肝俞 (UB-18)

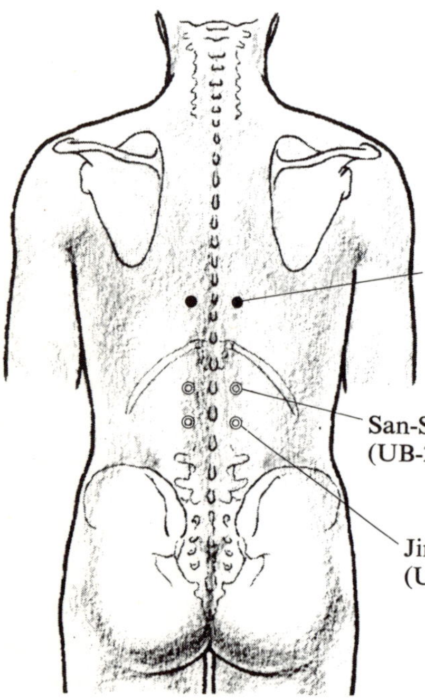

An old saying in Japan states that "the skin is the mirror (reflecting the condition) of the internal organs." It is true that when the functioning of the organs are impaired by fatigue, the effects appear immediately on the skin. The reason normal skin is slightly moist and shiny is because the amount of sweat and oils being excreted by the skin is at just the right level. Since the autonomic nerves controlling the excretion of sweat and body oils are connected with those nerves which control the internal organs, whenever a disfunction occurs in the internal organs, the excretion of body oils and sweat also becomes abnormal, and the skin loses its healthy shine.

The obvious thing to do to keep one's skin healthy and beautiful, therefore, is to improve one's physical condition. One of the best tsubos for improving one's overall physical condition is Kan-Yu 肝兪 (UB-18), located on both sides of the spine just below the level of the bottom of the shoulder blades. Even in modern medicine the liver is regarded as a vital organ which can affect one's overall physical condition for better or for worse. In Oriental medicine, special importance is attached to the liver as the place where one's soul resides. Kan-Yu is an important tsubo for checking the functional condition of the liver, as well as being very important for improving liver function when it becomes impaired.

The tsubos San-Shō-Yu 三焦兪 (UB-22) mentioned above and Jin-Yu 腎兪 (UB-23) just one finger width below can also be used along with Kan-Yu to improve one's overall physical condition. As already explained, San-Shō-Yu is a tsubo associated with the triple heater meridian which serves as the source of heat in the body. Jin-Yu has already been introduced as a vital tsubo of the kidney meridian where the basic energy acquired by birth, or the life force present in a person from birth, is stored. Kan-Yu is the main tsubo to be pressed for rough skin, and San-Shō-Yu and Jin-Yu are used as supplemental tsubos.

The tsubos on the back are generally hard to locate precisely for anyone except experts. Therefore, there is no need to worry too much about their exact location. As a more simple approach, just giving finger pressure along the spine from between the shoulder blades down to the hip bone serves to stimulate the three tsubos listed. Of course, this treatment is hard to do for yourself, so have someone press these tsubo for you. The key point in effectively treating these tsubo is to point the four fingers, aside from the thumb which is pressing the tsubo, up toward the head and to use these fingers to massage and relax the back muscles while pressing with the thumbs.

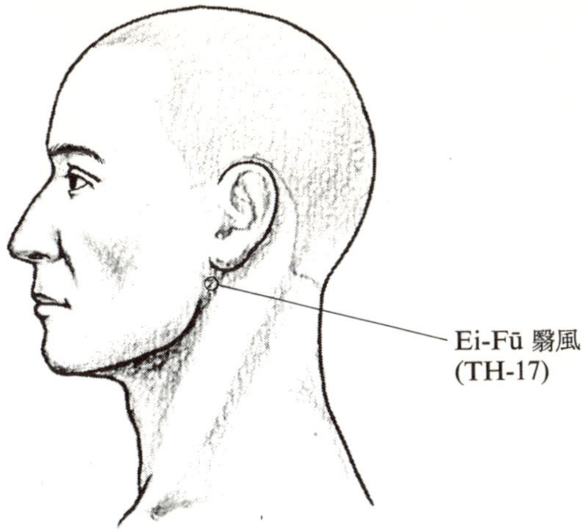

Finger pressure on the tsubo Ei-Fū 翳風 (TH-17) is also very effective in helping dry and rough skin.

K. Eczema on the face——Dai-Tsui 大椎 (GV-14)

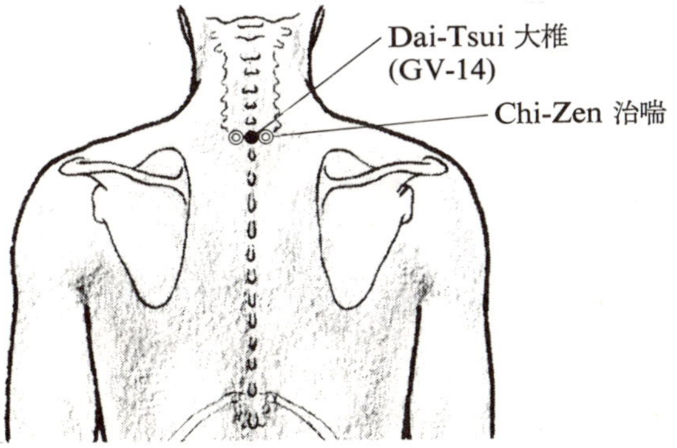

Pimples on the face are one sign of puberty and this is a relatively normal occurrence caused by temporary imbalances in hormone secretion, and there is no need for concern because it usually goes away by itself. There are people past their puberty, however, whose faces break out during the change of seasons, or when they become very fatigued. This is definitely the result of an allergic reaction. As already mentioned, those people with allergic conditions tend to get migraine headaches more easily, and fatigue is quite often manifested as skin allergies, or eczema. Since eczema is caused by an allergic condition, it is necessary that tsubos effective in changing the physical constitution of people be treated. The tsubo most effective for this purpose is Dai-Tsui 大椎 (GV-14) located at the bottom on the back of the neck. Have someone give finger pressure around the base of your neck at the back. There is a point around the top of the spine level with the top of the shoulders which feels tender with the slightest amount of pressure. This is the tsubo Dai-Tsui effective for allergic conditions. There is another tsubo half a finger width to the outside of Dai-Tsui called Chi-Zen 治喘. This tsubo is an extra point not among the traditional acupuncture points. Chi-Zen is a tsubo recently discovered in China and it is especially effective for asthma, just as its name, Chi-Zen (cure ashma) implies. Asthma is another condition caused by an allergic reaction. It can thus be understood how Chi-Zen is a remarkably effective tsubo for alleviating allergic conditions.

The treatment for such allergies should consist of finger pressure to Dai-Tsui and Chi-Zen. If there is no one around to give finger pressure treatments, one can place adhesive tape with metal grains (available in Japan) on the tsubos. There are some people in which this tape causes skin rashes, so instead of this, a person can get the adhesive tape of one's choice and tape a miniscule wad of tinfoil on these tsubo. Sometimes this will come off in a day or two, but you can simply put on another one. In addition to these measures, if possible, it is more effective when the tsubos Ken-Ryō 顴髎 (SI-18) and San-Chiku 攅竹 (UB-2) on the face are pressed. Both of these tsubos serve to improve the color and circulation in facial skin and muscles

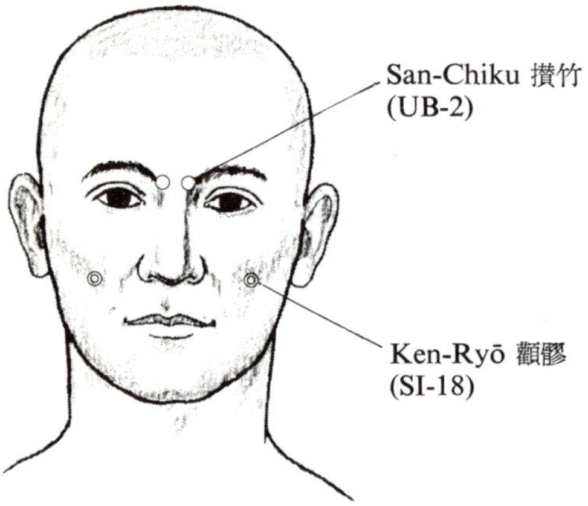

L. Freckles and facial blemishes——Shi-Haku 四白 (ST-2)

Freckles and facial blemishes often appear in girls especially after they reach puberty. There are many causes for the appearance of freckles such as the influence of ultraviolet light, pregnancy, gynecological disorders and impairment in the adrenal function. Also, at times, physical and mental overwork can cause the sudden appearance of freckles or facial blemishes. It is an obvious point, but facial skin receives the direct impact of the climate such as heat and cold and humidity. For

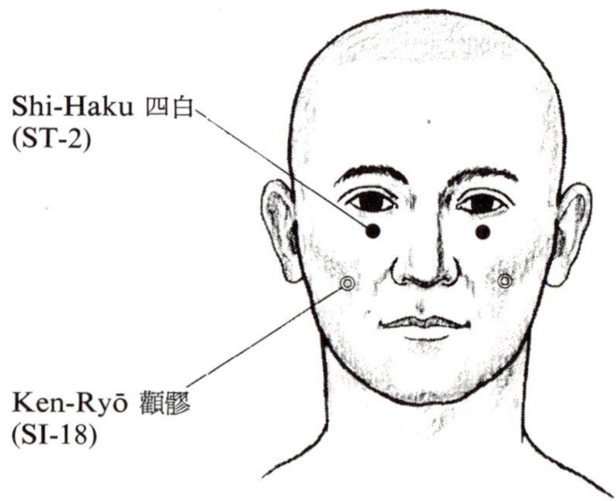

this reason, the circulation and nutrition in the facial skin becomes diminished more easily, and overwork aggravates this to cause freckles and blemishes. It is impossible to make freckles and blemishes go away immediately, even with tsubo therapy. Nevertheless, it is possible to alleviate these gradually when the right tsubos are treated.

Feeling just below the eyes, there is a bony ridge right beneath the skin. The tsubo Shi-Haku 四白 (ST-2) is located another one centimeter below this rim to either side of the nose. This is a place where freckles and facial blemishes appear most readily, and Shi-Haku also happens to be the most effective place to treat this condition. When freckles and blemishes become a cause for concern, press Shi-Haku very firmly, strong enough to where the pressure can be felt in the eyes. Freckles or facial blemishes resulting from overwork and stress can be cured by continuing this treatment patiently. When freckles and blemishes appear not only under the eyes, but all over the face, also apply pressure on the tsubo Ken-Ryō 顴髎 (SI-18) located below and slightly to the outside of the cheek bone. This is a very beneficial tsubo for women who wish to improve their appearance by increasing nutrition in the facial muscles and skin around their mouth.

Since freckles and blemishes appear most easily when a person is in poor physical condition, adding tsubos on the abdomen and lower back in the treatment makes it more well rounded. To do this, have someone press the tsubos Jin-Yu 腎兪 (UB-23) and Kō-Yu 肓兪 (KI-16). As mentioned before, Jin-Yu is an important tsubo for vitalizing one's life force. Kō-Yu located right next to the navel is also a tsubo which is said to "alleviate a kidney deficient condition" in Oriental medicine which, in other words, means that Kō-Yu is effective in restoring one's vitality.

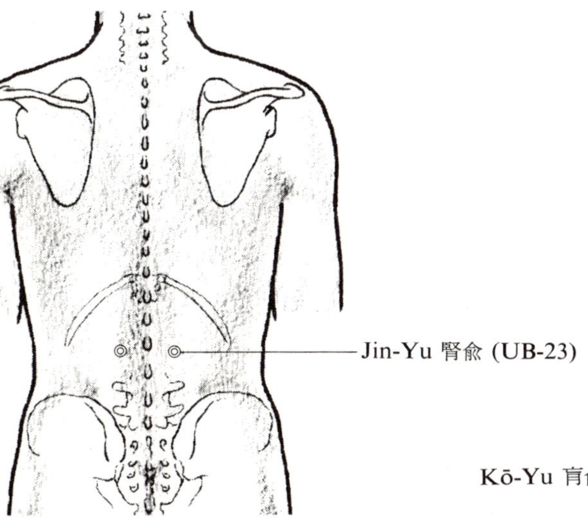

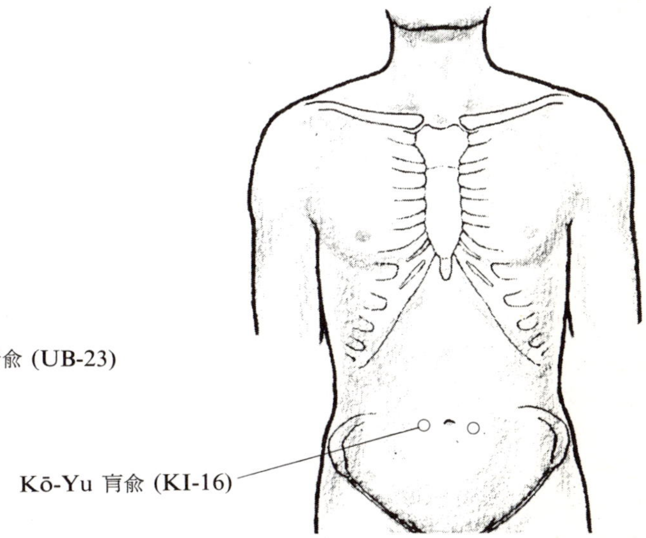

M. Face feeling hot and flushed——Kyaku-Shu-Jin 客主人 (GB-3)

Normally, when people become tired, their faces lose color and become pale, but there are people whose faces become flushed instead, as if they had been drinking alcohol. Whether a person's face is pale or flushed, these symptoms both result from the same root cause, which is an imbalance in the distribution of blood through the body. What happens is that, when these people get tired, their autonomic nervous system which controls blood circulation in facial skin becomes overactive, or otherwise underactive, to produce these states.

When your face becomes flushed, use your index fingers to press the tsubo located in front of the top of where the ear attaches to the head. You should feel a pulsation here. This tsubo is Kyaku-Shu-Jin 客主人 (GB-3), which is otherwise known as Jō-Kan 上関, and it is regarded as an important point for controlling blood circulation in the facial skin. Therefore, when lack of sleep or accumulated stress causes the face to become hot and flushed, the tsubo Kyaku-Shu-Jin should be treated. The best way to press this tsubo is to use the middle fingers and apply strong pressure so that it can be felt to the center of one's head. If this treatment is not sufficient, also apply pressure on Ken-Ryō 顴髎 (SI-18), discussed in the previous section, and Yō-Haku 陽白 (GB-14) which is located on the forehead. Yō-Haku is thought of as being located at the vertex of a right triangle with the eyebrow as its base. *Yō-Haku* 陽白 (yang white) is used often to treat facial neuralgia, but just as its name implies, it is known as being very effective for regulating blood circulation in the face and restoring normal facial color when a person has a flushed face.

There is another tsubo very efficacious for this purpose which can be treated easily any place and any time. This tsubo Rō-Kyū 労宮 (HC-8) is located in the palm of the hand between where the middle finger and ring finger touch when making a fist. The character *Rō* 労 means fatigue, and *Kyū* 宮 means a house or residence, so it is a place where fatigue resides or accumulates. Rō-Kyū is a vital tsubo which controls the

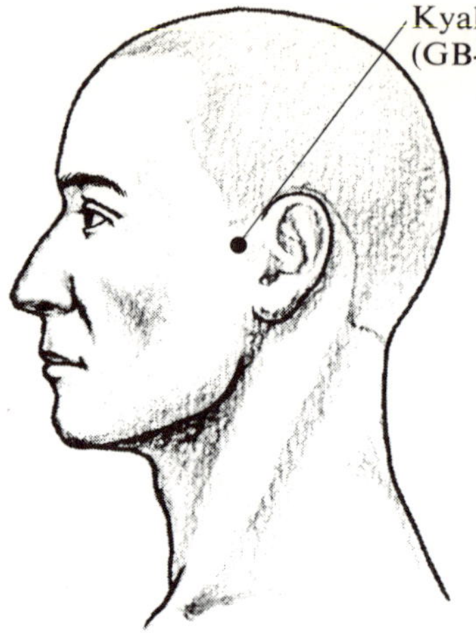

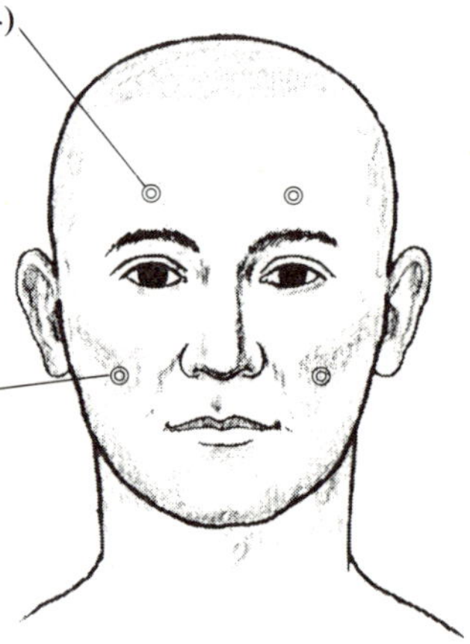

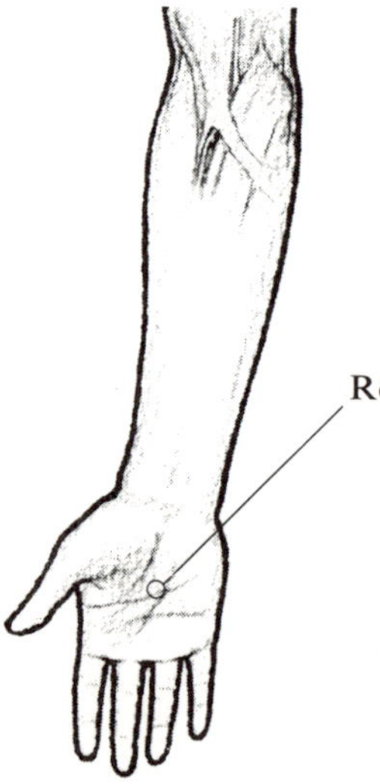

circulation of blood, especially above the base of the neck and in the face. In Oriental medicine this tsubo is designated as the place to treat symptoms of fatigue in the upper half of the body. Sometimes people find themselves massaging the palm of their hands without knowing it when they are tired, but this is an automatic response which is very appropriate from the standpoint of Oriental medicine.

IV. Face feeling drawn (facial paralysis)——Ei-Fū 翳風 (TH-17)

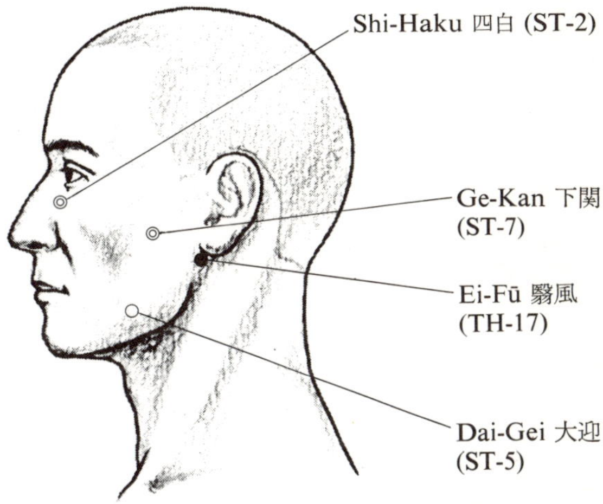

Facial skin differs slightly in its structure from other skin on the body in that the muscle tissue is intertwined with lower layers of the skin. The reason facial expressions such as laughing or crying can be made is because the skin of the face moves with the facial muscles which are controlled by the facial nerve. There are times when one's facial skin feels drawn and tight the morning after engaging in outdoor recreation in the winter, or after physical and mental strain has accumulated. Western medicine refers to this condition as Bell's palsy, or facial paralysis, while Oriental medicine refers to it as *Kō-Gan-Ka-Sha*. This condition occurs because the function of the facial nerve becomes overexcited and it is unable to properly control the movements of the facial muscles.

When this condition occurs, put your thumbs on the previously discussed tsubo, Ei-Fū 翳風 (TH-17), located right behind the earlobes, and press strongly toward the lower jaw. Ei-Fū is an important tsubo where the blood vessels going to the cranium branch off to supply the brain and the facial area respectively, and also, the facial nerve comes out from behind the ear at this point to go to the face. Ei-Fū has been used since times past as a special tsubo for tension in the face which comes from fatigue, and for trigeminal neuralgia which causes severe facial pain, and today, it is also used as a point for beauty massages.

Although the face may feel drawn and tight all over, the symptoms of facial paralysis do not usually appear over the whole face when paralysis occurs. Normally, the most apparent symptoms are around the eyes, the cheeks or the mouth. When tension in facial skin is mostly around the eyes, in addition to treating Ei-Fū, use Shi-Haku 四白 (ST-2); when the tension is between the cheeks and the ears also use Ge-Kan 下関 (ST-7) below the cheek bone, and when the tension is around the mouth also use Dai-Gei 大迎 (ST-5) which is over the base of the second molar.

Even better results may be obtained for facial paralysis by looking into the mirror and making all sorts of expressions such as crying, laughing, or that of anger. This serves to exercise various facial muscles. This exercise in addition to the above treatments should return the face to normal in a short period of time. The important point is to continue these treatments patiently until the symptoms disappear completely.

O. Swelling of face (facial dropsy)——Ken-Ryō 顴髎 (SI-18)

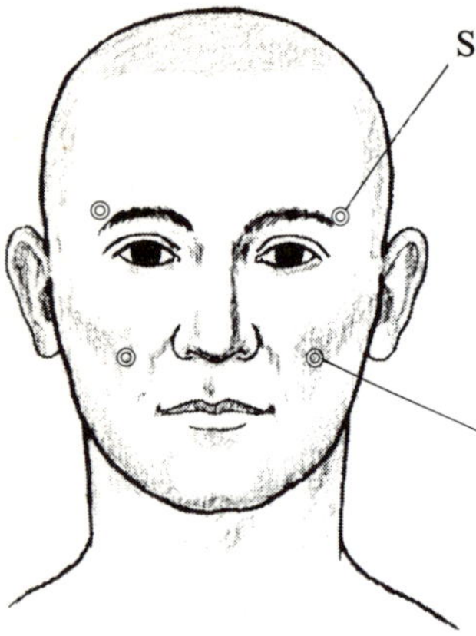

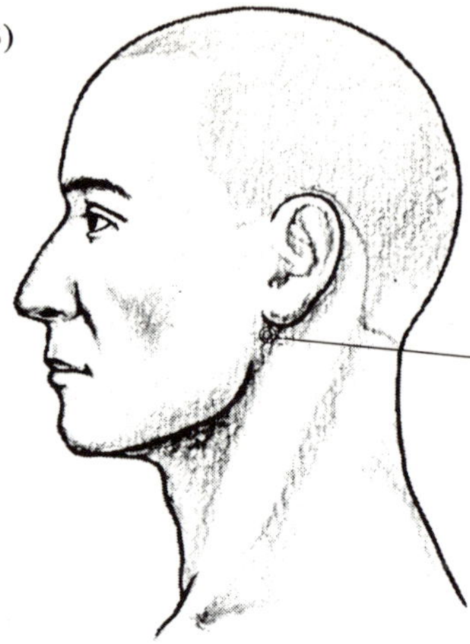

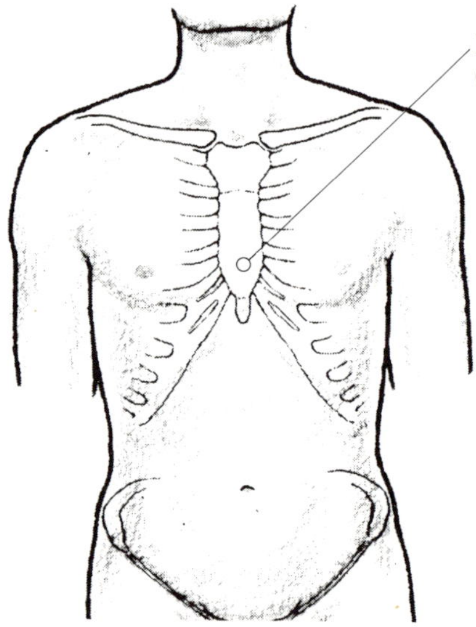

There are cases where a person's face becomes swollen and rounded like the full moon when steroids (a drug to stop pain in joints) are taken over a long period. This symptom is commonly referred to as "moon face," and this type of facial dropsy due to serious causes must be treated by medical specialists. Even among healthy individuals, however, there are people whose faces seem to become swollen and flushed the morning after having been exhausted by such things as working a long day at a desk.

As explained in the previous section, the facial nerve controls the facial muscles. Swelling occurs with mental and physical fatigue by the facial muscles and skin losing their tone and becoming loose due to a disfunction of the facial nerve. Swelling of the face is caused most often by fatigue, and generally, it is most pronounced around the cheeks. For this condition, treat the tsubo Ken-Ryō 顴髎 (SI-18) which was introduced before. The swelling in the face should gradually subside when this tsubo is pressed firmly toward the center of the face using the middle fingers.

There are cases where swelling occurs around the eyes and the eyes seem slightly feverish. In this case, also press the tsubo Ei-Fū 翳風 (TH-17) and Shi-Chiku-Kū 絲竹空 (TH-23) which is just to the outside of the eyebrows. Shi-Chiku-Kū is often used for facial paralysis, spasms and trigeminal neuralgia, but it also has a notable effect in relieving swelling of the face caused by fatigue, especially that around the eyes.

Another tsubo that may be pressed with good results for swelling in the face stemming from fatigue is Dan-Chū 膻中 (CV-17) which is in the center of the sternum, right between the two nipples. Dan-Chū is a vital tsubo located right over the heart which controls circulation throughout the whole body. The area around this tsubo is designated as a "Head's zone," after the English physiologist Sir Henry Head. In Oriental medicine this same area is used to provide treatments for pains resulting from heart problems, and also for a general lack of vitality. Light stimulation to these points improves the circulation in the face and alleviates swelling in the face.

P. Face feeling hot with chilling of feet——San-Shō-Yu 三焦兪 (UB-22)

Put this book down for a moment and feel your forehead and then your feet. If the temperature of your forehead, feet and hands are about the same, you can be considered as being healthy. There are times, however, when only the tips of the toes feel as cold as ice. This is a sign that fatigue has accumulated, and that one's physical condition has deteriorated.

The symptom of the face being flushed has already been discussed in a previous section, but it may be stated with certainty that usually, when the face feels flushed and hot, the feet in contrast become chilled. This is called a "top hot and bottom cold condition" in Oriental medicine. As you may well know, the body temperature of warm blooded animals including human beings is constantly maintained at 37 degrees centigrade. The circulatory system of our body can be divided roughly into the peripheral circulation which flows right beneath the skin, and the visceral circulation which supplies the cranial, thoracic and abdominal areas. Warm blooded animals have thus acquired the ability to automatically regulate their circulation and to adjust the body temperature to whatever environment they are in. Therefore, the "top hot bottom cold condition" means that the circulatory system is not functioning as it should.

The first thing that must be done when the face becomes flushed and hot, and the feet are chilled, is to send the chilled blood of the feet up to the head. The specially effective tsubo for this purpose is San-Shō-

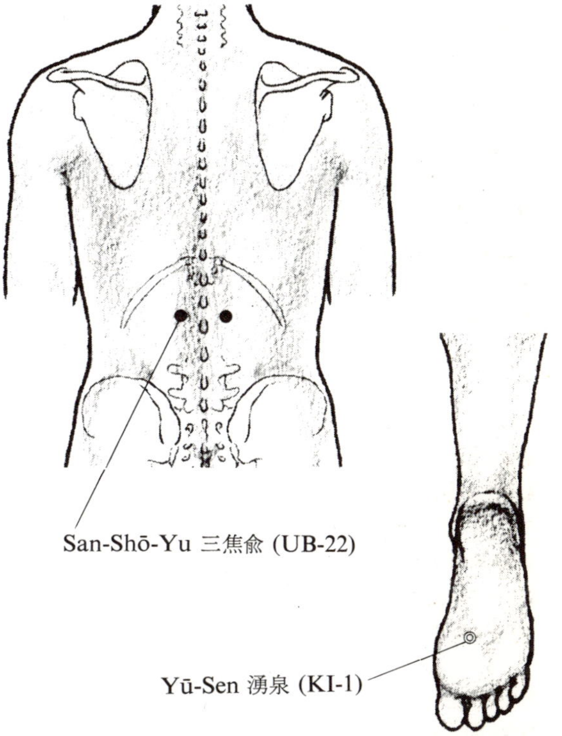

Yu 三焦兪 (UB-22) which has already been introduced, and this tsubo has to be pressed thoroughly to be effective. In Oriental medicine the human body is regarded as being a self contained cosmos containing parts corresponding to "heaven, man and earth" (top, middle, and bottom sections). The tsubo San-Shō-Yu is regarded as an important tsubo which regulates the distribution of heat (blood circulation) through this "heaven, man and earth" union of our body.

In addition to pressing San-Shō-Yu, also give thorough thumb pressure to Yū-Sen 湧泉 (KI-1) in the sole of the foot, as well

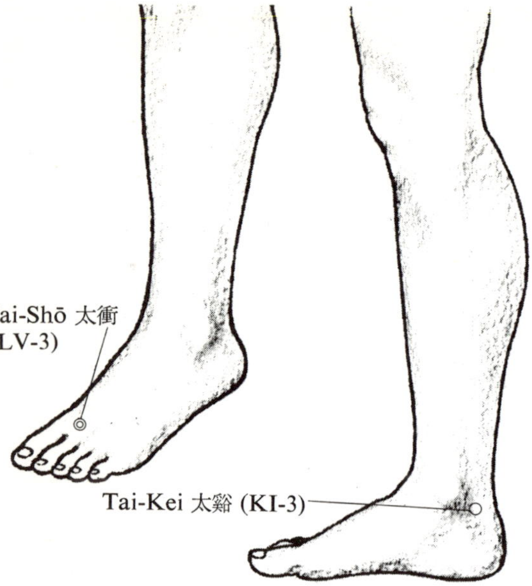

as to Tai-Shō 太衝 (LV-3) which is on the back of the foot at the highest point in the web between the big toe and the second toe. Both these tsubos are regarded as being effective against blood rising to the head, and pressure on these tsubos alone is often enough to bring relief from chilled feet and feverishness in the face. As explained before, the name *Yū-Sen* means a spring where life force wells up. Therefore, shiatsu on this tsubo is effective in preventing a general loss of vitality.

Also, there is a tsubo called Tai-Kei 太谿 (KI-3) behind the inner ankle bone. If possible, this tsubo too should be pressed quite strongly because it gives good results in relieving chilling of the extremities in general.

2. Treating Symptoms of the Eyes, Ears, Nose and Mouth

A. Bloodshot eyes——Sei-Mei 睛明 (UB-1)

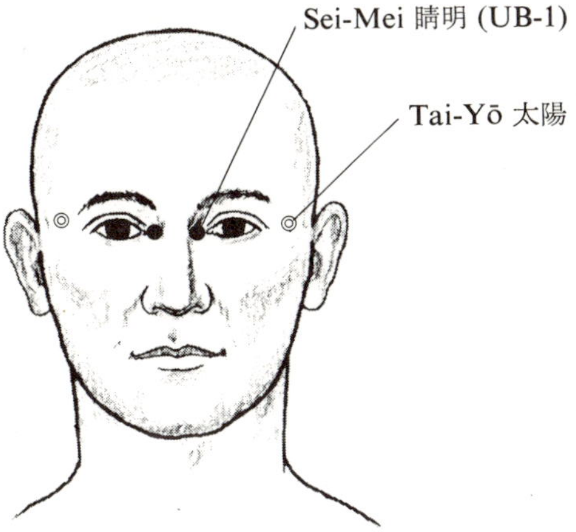

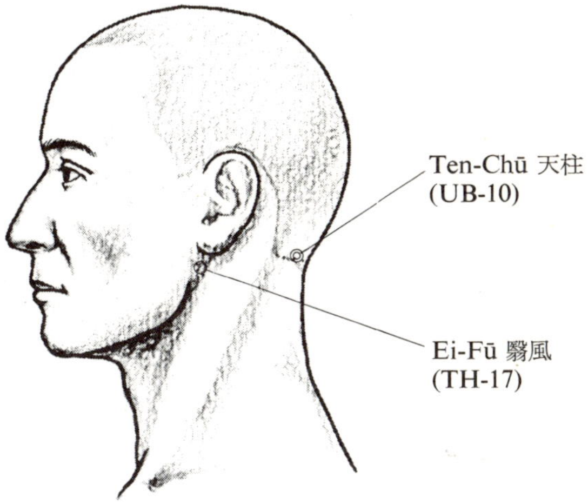

Everyone gets bloodshot eyes now and then after staying up late in the night reading a book, or playing an all-night poker game. There are two mucous membranes which cover the eyes; they are the palpebral conjunctiva on the back of the eylids, and bulbar conjunctiva which cover the eyeballs. Fatigue in the eyes first appears as congestion in the blood vessels of the conjunctiva. The best way to prevent eye fatigue is obviously to avoid staying up late, and to faithfully follow the dictum "early to bed and early to rise." In the busy pace of today's society, however, this type of lifestyle is not always possible. For this reason the method for relieving tired and bloodshot eyes is presented here.

As the first tsubo to remove congestion in the eyes, there is Sei-Mei 睛明 (UB-1) which is located on the bone to the inside corner of the eyes. As the name *Sei-Mei* (clear light) implies, it is a tsubo which restores clarity and brightness to the eyes. When your eyes are congested and bloodshot, use your index fingers to press these points, then move these fingers back and forth slightly and this will make the eyes much clearer and will add a sparkle to them.

Often when our eyes become tired after reading or watching television, we find ourselves pressing the area between the inside corner of the eyes and the bridge of the nose without knowing it. This is because people instinctively know the tsubo for relieving tired eyes. Bloodshot eyes can also be relieved faster by slowly pressing around the rim of the bone surrounding the eyes on both the upper and lower sides starting at Sei-Mei. Another tsubo that can be recommended for relieving bloodshot eyes is the tsubo Tai-Yō 太陽 (extra tsubo), to the back of the point between the outer corner of the eye and the eyebrow. A small hollow point can be located by pressing slightly to the outside of the point between Shi-Chiku-Kū 絲竹空 (TH-23), a tsubo discussed before, and Dō-Shi-Ryō 瞳子髎 (GB-1) on the outer corner of the eyes. Finger pressure should be applied on these points by pressing them together from both sides. Tai-Yō is a tsubo recently discovered in China. It has quite a remarkable effect in relieving fatigue in the eyes and eyestrain.

When the above treatments are not completely effective in curing the bloodshot eyes, give thumb pressure with a kneading action on Ten-Chū 天柱 (UB-10), pushing upward toward Hyaku-E 百会 (GV-20). Ten-Chū has long been known for its effectiveness in helping eye conditions, and it is used in acupuncture to cure bloodshot eyes. Pressure to Ei-Fū 翳風 (TH-17) is also effective for this same purpose.

B. Excessive tears and mucus from eyes——Shō-Kyū 承泣 (ST-1)

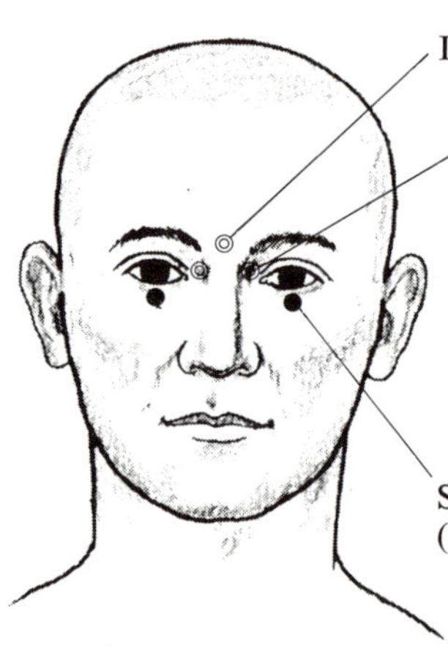

As explained in the previous section, fatigue in the eyes first appears as congestion in the eyes, but when a person continues to stay up late and lose sleep to accumulate fatigue, tears start to come to one's eyes when one is not even sad, and also mucus from the eyes increases substantially. It may be assumed, especially when mucus comes out of the eyes, that such a person is very fatigued. When a middle-aged person has a discharge of mucus from the eyes in the morning, and also the person's head is not clear just after waking up, it is proof that the person has high blood pressure stemming from fatigue. Such symptoms can also be alleviated by doing simple tsubo treatments in the morning, and this will make the discharge of tears and mucus stop and the eyes will clear up.

The tsubo used to help this condition is Shō-Kyū 承泣 (ST-1) located right under the eyes. There is a place directly under the pupils on the rim of the bone around the eyes, which when pressed firmly toward the back, causes a sensation to run from the middle of the eyes to the cheeks. The point where this pain is produced is the location of Shō-Kyū. The name of this tsubo means the place where crying is received, and this indicates that Shō-Kyū is to be used when excessive tears become a problem. Just pressing this tsubo with the index fingers, amazingly enough, causes the discharge of tears and mucus to cease. When the discharge is excessive, the supplemental use of the tsubo Sei-Mei 睛明 (UB-1) discussed in the last section is recommended. Sei-Mei is used quite often as the tsubo effective for all symptoms of the eyes. Furthermore, even better results are possible by using the tsubo called In-Dō 印堂 (extra tsubo).

This may be off the subject, but Sei-Mei is also used to treat children's convulsions and tantrums. *Kan-no-Mushi*, or convulsive fits in children are where young children become hypersensitive and irritable so that the slightest thing makes them unhappy, or starts them crying or throwing a tantrum. This type of behavior can be remedied through acupuncture and shiatsu. Of course, a specialist must be consulted for acupuncture, but shiatsu can be performed in one's own home. Therefore, even if a baby goes into a crying fit, just give finger pressure on Sei-Mei. Pressing this point lightly is usually sufficient to give good results for babies.

C. Dryness of eyes——Sei-Mei 睛明 (UB-1)

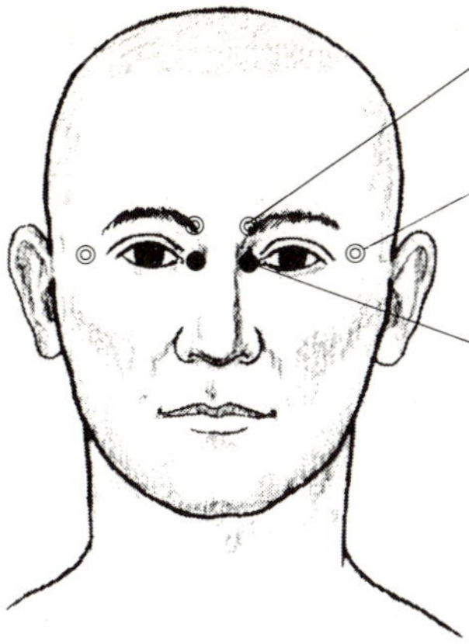

Usually when a person becomes fatigued, there tends to be more tears or mucus from the eyes, but there are people whose eyes become dry instead. The excretion of tears becomes abnormally low, and other symptoms appear such as the core of the eyes feeling sore. Pressing the tsubo Sei-Mei 睛明 (UB-1), beneficial for all symptoms of the eyes, is the most effective treatment in this case also.

The point which differs from treating a person for excessive tears or mucus, is that in this case, the tsubo is not to be pressed very hard. Even better results are possible when the tsubos Dō-Shi-Ryō 瞳子髎 (GB-1), in the hollow place behind the outer corner of the eye, and San-Chiku 攅竹 (UB-2), just to the inside of the eyebrows, are added in the treatment around the eyes.

The way to give shiatsu treatment around the eyes is to use the index and middle fingers to gently massage the upper and lower eyelids, beginning at Sei-Mei and working toward Dō-Shi-Ryō. After this apply finger pressure gradually on the edge of the bone around the eyes, working above and below from Sei-Mei to Dō-Shi-Ryō. The following three points need special attention when treating areas around the eyes; (1) Be careful not to apply direct pressure on the eyeballs, (2) direct the force of the finger pressure against the bone, and (3) increase pressure gradually instead of pressing hard all at once.

For giving finger pressure around the eyes, it is best to use the thumbs when pressing points above the eyes, and to use the index and middle fingers when pressing below the eyes. Finish treatments around the eyes by slowly pressing along the eyebrows from San-Chiku to Shi-Chiku-Kū 絲竹空 (TH-23) on the outside of the eyebrows. Treating the entire area around the eyes and covering many tsubos adds to the effect. Dryness of the eyes is relieved even faster when finger pressure is given to Ten-Chū 天柱 (UB-10) also.

In passing, it may be noted that growing numbers of women seem to be suffering from trigeminal neuralgia during puberty or after their menopause. The trigeminal nerve is a sensory nerve of the face which receives the sensations of pain and heat and cold. When this nerve is adversely affected, symptoms appear such as a sharp pain in the forehead and cheeks, congestion in the eyes, and copious tears. Pressing the tsubo San-Chiku slowly and firmly in three to five second intervals is effective for trigeminal neuraligia, and the pain gradually subsides.

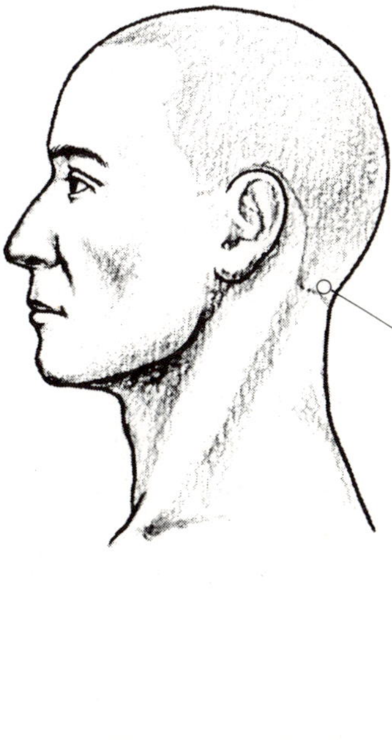

D. Dark rings under the eyes——Jin-Yu 腎兪 (UB-23)

Many middle-aged women come to my clinic saying words like the following, "I have problems with dark rings which form under my eyes in the afternoon. What can I do about it?" It is true that one of the common symptoms of fatigue among middle-aged women is rings under their eyes. No matter how carefully these ladies put on their makeup, by the time evening comes, they start looking haggardly with dark marks forming below their eyes.

One people get beyond their middle years, their muscles tend to lose tone and resiliency. As explained before, the facial muscles and skin are interwoven, so when facial muscles begin to droop with fatigue, the skin also sags to form what appears to be rings under the eyes. The best way to alleviate this problem is to maintain the body in a state where it never gets fatigued, and to work to rejuvenate facial muscles and improve the nutrition to the skin. Sleep is the most important thing for this. The tsubo specially effective for helping a person get good sleep is Jin-Yu 腎兪 (UB-23), which was introduced before. The muscles on both sides of the lumbar vertebrae in the area of this tsubo feel stiff and sore with the slightest pressure when a person is in a fatigued condition, and this is true also for women when they have lumbago, menstrual irregularity, or chilling of their feet. Therefore, the best thing to do when you have dark rings under your eyes is to ask someone you know to apply firm pressure on Jin-Yu so that you can sleep well and overcome fatigue.

Even greater benefits can be derived by receiving finger pressure on San-Shō-Yu 三焦兪 (UB-22), just above Jin-Yu, and on Kaku-Yu 膈兪 (UB-17), to either side of the spine almost level with the bottom of the shoulder blades. Explanations concerning San-Shō-Yu will be deleted since it was covered earlier. As for Kaku-Yu, it is a tsubo often used to adjust imbalances in physiological functions such as circulation and digestion and absorption.

Rings under the eyes is a symptom which causes a great deal of concern in women, so they tend to ask for a tsubo which is more efficacious. Generally, the place where rings form under the eyes most readily is right where the tsubo Shi-Haku 四白 (ST-2) is. Pressing Shi-Haku with the middle fingers and lightly massaging around this tsubo is usually quite effective for rings under the eyes.

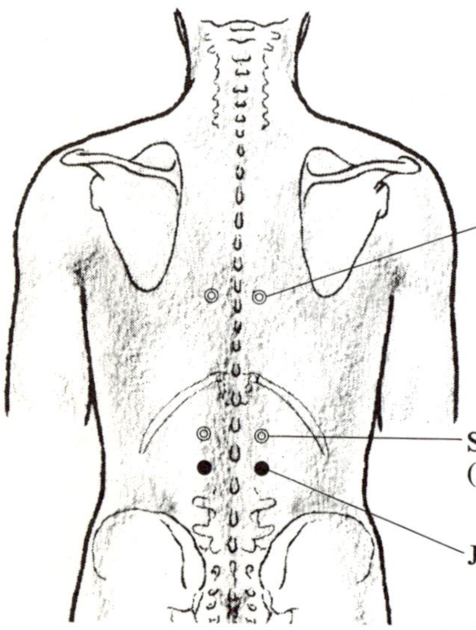

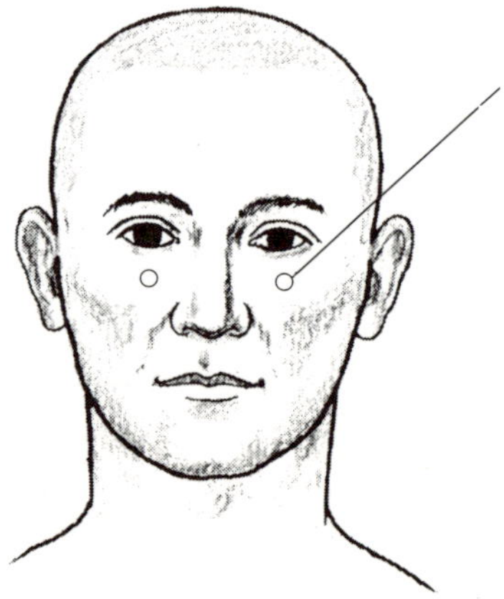

E. Glaring in eyes——Sei-Mei 睛明 (UB-1)

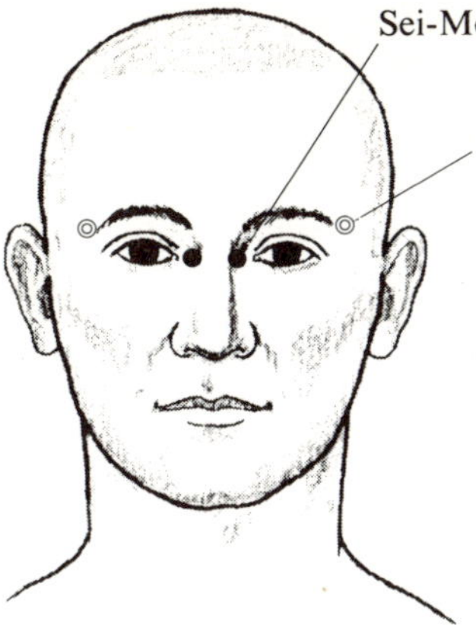

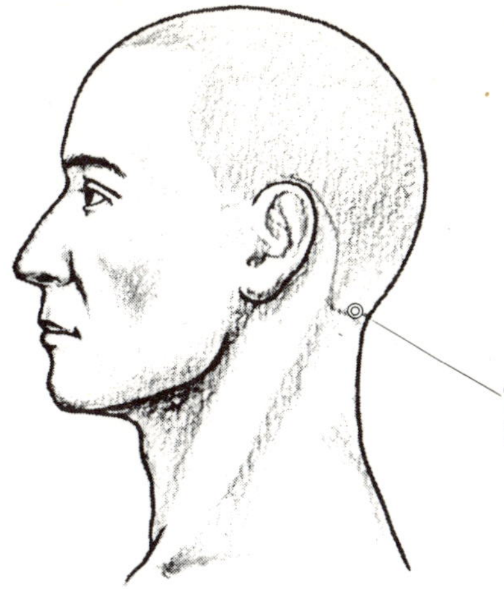

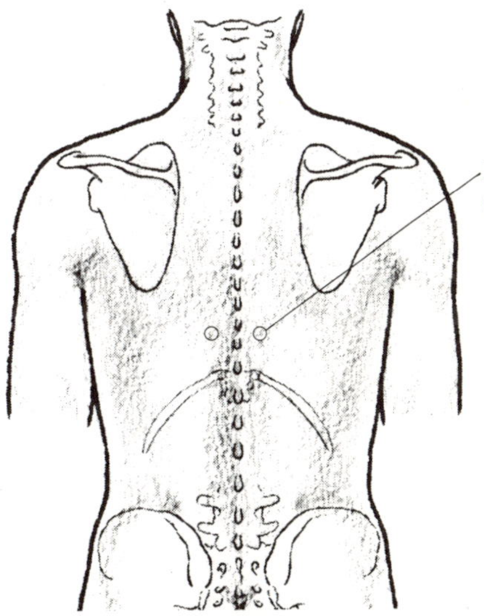

Most everyone has experienced situations where sunlight, or an electric light seems unusually bright. This is another symptom which tends to appear when a person's physical condition has deteriorated. Generally speaking, the deterioration of one's physical condition begins with weakening vision and progresses to one's teeth and ears, to finally affect one's sexual performance. The fact that aging starts with the weakening of one's eyesight, and progresses from teeth problems to a decline in sexual drive, indicates that fatigue affects the body more profoundly as one ages.

An unnatural amount of glaring in the eyes happens to be one of the symptoms of eyestrain which originates from general fatigue in the body. For this reason, the tsubo Sei-Mei 睛明 (UB-1), already listed as being effective for bloodshot eyes, as well as for excessive tears and mucus, is used in tsubo therapy. The way to go about this treatment is to first press Sei-Mei thoroughly and then to press the rim of the bone above the eyes to Dō-Shi-Ryō 瞳子髎 (GB-1). Next, press Shi-Chiku-Kū 絲竹空 (TH-23) rather strongly, and finish by giving strong pressure to Ten-Chū 天柱 (UB-10) from behind. This will relieve fatigue in the eyes and bring a surprising amount of relief from glaring in the eyes.

There is another tsubo called Kan-Yu 肝兪 (UB-18), on either side of the spine around the middle of the back, which is amazingly effective for symptoms of the eyes. It may seem strange that a tsubo on the back is used to treat symptoms of the eyes. This tsubo is used because there is a unique theory in Oriental medicine which holds that "the liver controls the tendons and opens to the eyes." This perspective is not so far fetched, even from the standpoint of Western medicine. As evidence for this, when liver conditions such as hepatitis of liver cirrhosis occur, jaundice appears in the whites of the eyes. Therefore, abnormalities in the liver do show up in the eyes. In Oriental medicine the liver is also regarded as being the main organ controlling the muscles and tendons in the body. This is why the tsubo Kan-Yu, known to regulate the function of the liver, is recommended when the body is fatigued. Therefore, stimulation should be given to Kan-Yu whenever visible signs of fatigue exist.

F. Eyes feeling tired (eyestrain)——San-Chiku 攅竹 (UB-2)

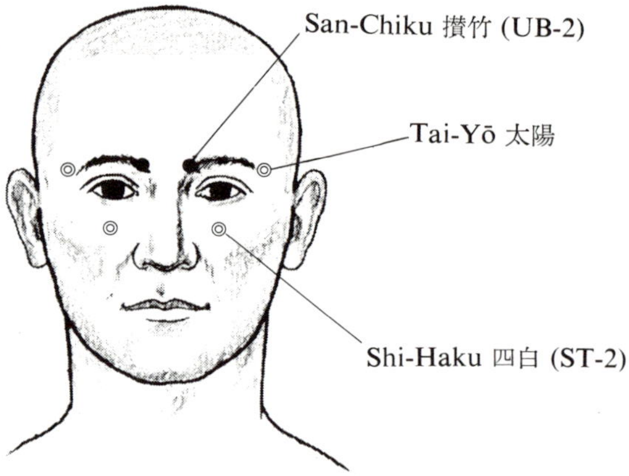

Various symptoms of fatigue appearing in and around the eyes have already been discussed; eyestrain, or the eyes feeling tired is another one. This symptom rarely occurs by itself. There are times when we find ourselves rubbing our eyes while talking to somebody. This is because our eyes feel tired and uncomfortable. At these times, there are usually other symptoms such as excess tears or mucus from the eyes, glaring in the eyes, pain deep in the eyes, heaviness over the head, tension from the back of the head down the neck, or a general feeling of weariness. Nevertheless, sometimes the symptom of discomfort in the eyes is the most prominent symptom, so the means of alleviating this symptom will be discussed.

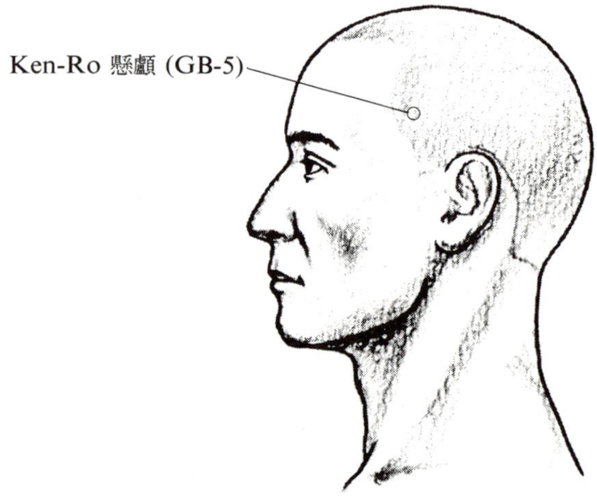

The character *San* 攅 of the tsubo San-Chiku 攅竹 (UB-2) means to gather or collect, and *Chiku* 竹 refers to a bamboo cane. This name came from San-Chiku being a place where harmful energy collects, as well as this tsubo being very effective for serious eye diseases which impair vision to a point where a person needs a bamboo cane to get around. To relieve the feeling of fatigue in the muscles surrounding the eyes, also use the tsubos Shi-Haku 四白 (ST-2) right under the eyes, and Tai-Yō 太陽 (extra tsubo) which is behind the point between Shi-Chiku-Kū 絲竹空 (TH-23) and Dō-Shi-Ryō 瞳子髎 (GB-1). Adding Ken-Ro 懸顱 (GB-5) in this treatment should give even better results.

Each of these tsubos can be pressed individually with the fingers, but it is usually more effective to give finger pressure and massage along the line connecting these tsubos. To treat the above symptom, begin by pressing slowly along the eyebrows from

San-Chiku toward Tai-Yō. Next, press along the rim of the bone around the eyes. Then give pressure to Ken-Ro and finish by lightly massaging the upper and lower eyelids. The important thing in this treatment is not to press very hard, but to massage lightly as if stroking the area. The effect is minimal when too much force is used and there is no benefit in exerting pressure on the eyeballs.

G. Poor eyesight——Moku-Sō 目窓 (GB-16)

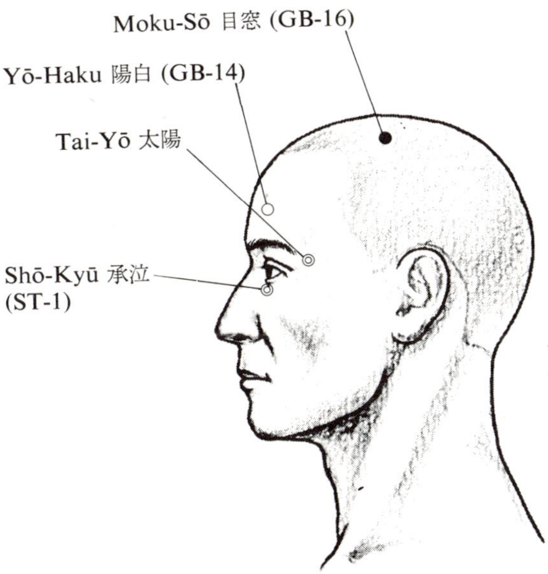

A person's eyesight generally gets worse as a results of serious eye diseases such as congestive glaucoma and uveitis, or otherwise, by eyestrain coming from overwork. The deterioration of vision which comes with serious diseases is usually accompanied by headaches or severe pain in the eyes. When such symptoms are present, the first thing necessary is to seek treatment from an eye specialist. If, however, there are no symptoms of pain in the eyes or headaches, and just the vision seems to have become blurred, it can be regarded as a symptom of eyestrain.

There is an old saying in Japan that "eating eels with eight eyes sharpens one's vision." This was probably thought to be good for the eyes because the eel had eight eyes. Nevertheless, this may not be entirely superstition even from a medical standpoint. Eels are eaten in great quantity in Japan during the summer season because this is believed to keep one from succumbing to the summer heat. The eel is, in fact, a very nutritious food ideal for overcoming fatigue. The approach in tsubo therapy is similar to this in that first the tsubos for relieving fatigue are treated to help the eyes.

The most effective tsubo for this purpose is Moku-Sō 目窓 (GB-16) which is on a line extending straight above the pupil of the eyes and four centimeters above the hairline. The name Moku-Sō means the "window of the eyes," and it is a well-known tsubo and a favorite since the old days for treating symptoms such as deteriorating vision and blurring vision. Pressing Moku-Sō strongly with the thumbs or index fingers should serve to clear up a person's vision. Additionally; treating the tsubos Shō-Kyū 承泣 (ST-1), Tai-Yō 太陽 (extra tsubo) and Yō-Haku 陽白 (GB-14), which have all been introduced before, should give even better results.

In these treatments, just giving finger pressure on individual tsubos is usually effective. More thorough finger pressure around the eyes, however, is recommended beginning at Sei-Mei 睛明 (UB-1) and working toward Tai-Yō around the top rim of the eyes, followed by that on the bottom rim passing Shō-Kyū and going to Tai-Yō. Fatigue in the eyes is quite often disregarded, but since it can affect one's overall physical condition, it is a good idea to treat such symptoms as soon as possible.

H. Swelling around the eyes——San-Chiku 攢竹 (UB-2)

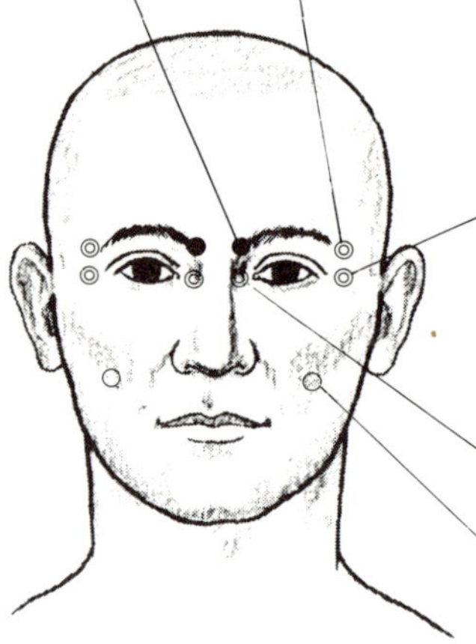

The eyelids tend to become swollen when sties or tarsal cysts form over the eyes. In such cases, there is also a throbbing pain around the eyes, or otherwise, there is discomfort even when the pain is minimal. If the area around the eyes is puffy and swollen without any pain or discomfort, it may be regarded that fatigue is showing up around the eyes.

Why is it that the area around the eyes sometimes becomes swollen when a person is fatigued? Try pinching up the skin of your arms or stomach. You can see how the skin and muscle are clearly separate. However, as explained many times before, in the face alone the skin and muscle tissues are intertwined. Therefore the tension of the facial muscles appears directly on the skin. The area around the eyes sometimes appears swollen because the muscles around the eyes become lose their tone with fatigue. For this reason, the treatment in this case should also concentrate on relieving the fatigue in the muscles around the eyes.

The truth of the matter is, it is very hard to select one single tsubo which is specially effective for swelling around the eyes. If one were to be named anyway, it would be San-Chiku 攢竹 (UB-2) which has been known from times past as a tsubo for curing swollen eyes. There are people who massage above their eyes with their fingers, but it is actually more effective to give firm pressure to San-Chiku using both thumbs. In this case also, instead of pressing San-Chiku only, apply massage and finger pressure between the various tsubos.

Since ways to do this have been discussed before, this will not be explained again, but do not forget to give finger pressure and massage to the top of the eyes from San-Chiku to Shi-Chiku-Kū 絲竹空 (TH-23), and on the bottom of the eyes from Sei-Mei 睛明 (UB-1) to Dō-Shi-Ryō 瞳子髎 (GB-1). In situations where the swelling extends down to the cheeks, also press the tsubo Ken-Ryō 顴髎 (SI-18) which is located slightly below and to the outside of the highest point of the cheek bone.

I. Dulling of sense of smell——Ko-Ryō 巨髎 (ST-3)

When people become fatigued and their physical condition deteriorates, their vision and hearing are weakened, and also, as another symptom of fatigue peoples' sense of smell become dulled and they lose the ability to smell things. The mechanism by which we are able to smell things depends on microscopic particles from the substances giving off smells entering our nostrils with respiration and stimulating olfactory cells deep in our nasal cavity.

The most common problem is where the

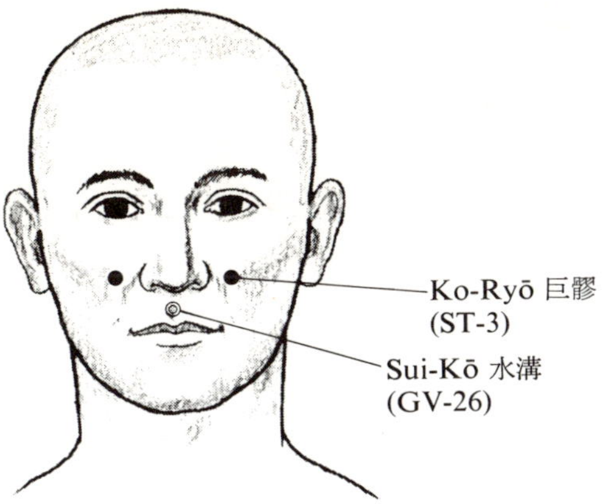

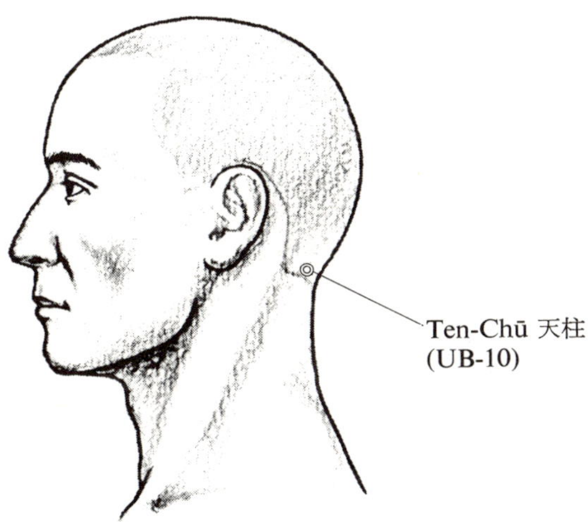

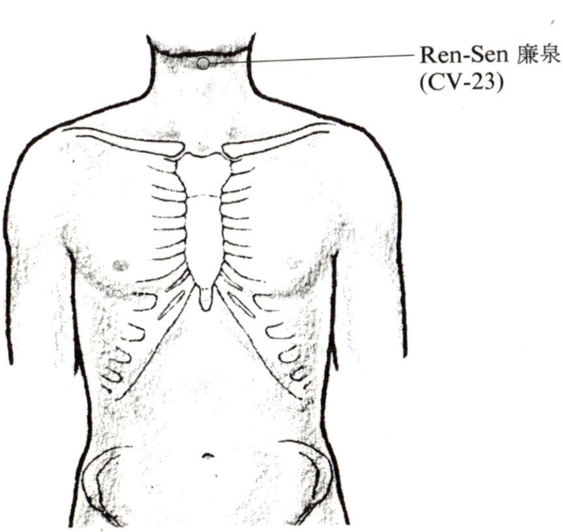

particles carrying the smell are unable to reach the olfactory cells. This occurs in diseases such as allergic rhinitis (inflammation of the mucous membrane of the nose), but the condition experienced most commonly is nasal obstruction accompanying a cold. The second most common cause for loss of smell is the disfunction of the olfactory cells, and this occurs with inflammation of the nasal tract by colds, or otherwise with mental and physical overwork. The tsubo most important in the latter case is Ko-Ryō 巨髎 (ST-3) which is located to either side of the nose.

The line or furrow going from the nose to the corner of the month is called the nasolabial sulcus in Western medicine. This is called *Ko-Bun* in Oriental medicine. The character *Ryō* 髎 means the edge of a bone. Ko-Ryō was thus named because it is just to the side of the furrow below the nose. This tsubo has been known since the olden days as being effective for symptoms in the nose. When this tsubo is pressed firmly, there is a penetrating sensation which goes to the nose, and amazingly enough, one's sense of smell will be sharpened after this.

In addition, give pressure to Sui-Kō 水溝 (GV-26), the tsubo right in the middle of the groove at the median line of the upper lip (philtrum), and also to Ten-Chū 天柱 (UB-10) on the back of the neck. Both of these tsubos are effective for symptoms of the nose, and they are naturally also effective for any impairment in the function of the olfactory cells. There is another tsubo right above the Adam's apple called Ren-Sen 廉泉 (CV-23) which should also be pressed. This tsubo is generally used when one becomes tongue tied, but it is also said to be related with one's sense of smell. Therefore, this tsubo should be pressed thoroughly together with the others mentioned. This should be very effective in restoring the impaired function of the olfactory cells.

J. Sores around the mouth——Chi-Sō 地倉 (ST-4)

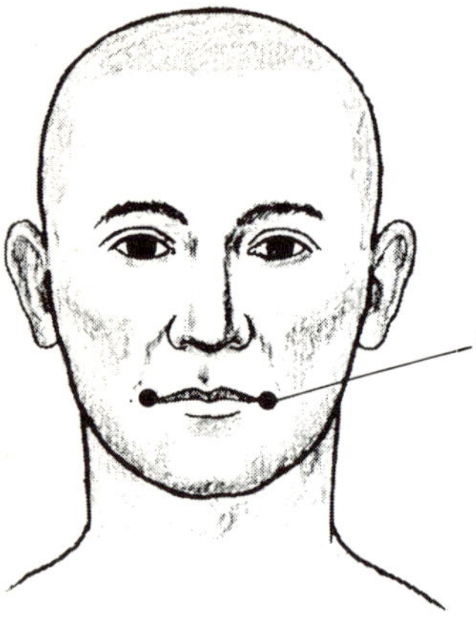

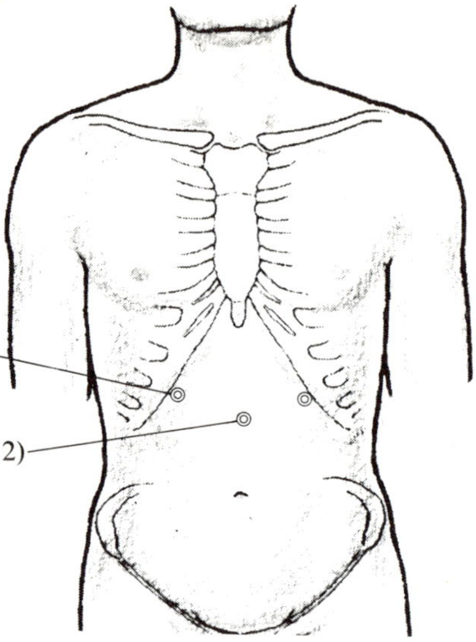

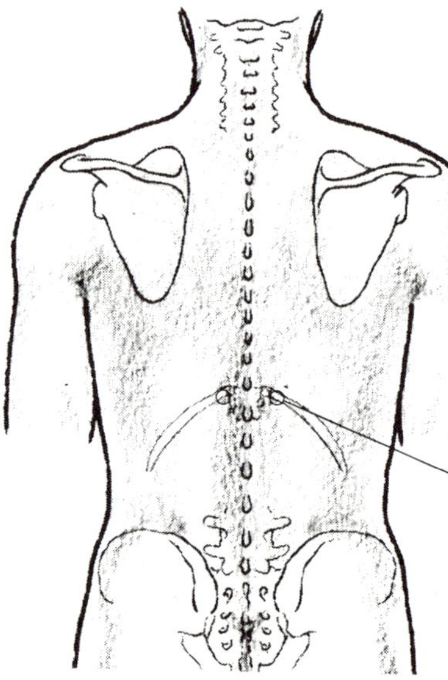

In the wintertime, almost everyone's lips seem to become chapped to some extent, but there are those who have dry lips with sores even in the warmer seasons. This can also be evidence that the person's stomach is weakened due to overindulgence in eating and drinking. In times when one's stomach function continues to deteriorate and problems occur in other digestive organs, this causes "cold sores," or festering sores, to form around the corners of one's mouth.

The specially effective tsubo used often for this condition is Chi-Sō 地倉 (ST-4) which is located on both corners of the mouth. In Oriental medicine the five traditional grains (rice, oats, foxtail millet, Chinese millet, and common millet) as well as food in general, is called the "energy of earth." From the mouth, or Chi-Sō, earth's energy represented by the five grains are taken into the body and sent to the stomach (also called *Tai-Sō*). When there are symptoms in the stomach, some sign of this almost always appears around Chi-Sō. Therefore, when there are stomach problems, or various symptoms of a weak stomach such as sores around the mouth, thorough finger pressure is recommended on the tsubo Chi-Sō.

Other tsubos that should be pressed to regulate the condition of the stomach are Shō-Man 承満 (ST-20), at the tip of the eighth rib to either side of the pit of the stomach, and Chū-Kan 中脘 (CV-12), right between the pit of the stomach and the navel. Shō-Man (accept fullness), just as the name implies, is a tsubo effective when the stomach feels distended and there is a stifling sensation in the pit of the stomach.

Chū-Kan, because it is located over the center of the stomach, is very well known as a specially effective tsubo for symptoms associated with stomach problems and stomach disorders as well as diarrhea and constipation.

An additional tsubo to be used in this case is Hi-Yu 脾兪 (UB-20) (spleen *yu*) located to either side of the eleventh thoracic vertebra. The spleen in Oriental medicine, unlike that known in modern medicine, refers to the pancreas which lies to the back of the stomach. This spleen is regarded as being the organ which functions in the absorption of nutrients obtained from the food digested in the stomach. For this reason, Hi-Yu is used for functional disorders in the digestive organs. Giving shiatsu to this tsubo in times when the lips have sores will work to alleviate them.

K. Throat feeling dry——Ko-Ketsu 巨闕 (CV-14)

Everybody gets a dry throat and becomes thirsty after strenuous exercises or physical labor. This is just the natural physiological response to dehydration in which the body demands the replacement of the water that was lost as sweat. There are cases, however, even when a person has not been working so hard, where the throat feels dried up and a person drinks water constantly. This sensation of thirst, instead of being a problem in the mouth or throat, may be regarded as a manifestation of fatigue in the digestive organs, or as a type of functional disturbance.

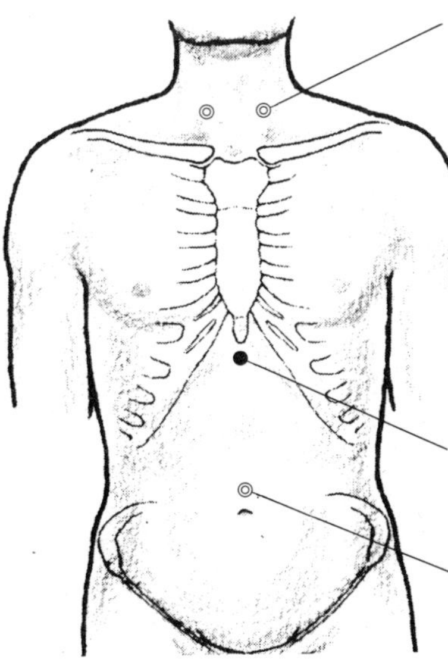

The most effective tsubo for relieving this condition is Ko-Ketsu 巨闕 (CV-14) which is located in the pit of the stomach. More precisely, this tsubo is located three centimeters below the tip of the sternum in the center of the chest. Any hardness or stifling sensation around this tsubo is referred to as "obstruction and hardness in the epigastrium" in Oriental medicine, and the resiliency of this area is regarded as being an indicator of a person's health. If the pit of the stomach feels tense and hard to the touch, it is a sign that the person is fatigued, even though there may be no apparent symptoms. The best policy in this case is to get plenty of rest and relaxation right away. Ko-Ketsu is used primarily for treating high blood pressure and heart diseases, but when it is pressed thoroughly, it can also be surprisingly effective in alleviating dryness in the throat due to gastrointestinal problems.

In addition to this, specialists of Oriental medicine use Sui-Bun 水分 (CV-9) just above the navel and Sui-Totsu 水突 (ST-10) to either side of the Adam's apple, to treat the above symptom. In Oriental medicine, it is maintained that food, after being digested and absorbed by the work of the stomach and spleen, is separated into fluid and solid wastes at Sui-Bun (separate water). Ostensibly, when the function of Sui-Bun weakens, symptoms such as dryness in the throat and frequent urination result. Sui-Totsu is another tsubo which is very effective for excessive thirst, or hoarseness. Therefore, be sure to give thorough finger pressure to these two tsubos in addition to that of Ko-Ketsu.

When a person's throat becomes dry because of fatigue in the digestive organs, it is also important to relieve the general fatigue, so it is a good idea to treat Jin-Yu 腎兪 (UB-23) on the back of the waist. Jin-Yu is especially effective for relieving fatigue in general and revitalizing one's energy throughout the whole body.

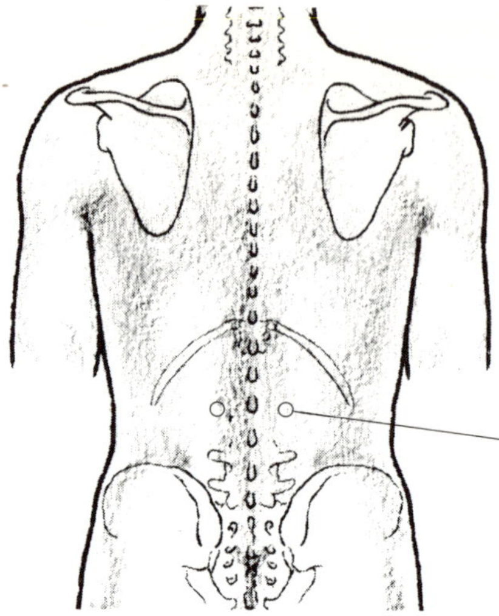

L. Loosening of upper teeth——Ge-Kan 下関 (ST-7)

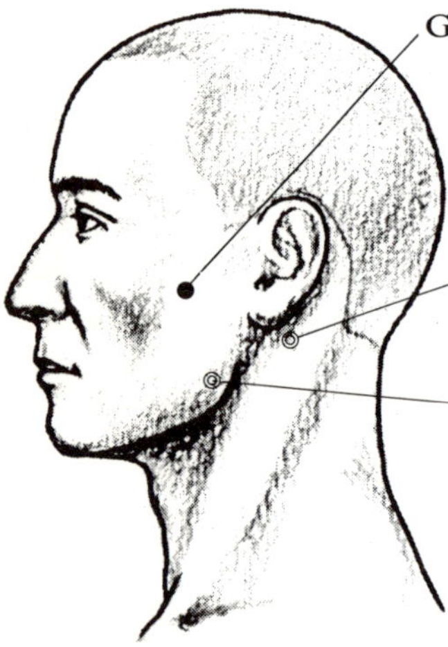

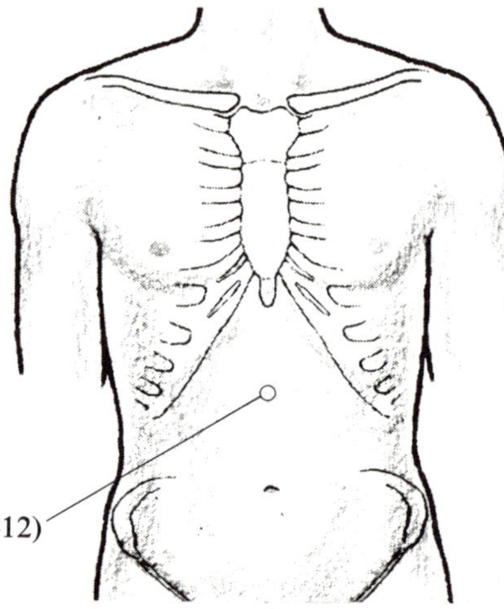

The term "loose teeth" is generally applied when one cannot bite down as usual, or when this causes one pain. If there is a throbbing pain or swelling in the gums, cavities or gum diseases could be the cause, so the best thing to do is to see a dentist. Oral diseases result from bacterial infections so the cause must be removed before a cure can be effected. There are cases where one feels like his teeth are becoming loose although there is no problem with the gums or teeth. For some people, getting behind on sleep over a period of time causes a feeling as if their teeth were set on end. This is not a pleasant feeling at all. This symptom results from a disturbance in the trigeminal nerves which control sensations on the face.

Finger pressure on the tsubo Ge-Kan 下関 (ST-7) located below the cheek bone (zygomatic arch) is very effective in relieving such discomfort. Ge-Kan was introduced before, and it is located just to the front of the ear, and it is easy to find even for novices because this point pokes up when the mouth is opened and forms a depression when the mouth is closed. Other tsubos important for regulating the nerves which go to the teeth are Kyō-Sha 頰車 (ST-6), on the corner of the chin a little below the earlobe, and Kan-Kotsu 完骨 (GB-12) at the tip of the mastoid process behind the ear. These are both tsubos known to be particularly effective for pain in the lower jaw, gums and teeth. Therefore, when finger pressure to Ge-Kan alone does not relieve the feeling of looseness in the teeth, also give pressure to Kyō-Sha and Kan-Kotsu.

The best way to treat Kyō-Sha is to press rather hard with the fleshy part of the thumbs, pushing from the back corner of the jaws toward the front. Kneading this tsubo afterward with the thumbs as if drawing small circles should give remarkable results.

When the digestive function of the stomach is weakened, some symptom or discomfort is felt in the teeth almost without exception. For this reason, steps have to be taken to deal with the stomach condition also. The tsubo specially effective for regulating the function of the stomach and normalizing the digestive function is Chū-Kan 中脘 (CV-12), located right between the navel and the pit of the stomach, as explained before.

M. Loosening of lower teeth——Dai-Gei 大迎 (ST-5)

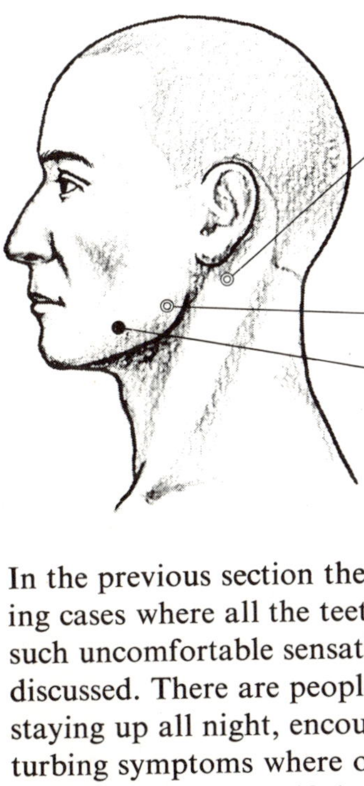

In the previous section the method for treating cases where all the teeth feel loose and such uncomfortable sensations persisting was discussed. There are people who, after staying up all night, encounter such disturbing symptoms where only the teeth in the lower jaw feel as if they were loose.

As explained before, the trigeminal nerve governs the sensations on the face such as pain, heat and cold. This nerve with main branches on either side of the face, as is inferred by a name like trigeminal, divides into three branches on both sides. The first branch goes to the forehead and around the eyes, while the second branch goes to the upper jaw, and the third branch goes to the lower jaw. Of these three branches, the third comes through the jaw bone to the skin of the lower jaw slightly below and to the inside of the corners of the mouth. The hole which this nerve comes through the jaw is called the mental foramen. The tsubo Dai-Gei 大迎 (ST-5) is located right over this hole. In relation to the teeth, this is just under the second premolar. The feeling of looseness in the lower jaw is caused by disturbances in the branch of the trigeminal nerve going to the lower jaw. Thus, finger pressure on Dai-Gei proves most effective in this case. When one feels a dull pain in this area in addition to the feeling of loose teeth, thorough pressure on Dai-Gei and the previously mentioned Kyō-Sha 頰車 (ST-6) should work to gradually ease the pain. Naturally, pressing Kan-Kotsu 完骨 (GB-12) along with the above tsubos will further improve the effectiveness of the treatment.

When treating these tsubos, massaging along the lines connecting the tsubos can be very effective. One way to do this is to first give finger pressure to individual tsubo, and

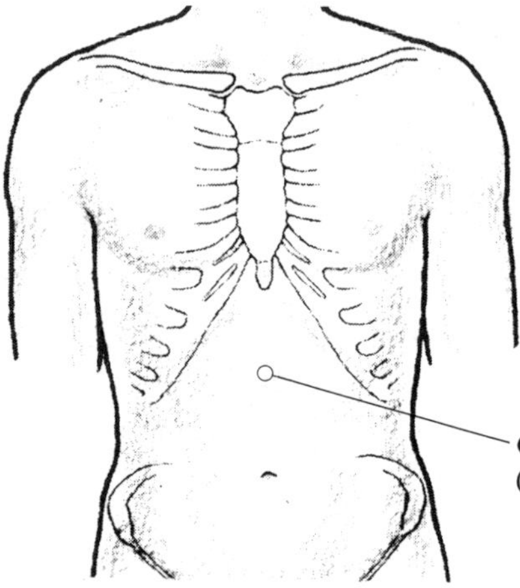

then to lightly press with the thumbs and index fingers beginning at Dai-Gei and working past Kyō-Sha up to Kan-Kotsu. Finish the treatment by stroking down this same path with both palms. Another way to stimulate this area would be to warm it by applying hot compresses or blowing hot air on it with a hair drier. The above mentioned symptoms also often come from fatigue of the stomach, so the effect should be enhanced by applying finger pressure on Chū-Kan 中脘 (CV-12) for good measure.

N. Roughness of tongue——Hi-Yu 脾俞 (UB-20)

The taste buds on our tongue are responsible for our being able to distinguish the tastes represented in Oriental medicine as the five basic tastes of sour, bitter, sweet, pungent and salty. When people become very fatigued, their sense of taste is usually dulled. The surface of the tongue becomes rough and one is unable to taste things, especially after the function of the digestive organs are impaired by eating and drinking too much, or otherwise, by smoking too much. Normally the surface of the tongue has a light coating of mucus, but when this coating becomes very thick and turns white or yellow in color, one's sense of taste is dulled and it is highly likely that the function of the digestive organs have weakened. You may think that a tsubo around the mouth is the most effective tsubo for this condition, but in fact, the most important tsubo in this case is Hi-Yu-脾俞 (UB-20) which was also mentioned for sores around the lips. Also treating Kan-Yu 肝俞 (UB-18) which is just above Hi-Yu, is even more effective for alleviating roughness on the surface of the tongue. In Oriental medicine the "spleen" is regarded as being the organ in charge of digestion and absorption, and the liver is regarded as being in charge of detoxifying the body. When a person's di-

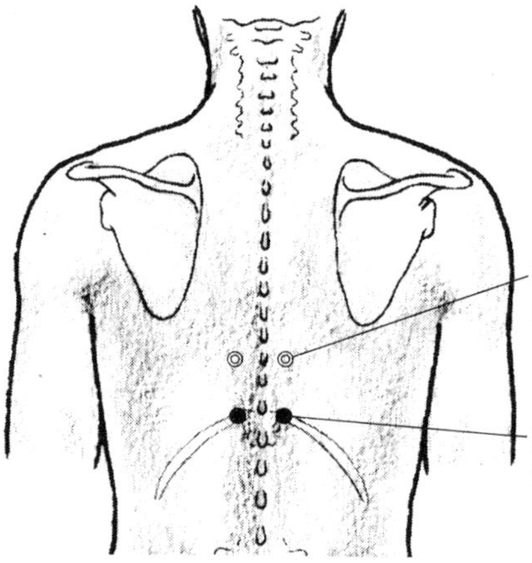

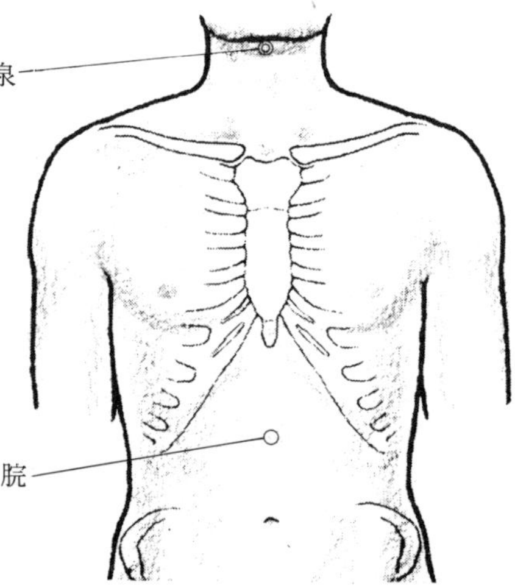

gestive organs are in bad shape, pressing around the middle of the back where Kan-Yu and Hi-Yu are located above and below respectively, often reveals a hard band of tension across this area.

These tsubos are hard to press all by yourself. Since, as already stated, there is no need to be overly concerned with the exact location of the tsubos, just get someone to give you strong finger pressure along the spine from between the shoulder blades down to the hip bone. It is also acceptable to have someone just massage from Kan-Yu down to Hi-Yu. As the tension down the back diminishes, the digestive organs will be restored to a healthy state and the roughness of the tongue will gradually return to normal.

The tsubos Ren-Sen 廉泉 (CV-23), right above the Adam's apple, and Chū-Kan 中脘 (CV-12), above the navel, are also said to be effective for roughness of the tongue. The important point in treatment is to regard the roughness of the tongue as just a symptom of problems in the digestive organs.

O. Ringing in the ears (tinnitus)——Tinnitus point

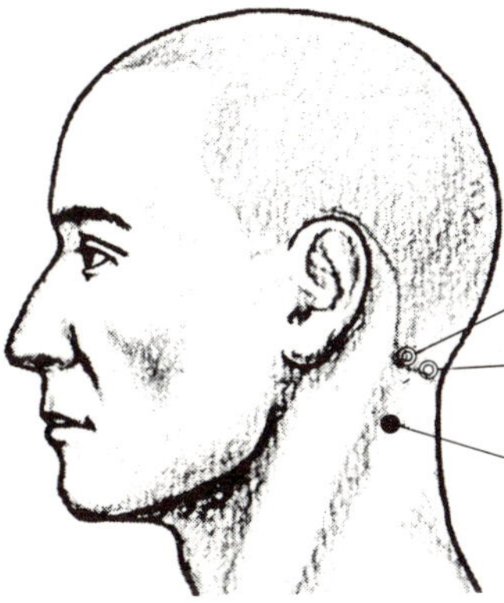

When a person is very tired after a long hard day at work, or after engaging in vigorous sports, sometimes upon waking up the following morning, one hears a ringing in the ears or a buzzing sound like cicadas. People past their prime often are troubled by tinnitus even when the amount of fatigue is slight. This symptom is almost always accompanied with stiffness or tension from the side of the neck down to the shoulders. This could even be coined as "cervical tinnitus." This means that the muscular tension in the side of the neck and the shoulders is causing the tinnitus.

When this is the case, use the fleshy part of your thumb to firmly press the point just one finger width below the tsubos Ten-Chū 天柱 (UB-10) and Fū-Chi 風池 (GB-20) discussed before. There should be a point where the ringing in the ears disappears all of a sudden, or instead grows even louder. There is no need to be concerned even if the ringing becomes louder because once the muscular tension in the neck is completely relieved by finger pressure and massage on this tsubo, the noise will gradually subside. This is not a traditional tsubo, instead it is one which we discovered in our clinical practice. It is simply called the *tinnitus point.* Probe for this point down below the tsubos Ten-Chū and Fū-Chi. Be sure to apply thorough finger pressure on Ten-Chū and Fū-Chi as well.

People often ask me, "Just how to locate tsubos precisely." Truth of the matter is, even specialists in this field do not have a hard and fast rule for accurately locating all the tsubos. The main point is to get a general idea of where the tsubo is located, and to feel this area lightly with the fingertips until a tender spot where the skin feels somewhat rougher is found. In simple terms, this point corresponds to the tsubo. Use the figures provided to get a rough idea of where the tsubos are located and then press around in this area until you find the spot.

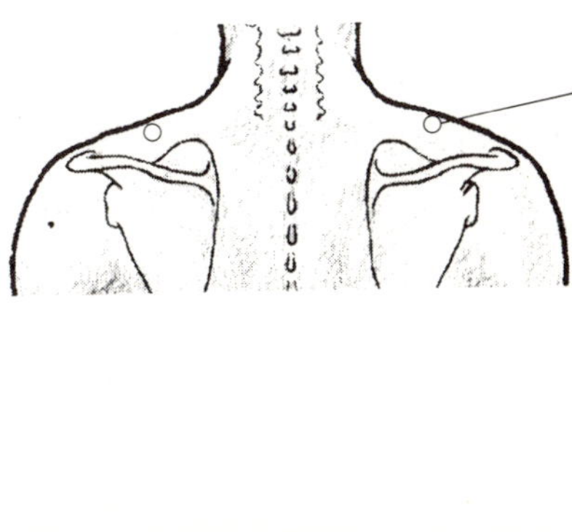

As mentioned at the start, since tinnitus is most often accompanied with shoulder tension, in addition to treating the tinnitus point, it is important to give finger pressure and massage to the tsubo Ken-Sei 肩井 (GB-21) located on top of the shoulder just between the base of the neck and the tip of the shoulder.

P. Hearing problems——Ten-Yō 天牖 (TH-16)

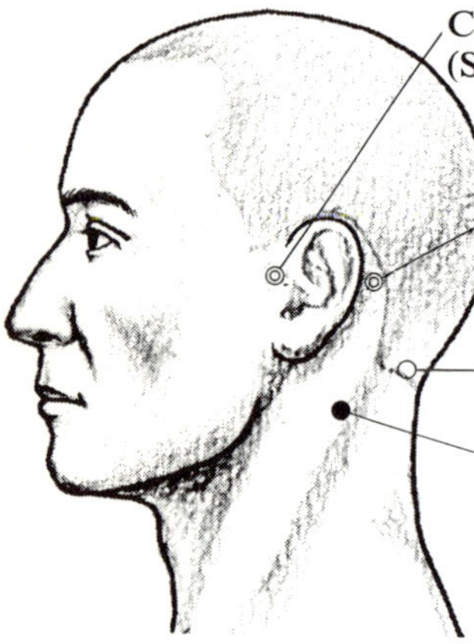

Hearing problems can be divided roughly into the two types of either sound perception disfunctions or sound conduction disfunctions. Curing hearing problems which are caused by sound perception disfunctions, which are diseases in the auditory center of the brain responsible for recognizing and picking out sound signals, is not an easy matter for Western medicine, let alone for Oriental medicine. For sound conduction disfunctions that are problems of transmitting the sound to the auditory center, however, shiatsu treatments on the appropriate tsubo can be very effective because the problem is often caused by nothing more than fatigue.

How then do sound conduction disfunctions occur? To explain this simply, the direct cause is fatigue accumulating in the splenius capitis muscle which is on the side of the neck near the back. The Eustachian tube which is an air passage between the ear and the throat is compressed when the splenius capitis muscle gets tense with the loss of vigor in the body. The normal balance of air pressure between the inside and outside of the eardrum is lost because of this and the eardrum does not vibrate as it should.

This type of sound conduction disfunction is most common among the middle-aged and elderly, and is not seen very often in young people except in cases of occupational diseases such as with flight attendants. In older people with this problem, when there is accumulated fatigue, generally they do not have any problem hearing in the morning, but once evening comes their hearing suddenly becomes very poor and they often hear a loud buzzing sound in their ears like that of cicadas.

For this type of hearing problem stemming from fatigue, the tsubo Ten-Yō 天牖 (TH-16), located just to the front of the previously mentioned tinnitus point, is very important. When this area is pressed firmly with one's middle fingers, the tension in the splenius capitis muscle is relieved and hearing is gradually restored. Chō-Kyū 聴宮 (SI-19), located to the front of the tragus (the fleshy protrusion at the front of the ear which covers the opening), and Kyō-In 竅陰 (GB-11), to the back of the ear, are also effective for sound conduction disfunctions. Chō-Kyū (hearing palace) as its name implies, is a very important tsubo used for every kind of ear disease. Apply thorough finger pressure on this tsubo along with Ten-Chū 天柱 (UB-10).

As explained before, Kyō-In is a specially effective tsubo for dizziness and tinnitus. This point, aside from finger pressure treatments, is a good place to affix metal grains with adhesive tape (available in Japan). Just this can yield surprising results.

3. Treating Symptoms of the Neck, Shoulders and Back

A. Stiffness in back of neck——Ten-Chū 天柱 (UB-10)

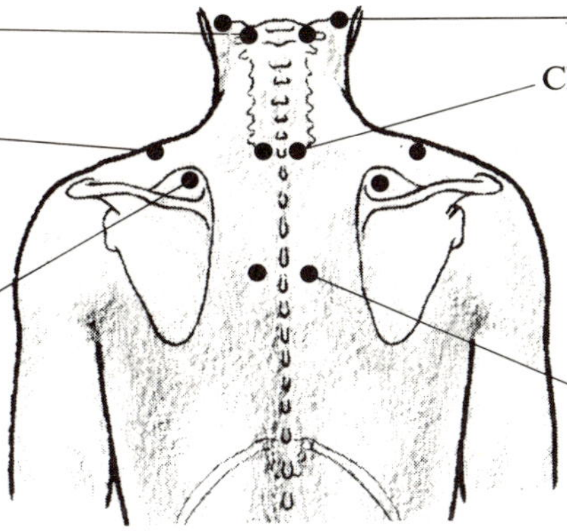

When we attend lectures and have to listen too long and complicated explanations, sometimes our head becomes heavy and it starts to nod up and down until finally we fall asleep. This is the work of our natural defense mechanism which relaxes our tense muscles without our being aware of it.

Man has evolved to become the supreme animal by his superior mental faculty and the upright posture which freed the arms for manipulating his environment. The upright posture unique in the animal kingdom forces man to support his head which weighs around four kilograms with nothing more than the cervical vertebrae and the muscles between the neck and shoulders. In addition, the muscles of the shoulders have to support the weight of the arms which amount to one eighth of one's total body weight. Therefore, the tendency in man for tension to accumulate in the back of the neck may be regarded as a price that we have to pay for evolving this far.

The cervical vertebrae are connected by thick cord-like structures called ligaments. There is a tendency for calcium deposits to form here in older people, and this causes the ligaments to harden. This adds to the tension in the back of the neck, and eventually the neck becomes very inflexible, and one becomes unable to bend it forward. This is the reason why tension or stiffness in the back of the neck should be taken care of right away. One must pay attention to retain the resiliency in the muscles between the neck and shoulders so as to forestall the debilitating effects of aging. The first thing that needs to be done for this purpose is to remove the tension in the muscles on both sides of the cervical spine, the ligaments in the neck, and the muscles between the shoulder blades. In this case, instead of just pressing individual tsubo, massaging between the lines connecting the tsubos is more effective.

One method is to first massage from Ten-Chū 天柱 (UB-10) to Kyoku-En 曲垣 (SI-13), and then from Fū-Chi 風池 (GB-20) to Ken-Sei 肩井 (GB-21), and finally from Chi-Zen 治喘 (extra tsubo) to Ketsu-In-Yu 厥陰兪 (UB-14). Follow this sequence up with light massages along these lines using the fleshy part of the thumbs as if drawing small circles. When you fail to treat tension in the back of the neck soon after it occurs, it will eventually become chronic. The important thing is to treat this tension yourself at the earliest opportunity so that the symptom does not persist.

B. Stiffness in side of neck toward the back——Ken-Sei 肩井 (GB-21)

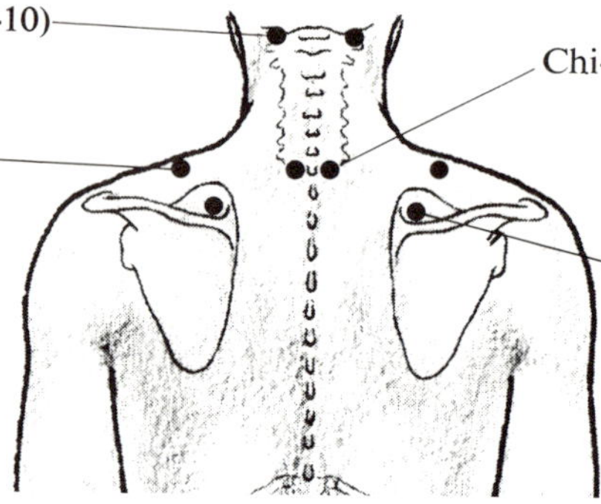

As stated in the previous section, human beings hold their head up, which weighs around four kilograms, with only the cervical vertebrae for support. The head and trunk are also connected by muscles such as the trapezius muscle which is the big hard muscle in the nape of the neck, and the levator scapulae muscle under the trapezius muscle. The trapezius muscle holds up the shoulders and arms while the levator scapulae muscle connects the back of the skull with the shoulder blades. These muscles must remain in a constant state of tension while a person is standing up. Also, these muscles have to work whenever the neck is moved in any direction. As a result, the trapezius and levator scapulae muscles are the most likely to become fatigued and hardened with tension. Fatigue in these muscles takes the form of stiffness in the back of the neck.

When the amount of tension is minimal, one can obtain a measure of relief just by rotating the head or turning it from side to side. Treatments on the specially effective tsubos becomes necessary when the tension is great enough for there to be pain. The first thing that needs to be done before pressing the tsubos is to relax the muscles in the area. The best way to do this is to lie down for a while and rest these muscles. While doing this, a hot towel can be wrapped around the neck and a plastic sheet can be placed over this to contain the heat and warm up the neck area. Doing this for fifteen to twenty minutes will serve to greatly enhance the effect of the tsubo treatment.

Once the back of the neck becomes relaxed and the muscles have become softer, begin by pressing Ten-Chū 天柱 (UB-10) on both sides. Then press Kyoku-En 曲垣 (SI-13) at the top of the scapula toward the inside. Follow this with pressure on Ken-Sei 肩井 (GB-21) at the midpoint between the neck and the shoulder, and on Chi-Zen 治喘 (extra tsubo), a little to the inside from Kyoku-En. In this case, each tsubo may be pressed individually, but to remove the tension completely, it is best to massage along the lines connecting these tsubos. One way to do this is to apply firm pressure with your thumbs or four fingers using a slight kneading action between Ten-Chū and Kyoku-En, Ten-Chū and Ken-Sei, as well as Ten-Chū and Chi-Zen.

C. Stiffness in side of neck toward the front——Ten-Sō 天窓 (SI-16)

When you draw your chin in and turn your head to one side, a thick muscle stretches from below the throat to below the ear. This is the sternocleidomastoid muscle. It is a very important muscle which connects the head to the trunk along with the trapezius and the levator scapulae muscles mentioned before. The main function of the sternocleidomastoid muscle is to bend the head forward. This muscle becomes fatigued and stiff when a person remains bent over for long periods. This is why the longer a person works at a desk, the more this muscle becomes stiff and sore to the front of the neck.

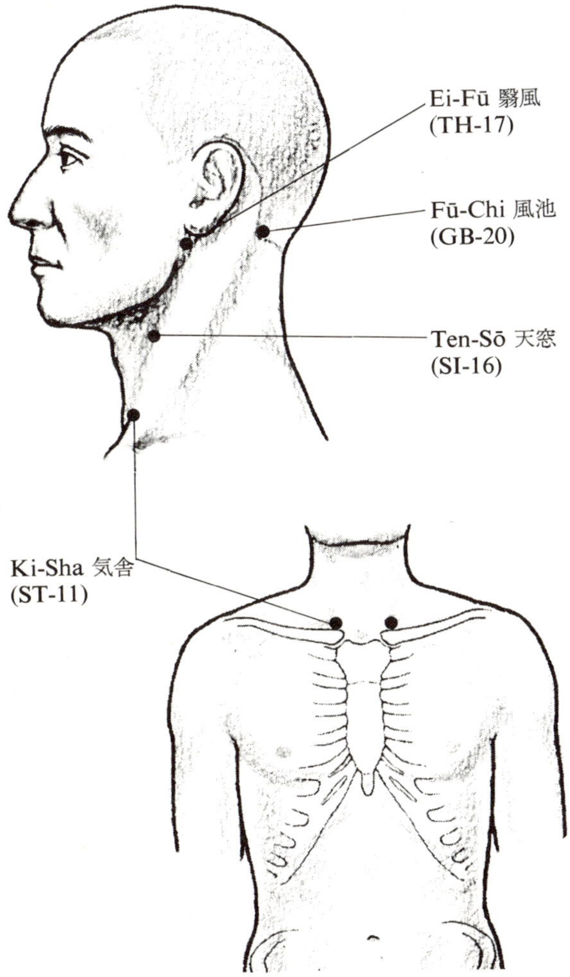

As already noted, underneath the sternocleidomastoid muscle pass vital nerves and blood vessels which connect the head and trunk. For this reason, when circulatory disorders such as high blood pressure occur, there is a tendency for tension to appear in this muscle. When the sternocleidomastoid muscle is stiff and sore, one's body becomes fatigued that much faster, and other symptoms such as feeling hot in the head and cold in the feet appear. Therefore, it is important to treat the sternocleidomastoid muscle as soon as it begins to feel sore, so as to maintain its tone and resiliency.

The specially effective tsubos for this purpose are Ei-Fū 翳風 (TH-17) and Fū-Chi 風池 (GB-20) as mentioned before, Ten-Sō 天窓 (SI-16) which lies to the back of the midpoint on the sternocleidomastoid muscle, and Ki-Sha 気舎 (ST-11), to either side of where the knot in a necktie goes (above the clavicle). It goes without saying that in this case also, instead of pressing each tsubo individually, it is best to massage along the lines connecting the tsubos. The best treatment would be to massage the entire sternocleidomastoid muscle by firmly grasping it with the thumb and four fingers starting around Ei-Fū and Fū-Chi and working past Ten-Sō down to Ki-Sha. The effect is enhanced by moving the head around for a person, going forward and backward as well as sideways. The important thing to remember in moving a person's head back and forth is never to force it.

The tsubo Ki-Sha is located close to the lymph glands in the supraclavicular fossa which has a deep connection with the function of the stomach, so aside from stiffness and "cricks in the neck," Ki-Sha is effective for stomach symptoms such as nausea.

D. Stiffness in side of neck——Ten-Chū 天柱 (UB-10)

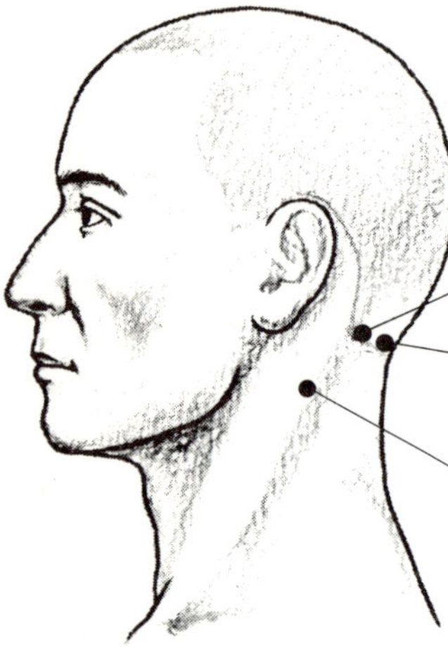

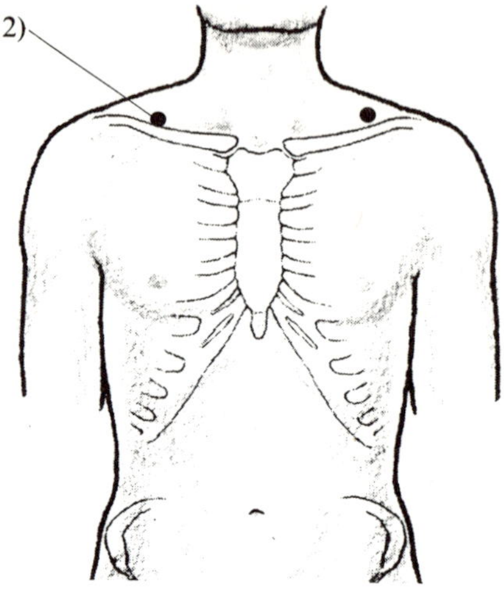

There are two more muscles in the side of the neck aside from those already mentioned. One is the scalenus muscle, and the other is the splenius capitis muscle, once mentioned in reference to hearing problems. These muscles sometimes become very stiff and sore depending on a person's posture. In such cases, feeling the area in the back of the head between the ears reveals great rigidity in these muscles, and they feel tender with only slight pressure from the fingertips. Tension in this area is also often associate with other symptoms like headaches, tinnitus and hearing problems.

Tension or stiffness in muscles in simple terms is hardening caused by metabolites such as lactic acid accumulating in the blood and chemically bonding with calcium to create a loss of elasticity in the muscles. Further, this irritates the nerves running through the muscle in all directions, and produces a sore or heavy sensation. Therefore, to remove tension and restore the muscles to a soft and pliable state once more, first the circulation in the area must be improved. To treat muscular tension as detailed above, massaging the area between the tsubos shown in the figure, Ten-Chū 天柱 (UB-10), Fū-Chi 風池 (GB-20), Ten-Yō 天牖 (TH-16) and Ketsu-Bon 欠盆 (ST-12), is recommended. Massaging will improve circulation in this area which will serve to remove the metabolic wastes in the muscles. This process can be facilitated considerably by applying hot compresses on the back and side of the neck before massaging.

A simple way to apply hot compresses is to soak a thick towel in hot water (around forty-five degrees centigrade) while holding both ends, and wringing this out lightly before placing it on the neck. There are people who soak a whole towel in hot water to make compresses, but this makes it too hot to wring out. Waiting for the towel to cool down before wringing it is not good because then the effect of the hot compress is lost. The best way is hold the ends of the towel and soak the middle of the towel while the water is still good and hot. Apply hot compresses two or three times first, and this should double the effectiveness of the treatment.

E. Raspy feeling in the throat——Ten-Totsu 天突 (CV-22)

Teachers, newscasters and television entertainers who have to constantly use their voice in their profession are the first to complain of a raspy feeling in their throat accompanied with dryness and pain. This could almost be called an occupational disease caused by the overuse of the vocal cords. Normal people also occasionally experience this uncomfortable sensation where one's voice sounds as if phlegm is caught somewhere in the throat. This symptom is most common at the onset of a cold, but sometimes it comes from physical and mental fatigue as well.

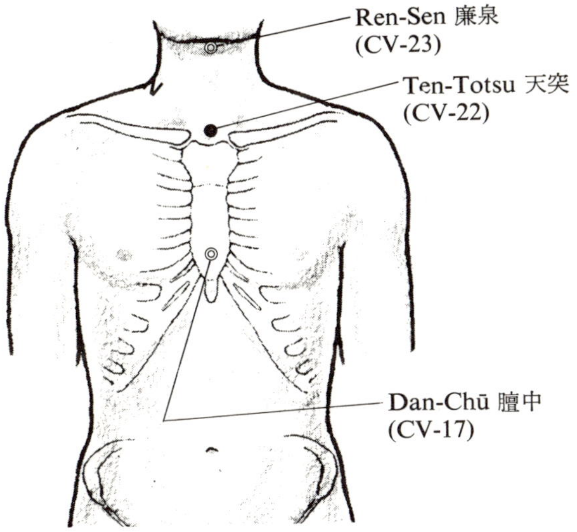

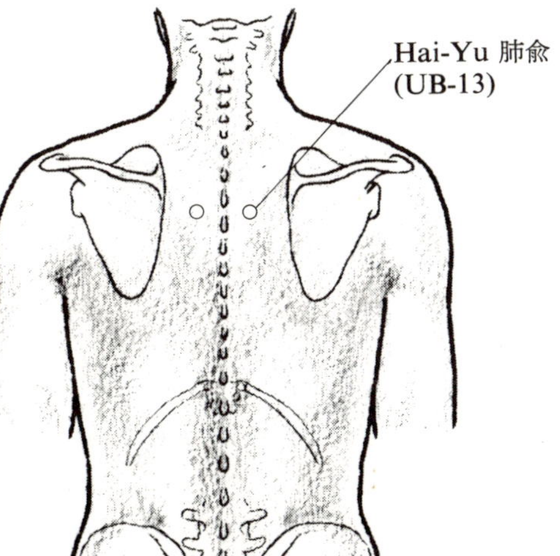

The specially effective tsubos used in such cases are, Ren-Sen 廉泉 (CV-23), Ten-Tostu 天突 (CV-22) and Dan-Chū 膻中 (CV-17), all on the anterior medial line, going from the throat down toward the pit of the stomach. The most important tsubo is Ten-Totsu which is above the sternum and between the clavicles. This tsubo, just under where the knot of a tie goes, is easy to locate because hooking the index finger around the top of the sternum and pressing down usually produces a penetrating sensation. In the past, acupuncture was performed at this point to treat pain in the throat caused by tonsillitis.

Of course, there is no need for acupuncture just to cure raspiness in the throat which comes from simple fatigue. Applying pressure on Ten-Totsu should be enough to provide quick relief. Pushing straight toward the throat when pressing Ten-Totsu will make it hard to breathe, so the best way to stimulate this tsubo is to hook the index finger around the sternum and to press down and back toward the sternum.

The tsubos Ren-Sen and Dan-Chū have both been discussed before, and they are used most often for symptoms occurring between the throat and the pit of the stomach such as shortness of breath, palpitations and coughing. Therefore, it is ideal to treat Ren-Sen and Dan-Chū along with Ten-Totsu when there is a raspy feeling in the throat.

When the throat feels raspy, aside from it being a manifestation of fatigue in the throat, it is safe to assume that there is some problem in the respiratory system as well. This is why also getting someone to press Hai-Yu 肺兪 (UB-13) firmly will yield the desired effects much faster.

F. Hoarseness——Sui-Totsu 水突 (ST-10)

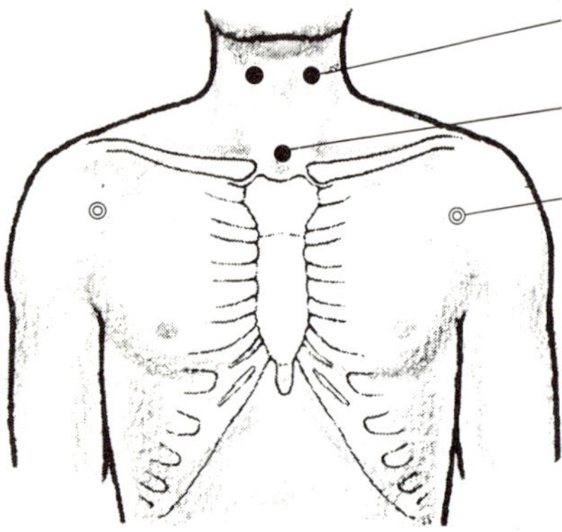

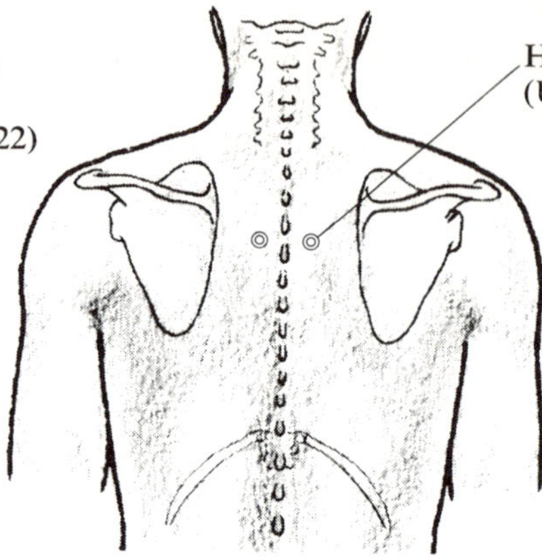

When the raspy feeling in the throat discussed in the previous section is ignored long enough, one becomes hoarse. When this happens, one's throat also feels dry and sore. Although hoarseness is accompanied with pain in the throat, sometimes this goes beyond the bounds of simple fatigue or colds, and the pain could be caused by serious diseases like tuberculosis or cancer of the larynx. Therefore, it is best to consult a specialist when the pain is specially strong. Hoarseness which comes from simple fatigue, on the other hand, can be treated successfully with tsubo therapy.

When our voice becomes funny, we usually feel for our Adam's apple without thinking too much about it. This happens to be right where there is a tsubo specially effective for hoarseness. The tsubo Sui-Totsu 水突 (ST-10) is located two finger widths (using the index and middle fingers) in front of the midpoint of the sternocleidomastoid muscle to either side of the neck. As explained before, this tsubo is used to treat dryness in the throat and excessive thirst, but it is also used in Oriental medicine to cure conditions where "one's voice becomes like waterfowl." Waterfowl means birds like ducks, so this tsubo is effective for sore throats and hoarse voices that sound like a duck. Therefore, in such cases, it is wise to press the tsubo Sui-Totsu on either side of the neck using the thumb and four fingers. This will serve to clear the throat, and one's voice will become more normal. Also, pressing Ten-Totsu 天突 (CV-22) in this case should increase the benefit.

In addition to this, treatments must be given to normalize the overall condition of the respiratory organs, in the same manner as when there is a raspy feeling in the throat. Hai-Yu 肺兪 (UB-13) on the back and Chū-Fu 中府 (LU-1) below clavicle to the outside are the tsubos used for this purpose. Gently pressing these tsubos will bring relief especially when, along with hoarseness, there

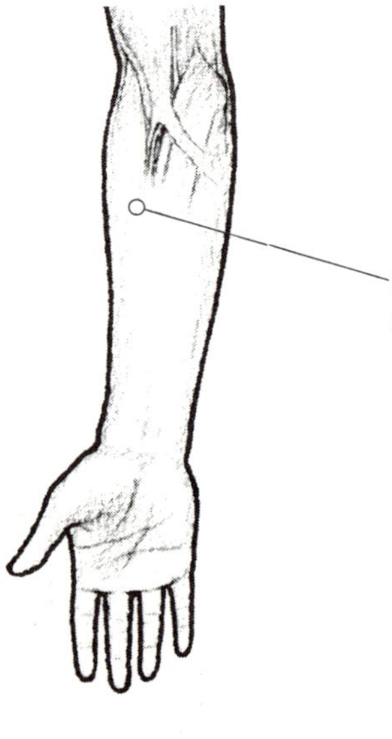

are symptoms such as discomfort in the chest and shortness of breath.

Another tsubo convenient to keep in mind for times when your voice suddenly gives out is Kō-Sai 孔最 (LU-6). This tsubo is located on the place one third the distance to the wrist from the elbow. Kō-Sai is the tsubo known as being specially effective for acute symptoms of the respiratory organs such as sudden coughing fits. It is also very effective for conditions where one is hoarse and coughing out phlegm.

G. Hiccoughing——Ten-Tei 天鼎 (LI-17)

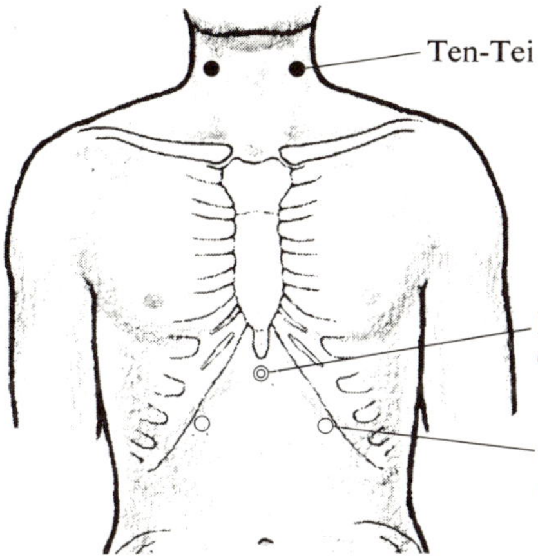

There is an interesting belief in some parts of Japan concerning how to stop hiccoughing. According to this, a hiccoughing person is given a bowl of water with a pair of chopsticks crossed over it, and is supposed to drink the water all at once from between the chopsticks. This may seem like a pointless ritual, but it cannot be completely dismissed as just superstition. The reason for this is that hiccoughing in physiological terms is spasms in the diaphragm which may even be regarded as one kind of abnormal respiration. The normal rhythm of breathing is reestablished and the hiccoughing stops when a person's breathing is temporarily suspended by drinking water quickly, or when surprised by someone.

Sometimes when a person is extremely tired, however, nothing seems to be able to stop the hiccoughing, and this simple symptom can become quite disconcerting for a person. There is no method available even from modern medicine which can stop hiccoughing instantly. This is where tsubo therapy can show amazing results. The specially effective tsubo for hiccoughing used often since the old days is Ten-Tei 天鼎 (LI-17) which is located in front of the midpoint of the sternocleidomastoid muscle, just to either side of the throat. The vagus nerve which goes from the brain to the diaphragm passes beneath the sternocleidomastoid muscle and down both sides of the esophagus to go past the pit of the stomach. Ten-Tei is the tsubo which lies on a focal point of this nerve pathway. Therefore, gently pressing Ten-Tei with the fleshy part of one's thumbs or index fingers will mysteriously cause the hiccoughing to stop.

For stubborn hiccoughs which still do not stop, supplement the above treatment with pressure to Kyū-Bi 鳩尾 (CV-15), at the bottom of the sternum, and Fu-Yō 不容 (ST-19), right below the eighth rib. Both of these tsubos are usually used to relieve symptoms in the chest under the rib cage. Applying pressure on these points will stop the hiccoughing before you know it.

Aside from the above, there is yet another tsubo effective for stopping hiccoughing,

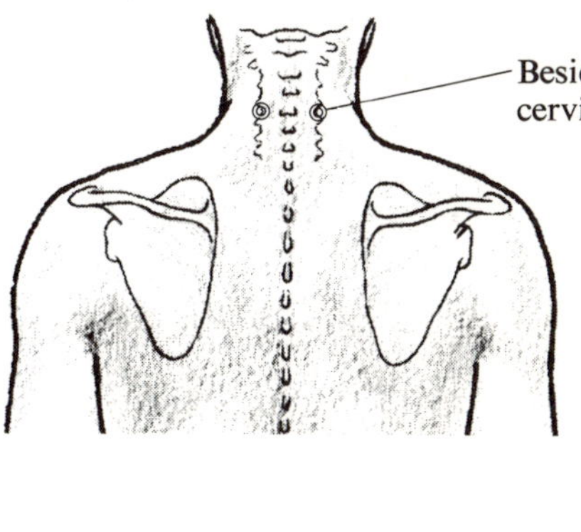

and although this may seem an unlikely place, it is located on the back of the neck. It is right between the back of the skull and the top of the shoulders. Press this area to either side of the fourth cervical vertebra using the index and middle fingers. Instead of simply applying pressure in this case, move the fingers back and forth slightly while applying pressure. This point is not a tsubo per se, but try pressing it whenever hiccoughing becomes a problem because it can sometimes prove unexpectedly effective.

H. Stiffness at base of neck——Kyoku-En 曲垣 (SI-13)

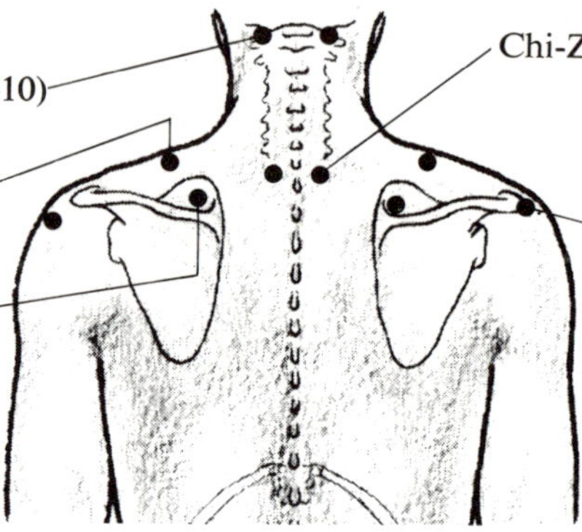

Sometimes we find ourselves rotating our head to dispell tension while working or studying. This is one sign of how the muscles down the nape of the neck are the most susceptible to fatigue. Since human beings hold up their heavy head with the cervical spine and the muscles of the neck, naturally, the circulation in the muscles in the nape of the neck is impaired when a forward bending posture is held for a long time. As a result, the supply of oxygen and nutrients necessary for the contraction of the muscles is not adequate. Also, the metabolites such as lactic acid accumulate in the muscles and they become tense and stiff. Therefore, performing simple exercises, or movements involving the whole body, or otherwise slipping into a warm bath, improves one's circulation and brings relief from muscular tension.

When, aside from stiffness at the base of the neck, one also has symptoms of general fatigue, lack of appetite and a sensation of heaviness over the head, this is a sign that a considerable amount of fatigue has accumulated. In this case, treat the tsubos shown in the figure. It is fine to press each tsubo individually, but if possible, even better results can be obtained by first massaging down from Ten-Chū 天柱 (UB-10) to Chi-Zen 治喘 (extra tsubo) and then again from Ten-Chū to Kyoku-En 曲垣 (SI-13), and once more from Ten-Chū past Ken-Sei 肩井 (GB-21) to Ken-Gū 肩髃 (LI-15). The best way to do this is to first gently stroke these areas with the palm of your hand and then to press along those lines using the thumb and middle finger.

Another very effective method is to place a towel soaked in lukewarm water on the base of the neck and blowing hot air on this with a hair drier. Applying a hot compress here is also good, but using a hair drier for this purpose is easier, and it is just as effective. A hair drier happens to be about the most convenient tool in tsubo therapy. It is especially effective for neck and shoulder tension which feels quite sore. Such soreness can be alleviated to an amazing extent just by carefully blowing hot air on this area so as not to cause a burn. The reason this is so effective is because the heat and the wind pressure provide an ideal massaging effect. Hair driers are actually used in our clinic with excellent results.

1. Neck immobilized by "crick in the neck"——Kan-Kotsu 完骨 (GB-12)

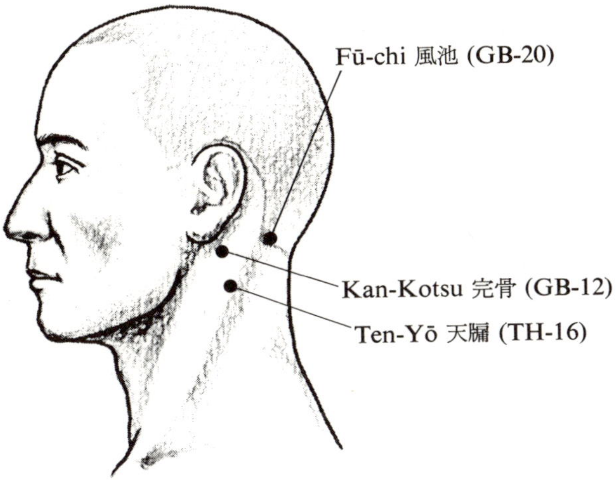

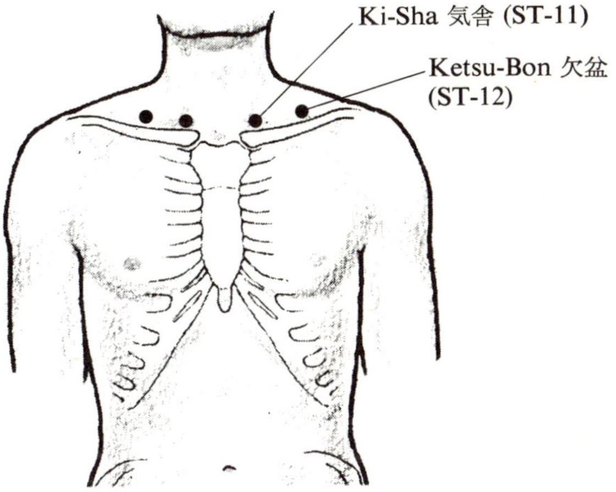

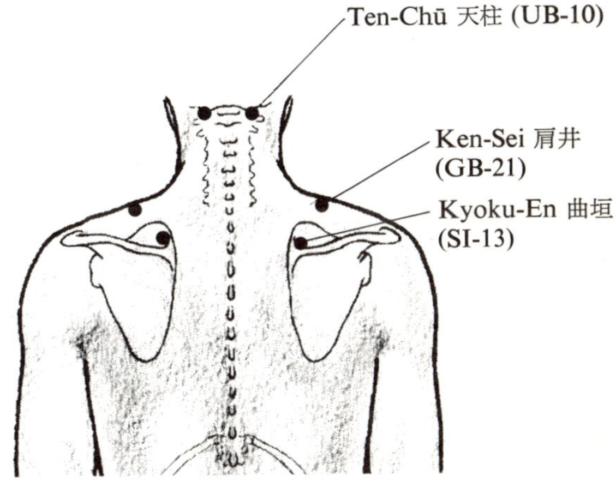

There are cases where people wake up in the morning and find that they cannot turn their head because a sharp pain shoots down the neck to the shoulders when they try to turn their head. This condition is sometimes referred to as a "crick in the neck," and in more specialized language it is called "acute cervicodynia."

How then do people get "cricks in the neck?" As already discussed previously, there are many muscles in the neck including the trapezius and sternocleidomastoid muscles. There is no problem so long as all these muscles are contracting and extending in the right direction. However, when one sleeps in an awkward position, or otherwise becomes overly fatigued, this direction of muscular movement can deviate to cause what is called a "crick in the neck."

When this happens, you must first find out which muscle has been affected. This can be determined by checking the tsubos shown in the figure and feeling the muscle under them. The muscle with the "crick" feels stiff and hard, and the slightest bit of pressure on it causes pain. If the stiffness and pain can be felt between the tsubos Kan-Kotsu 完骨 (GB-12) and Ki-Sha 気舎 (ST-11), it can be regarded as a "crick" in the sternocleidomastoid muscle. Likewise, stiffness and pain between Fū-Chi 風池 (GB-20) and Ketsu-Bon 欠盆 (ST-12) means the scalenus muscle; that around Ten-Yō 天牖 (TH-16) means the splenius capitis muscle; that between Ten-Chū 天柱 (UB-10) and Kyoku-En 曲垣 (SI-13) means the levator scapulae muscle, and that immediately around Fū-Chi means the trapezius muscle has been affected.

Once you find out which muscle is causing the problem, press this muscle just enough so that it does not hurt, and turn the head in the opposite direction from the "crick." Doing this several times will gradually correct the deviation in the position of the muscle and the pain should begin to ease. If the pain still persists, massage each tsubo while pressing them somewhat strongly. It is also effective to massage along the muscle with the fleshy part of the thumbs and four fingers in a circular movement. Another effective method is to heat the area using a hot compress or a hair drier.

Naturally, some "cricks in the neck" are not all that serious, and minor cases can be cured simply by rotating the head slowly in large circles, or bending the head down to either side.

J. Fatigue in shoulders——Ken-Sei 肩井 (GB-21)

Fatigue and the sensation of heaviness in the shoulders is a symptom normally grouped together with stiff shoulders, but there are many cases where a person feels fatigued and heavy from the back of the neck down to the back, without there necessarily being anything like tension or stiffness. This kind of symptom is especially common among truck drivers and taxi drivers, typists and key punchers, or otherwise, people who have jobs which require them to maintain a certain posture all day and to work with only their hands. This symptom is caused when the muscles in the back of the neck and the shoulders reach their limit of tension, and their elasticity and resiliency are lost.

In this case, if the symptoms are fairly minor, just the exercise of reaching the arms out over one's head and bending backward will release the muscular tension and the shoulders will feel quite a bit lighter. The best idea is to exercise lightly like this now and then during break time to keep these muscles from becoming too tense.

When the sensation of heaviness over the shoulders does not go away just by exercising, apply pressure on the tsubos Ken-Sei 肩井 (GB-21), Kyoku-En 曲垣 (SI-13), Ken-Gū 肩髃 (LI-15), Hi-Ju 臂臑 (LI-14) and Gō-Koku 合谷 (LI-4) which are shown in the figure. Apply firm pressure on these tsubos so that the sensation reaches to the center of the body. You should be able to feel the

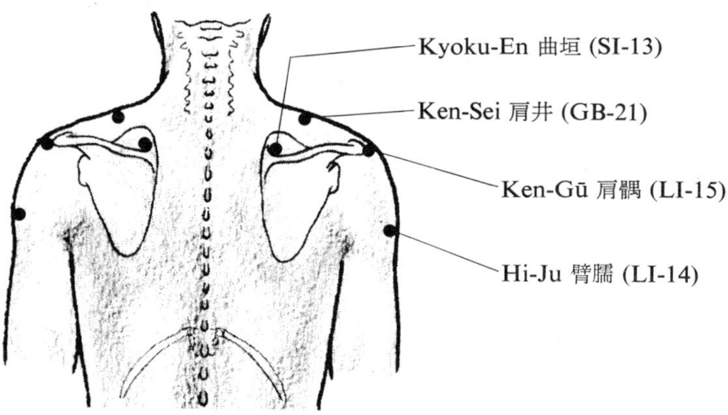

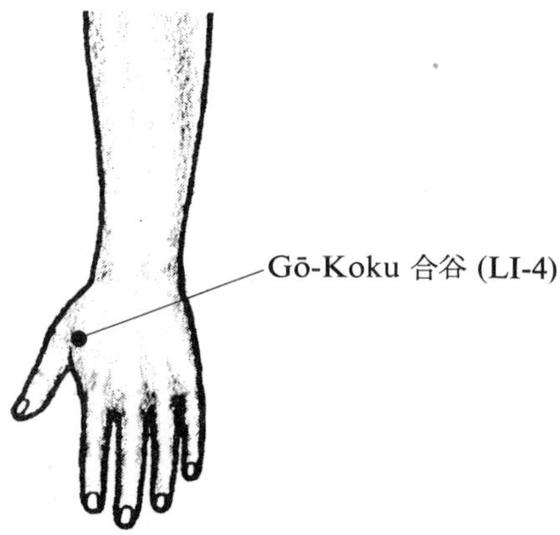

heaviness in the shoulders gradually dissolving. Each one of these tsubos mentioned are important, but among them, Ken-Sei, located at about the midpoint between the base of the neck and the tip of the shoulder, is known as being particularly effective for symptoms affecting the back of the neck and the shoulders such as stiff shoulders or "frozen shoulders." In *anma* massage of Japan there is even a "Ken-Sei technique" where the area between the neck and the tip of the shoulder is massaged with special emphasis on this tsubo.

Some of you may wonder why the tsubo on the arm named Hi-Ju is being treated when the symptom is on the shoulder. Hi-Ju happens to be located right over the path of the radial nerve which controls the movement of the thumb and index finger. It is therefore a very important tsubo for maintaining the proper functioning of the arm. As mentioned already in the beginning, fatigue over the shoulders comes from working with one's hands only. Considering the cause of this symptom, therefore, it can be understood why one should never overlook Hi-Ju in the treatment.

K. Stiffness between shoulder blades——Dai-Jo 大杼 (UB-11)

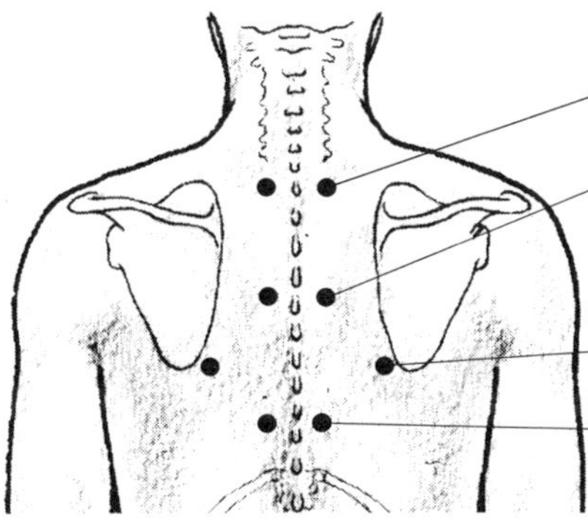

The spinal column is the pillar which supports the upright posture of man. The spinal column is composed of numerous vertebrae held together by ligaments, and it is able to freely move forward and backward and to either side by the action of the erector spinae muscles on both sides. This makes all movements like walking, sitting and standing possible. As long as we are awake, naturally, the erector spinae muscles have to remain in a constant state of tension. When fatigue builds up in these muscles, although symptoms of stiffness appear in the back of the neck as mentioned before, stiffness manifests just as readily between the shoulder blades. Especially since we often sit in chairs with soft cushioning these days, the tension in the erector spinae muscles is even greater, and this causes the area between the shoulder blades (the scapulae) to become very stiff and sore. This symptom often appears in people who have a weakness in their circulatory system and who tend to catch colds and get a bad cough.

The symptom of stiffness between the scapulae, aside from tension in the erector spinae muscles as mentioned, is also caused by tension in the rhomboid muscle connecting the inside edge of the scapulae with the spine. This tension must be removed in order to provide relief. The most important tsubos for this purpose are Dai-Jo 大杼 (UB-11), on either side of the first thoracic vertebra,

Ketsu-In-Yu 厥陰兪 (UB-14), on either side of the fourth thoracic vertebra, and Kan-Yu 肝兪 (UB-18), on either side of the ninth thoracic vertebra. To treat these tsubos, first apply hot compresses using a towel along the lines connecting these tsubos, and follow this with finger pressure and massage. This will improve the circulation and dissolve the stiffness to make one feel much better.

In addition to the above mentioned tsubos, there is one more tsubo which must not be overlooked when there is stiffness between the scapulae. It is Kaku-Kan 膈関 (UB-41), located to the inside of the tip of the scapula. When a person works at a job which requires the use of one's hands only, without movement of the shoulders, tension accumulates around this tsubo almost without exception. This is a symptom commonly seen among sculptors and calligraphers, but also, women with a passion for embroidering or wood carving come to our clinic quite often complaining of stiffness and soreness between their shoulder blades. Also, apply hot compresses between the tsubo Dai-Jo and Kaku-Kan in such cases to warm up the area well, and then give thorough finger pressure and massage.

L. Fatigue over whole back——Kan-Yu 肝兪 (UB-18)

Everyone gets a sensation of heaviness over the back sometime after becoming middle-aged. As one gets older the neck and shoulders tend to become stiff a lot easier. When tension accumulates in the neck and shoulders, this just naturally extends downward to eventually make the whole back feel heavy. Such sensations of heaviness can gradually be worked off by giving tsubo treatments for curing stiffness in the neck and shoulders as detailed in previous sections.

Although this condition is most common in older people, this does not mean that young people do not suffer from the same symptoms occasionally. The part called the middle of the back, or the area between the bottom of the scapulae down to the lowest rib, becomes tense and stiff in young people especially when they become fatigued and their digestive system is out of order, and this can lead to a feeling of heaviness over the whole back. Such symptoms also appear when a person is hung over. Sometimes, when the hangover is very bad, one can feel a distinct hardness in the middle of the back.

The important tsubos for alleviating the sensation of heaviness in the back are Ketsu-In-Yu 厥陰兪 (UB-14), Kan-Yu 肝兪 (UB-18), Jin-Yu 腎兪 (UB-23) and Kan-Gen-Yu 関元兪 (UB-26: on either side of the fifth lumbar vertebra) which are all on a single line on

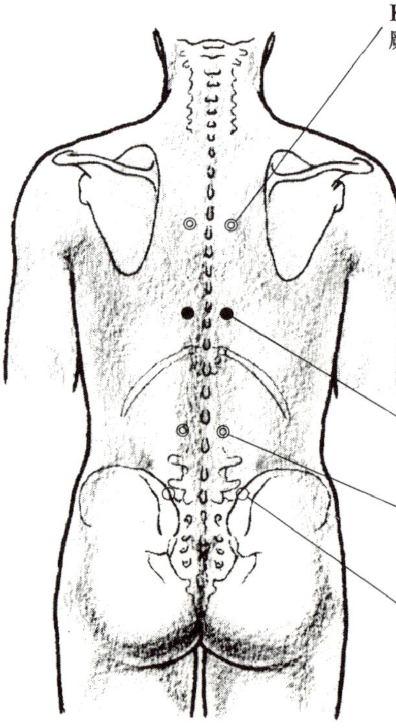

the back on either side of the spine. These are the specially effective tsubos for curing stiffness in the middle of the back. When there is a particularly heavy sensation over the back, try pressing the line connecting these tsubos on both sides of the spine. The muscles down the back are always very stiff and hard for these people and the slightest pressure can feel painful. This is proof that one has become fatigued and that the function of the digestive system has weakened. Sometimes there are other attendant symptoms such as high blood pressure, loss of vigor, swelling of feet and insomnia.

The thing to do is to treat the tsubos on the back, but of course, these cannot be reached by oneself. So therefore, lie face down and have another person give you a good massage on both sides of the spine. The effect is enhanced when each of the tsubos mentioned are pressed somewhat stronger during this massage on the back.

M. Arm cannot be raised——Ken-Gū 肩髃 (LI-15)

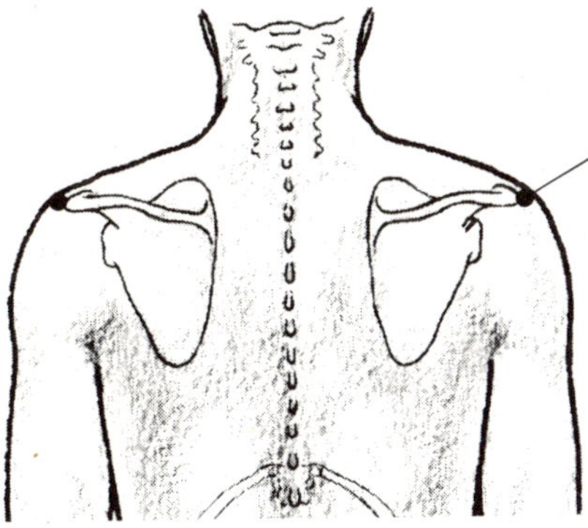

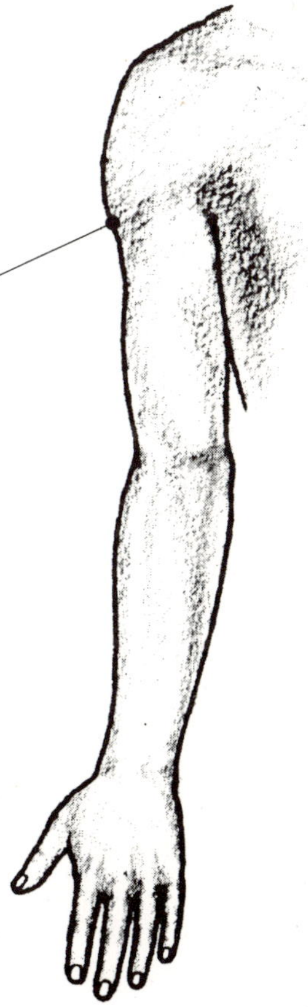

Many of us have had the experience, like the day after lifting heavy objects during a move, where trying to raise our arms causes a sharp pain in the shoulders which is almost enough to make one cry out. Great freedom of movement in the shoulder joint is one physical characteristic of man which not many other animals have, and for this very reason, we seem to experience more problems with our shoulders. Our ability to raise our arms out to the side is the work of the deltoid muscles. When we lift heavy objects, or otherwise force some movement with the arm that places a sudden load on the deltoid muscles, this causes mild inflammation which creates a condition where the shoulders cannot be raised. It is therefore important not to place too great a burden on the deltoid muscles. When this symptom does occur, however, the most important tsubos effective for this condition are Ken-Gū 肩髃 (LI-15), to the front of the tip of the shoulder, and Hi-Ju, 臂臑 (LI-14) located on the side of the upper arm just below where the deltoid muscle of the shoulder ends.

There is another shoulder problem where the arms can be lifted as far up as shoulder level, but cannot be raised over the head. This is a condition which is commonly encountered in "frozen shoulders," which occurs most often with people in their forties and fifties. There is a joint above our chest, under the knot of a necktie, where the sternum and clavicles join, and this is called the sternoclavicular joint. To the outside tips of the clavicles there are the acromioclavicular joints where the clavicles and the scapulae join. Unless these two joints operate smoothly, the arms cannot be raised any higher than horizontal. "Frozen shoulders" occurs because the muscles, ligaments, and tendons around the shoulder joint become more susceptible to inflammation as one advances in age. Naturally, young people also experience a similar condition when they overdo a sport or sustain an injury.

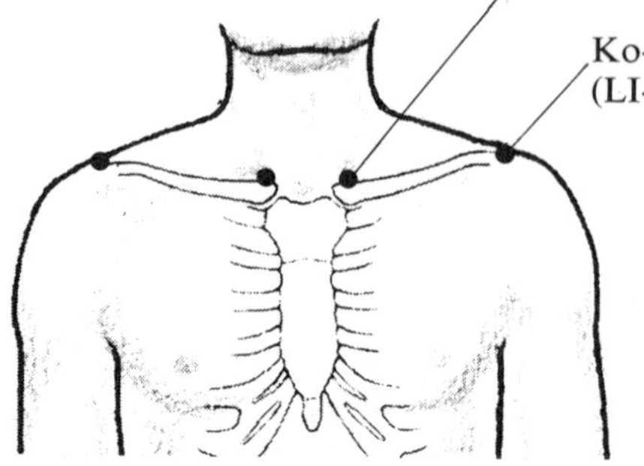

The tsubos effective for conditions where the arms cannot be raised above the level of the shoulders are, Ki-Sha 気舎 (ST-11), above the sternoclavicular joint, and Ko-Kotsu 巨骨 (LI-16), above the acromioclavicular joint. Aside from directly treating the tsubos Ken-Gū, Hi-Ju, Ki-Sha and Ko-Kotsu with finger pressure, giving a thorough massage around these tsubos will yield positive results in time. It is also important to move the arms up and down a bit while massaging, even though this may cause some pain.

N. Fatigue in lower back for the middle-aged——Dai-Chō-Yu 大腸兪 (UB-25)

Even when speaking of low back pain, there are a wide variety of causes including problems in the skeletal or joint structure, colds, neuralgia, digestive disorders, and urological diseases, so it is hard to generalize. The most common type of low back pain for middle-aged people, nevertheless, has to be what is known as a "slipped disk." This is an acute condition resulting mainly from abnormalities in the vertebrae or their joints, such as the displacement of intervertebral disks and spondylosis deformans.

There are, however, those who have no structural abnormalities, but still are beset with stubborn low back pain. This is referred to as the "myofascial syndrome," and it is caused by fatigue accumulating in the quadratus lumborum muscles. This muscle connects the twelfth rib to the pelvis, and as one ages, this muscle tends to become stiff and sore much easier. In addition, the ligaments which connect the spine and pelvis also start to show the effects of aging and lose their elasticity, and this makes the quadratus lumborum muscles that much more prone to fatigue and strain.

The main aim in treatment of the "myofascial syndrome," therefore, is to relieve the tension in the quadratus lumborum muscles and to remove the stiffness. The specially effective tsubos for this purpose are Jin-Yu 腎兪 (UB-23), Dai-Chō-Yu 大腸兪 (UB-25), and Kan-Gen-Yu 関元兪 (UB-26), along the spine on the lower back, as well as Yō-Kan 陽関 (GV-3) located between the

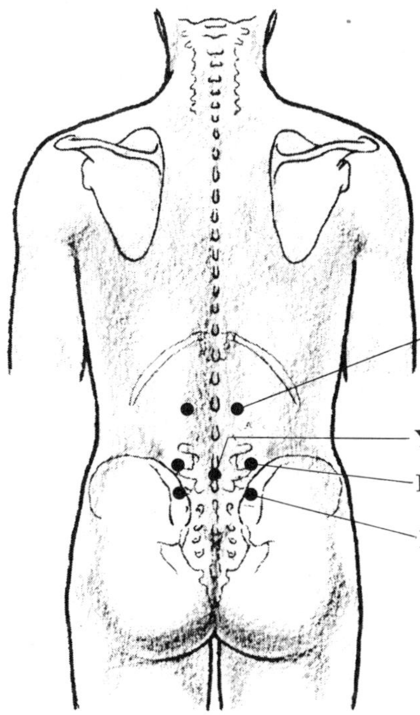

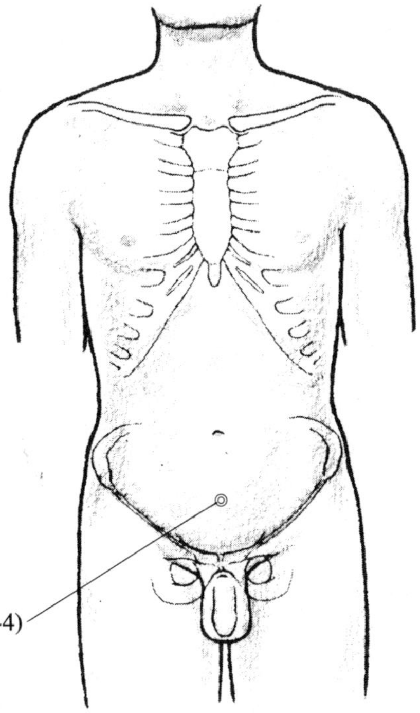

fourth and fifth lumbar vertebrae. The tsubos can be located simply by lying on your back and having someone press both sides of your spine with their thumbs. The tsubos are the places which are tender, but feel good when pressed. Receiving finger pressure around these tsubos is very beneficial, and getting massage treatments along the lines connecting these tsubos is also fine.

It should be noted that low back pain is not solely a problem in the lower back. Normally, when there is low back pain, there is also some tension in the rectus abdominis and transversus abdominis muscles. The reason for this is that, when the lower back is in pain, one has a tendency to stoop forward and this places an added burden on the abdominal muscles. The tsubo, Kan-Gen 関元 (CV-4), located four finger widths below the navel, is very effective for such tension in the abdominal muscles.

O. Low back pain from fatigue of digestive organs——Chū-Kan 中脘 (CV-12)

Generally speaking, the causes of low back pain can be largely divided into the following three categories. One is where deformities occur in the lumbar vertebrae due to aging, and in this case the surrounding ligaments and muscles become tense to put pressure on spinal nerves. This is the type of low back pain discussed in the previous section called "slipped disks." The next type of low back pain is caused by the muscles between the back and the hips becoming fatigued, and this condition has also been discussed already. The last type of low back pain is caused by organic disorders such as digestive problems or urological diseases. People with weak constitutions, especially, seem to suffer from low back pain stemming from digestive problems. In

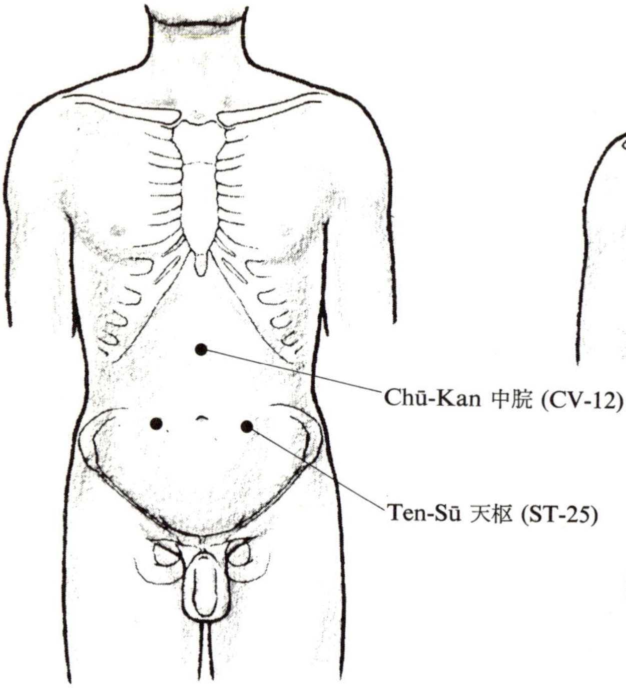

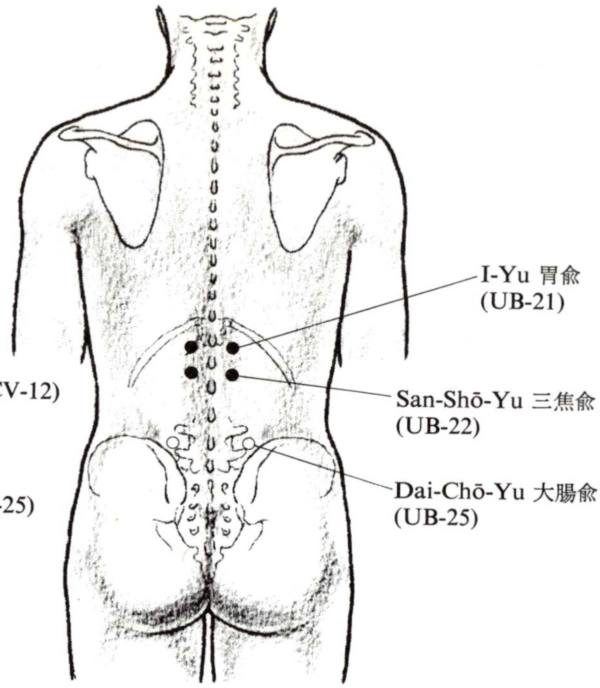

this case there are often other symptoms like a heavy or distended feeling over the stomach, nausea, lack of appetite, and a tendency to be constipated.

No matter how much the lower back may be treated to relieve the last type of low back pain mentioned, there is no real cure. The first priority in this case is to normalize the functioning of the digestive organs. The main tsubos for this purpose are Chū-Kan 中脘 (CV-12), below the pit of the stomach, Ten-Sū 天枢 (ST-25), on both sides of the navel, I-Yu 胃俞 (UB-21), to the side of the point below the twelfth thoracic vertebra, and San-Shō-Yu 三焦俞 (UB-22), just below I-Yu, as well as Dai-Chō-Yu 大腸俞 (UB-25), to the side of the point below the fourth lumbar vertebra. The way to treat these tsubos is to first lie down on your back and apply pressure over your whole abdomen using the palm of your hands, and then massage the lines connecting Chū-Kan and Ten-Sū thoroughly. Next lie on your stomach and get someone to press and massage the lines connecting I-Yu and Dai-Chō-Yu.

As their names imply, I-Yu and Dai-Chō-Yu (stomach and large intestine *yu* points) are important tsubos which regulate the function of the digestive organs. One of the basic principles in tsubo therapy when treating digestive problems is to judge the condition of the organs involved by comparing the reactions occurring on both sides of the body by checking Chū-Kan and Ten-Sū on the front, and I-Yu and Dai-Chō-Yu on the back. Furthermore, since there is chilling of the lower extremities in almost every case of low back pain resulting from digestive disorders, San-Shō-Yu should also be treated. If all the tsubos mentioned are treated thoroughly, the low back pain should gradually be eliminated and one can regain robust health.

P. Low back pain from general fatigue——Jin-Yu 腎兪 (UB-23)

Low back pain is a symptom common among the women beyond middle age, but this is not to say that young people never have backaches. In particular, there seem to be some young women who suffer from a condition where they cannot maintain one posture for very long because of pain in the lower back. For women, menstrual cramps are often accompanied with low back pain, and when there is no problem with the menses, this usually means that fatigue has accumulated in the quadratus lumborum muscle. As already mentioned before, the quadratus lumborum muscle connects the twelfth rib to the top edge of the iliac and serves to coordinate the muscles along the back, hips and legs. Since women often wear high heeled shoes, the quadratus lumborum muscle must remain in a constant state of tension which makes it fatigue that much faster. Furthermore, our means of transportation has become so convenient in recent years that we seem to be walking less and less, and this has caused the muscles in our abdomen and back to become weak which has only increased the amount of stress placed on the quadratus lumborum muscle.

The specially effective tsubo for this condition also happens to be San-Shō-Yu 三焦兪 (UB-22), Jin-Yu 腎兪 (UB-23) and Dai-Chō-Yu 大腸兪 (UB-25) which are lined up along the spine. The effect can be increased even more by also pressing Shi-Shitsu 志室 (UB-47), located two finger widths (using the index and middle fingers) to the outside of Jin-Yu. Begin by heating this area for about twenty minutes using hot compresses or heating pads. When the pain begins to ease, massage along the spine from San-Shō-Yu down to Dai-Chō-Yu, drawing small circles with the fingers, and then end with firm pressure on Shi-Shitsu.

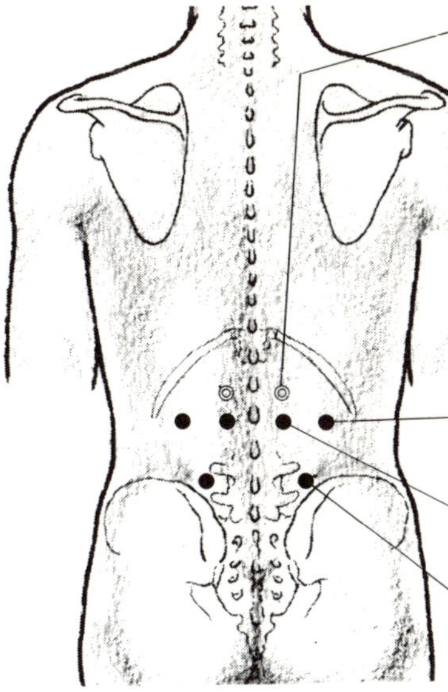

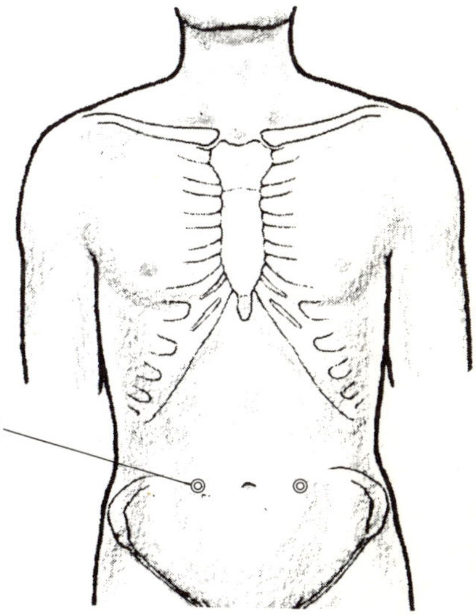

This will make the pain subside, and the person will feel much better.

Low back pain which comes from fatigue in the quadratus lumborum muscle is sometimes accompanied with pressure sensitivity on the abdomen. There are times when the area around the navel becomes hardened and sensitive to the slightest pressure. When this happens, give finger pressure and massage around Ten-Sū 天枢 (ST-25).

There is another specially effective tsubo which should be mentioned here, and it is Rin-Kyū 臨泣 (GB-41), located between the fourth and fifth metatarsal bones on the back of the foot. It may seem unlikely that a tsubo on the feet can cure low back pain, but nevertheless, applying finger pressure on this tsubo during break while at work can be amazingly effective.

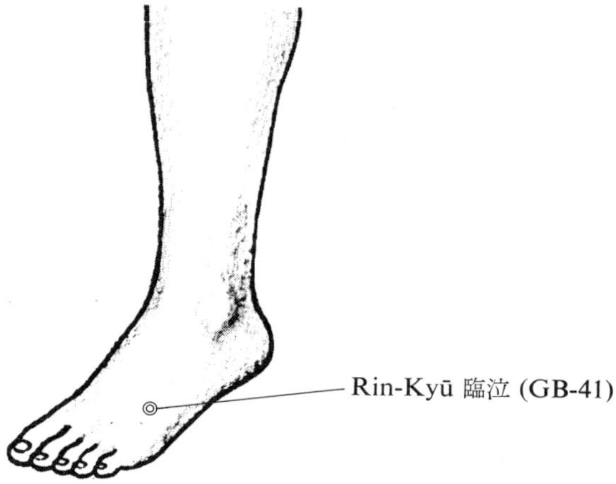

Q. Low back pain from obesity——Ten-Sū 天枢 (ST-25)

There seem to be some obese people who constantly go around thumping their lower back with their fist saying things like, "My back just always seems to ache." Any amount of fatigue immediately appears as low back pain in such people, and when they over exert themselves even slightly, they become unable even to sit up because the pain is so intense.

Our internal organs are held in position by the proper development of the abdominal muscles. When fat accumulates around the abdomen, however, it weakens the muscles holding the internal organs in place from

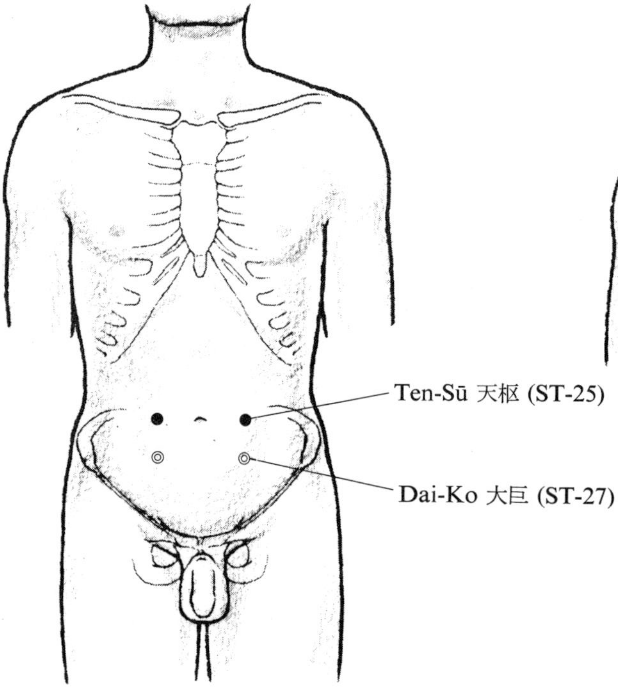

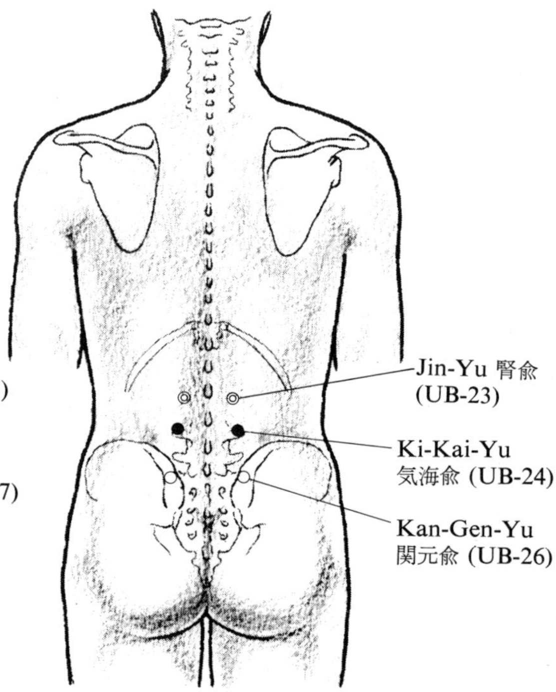

the outside, and the organs fall out of position. Naturally, this means that the organs begin to sag. Gastroptosis where the stomach's position lowers, is one example of this. The displacement of internal organs places an even greater burden on the lower spine and the back muscles, and this sometimes culminates in low back pain. When this is the case, the primary object is to get rid of the excess fat and to restore tone in the abdominal muscles. Therefore, along with tsubo therapy for removing fat, one must also do exercises to strengthen the abdominal muscles.

As for the tsubos to be treated, apply thorough finger pressure and massage along the lines connecting Ten-Sū 天枢 (ST-25) and Dai-Ko 大巨 (ST-27) on the stomach, and also that connecting Jin-Yu 腎兪 (UB-23), Ki-Kai-Yu 気海兪 (UB-24) and Kan-Gen-Yu 関元兪 (UB-26) on the back. Massage and finger pressure treatments on these tsubo just once or twice will not yield any results. It is important to continue these treatments faithfully everyday. There are many exercises one can do to strengthen the abdominal muscles. One can raise the arms over the head and then bend forward to touch the toes. Otherwise, one can lie on the back and sit up without using the arms, or conversely, remain lying on the back and lift the legs up while keeping them stretched straight out. The only thing about these exercises is that they will not have any effect unless they are performed a little every day over a long period. When a person perseveres with the above exercises and tsubo therapy, the fat around the abdomen will eventually come off and strength will be developed in the abdominal muscles. As a result, the sagging internal organs will return to the normal position by themselves, and low back pain should no longer be a problem.

4. Treating Symptoms in the Arms and Legs

A. Fatigue in the arms——Hi-Ju 臂臑 (LI-14)

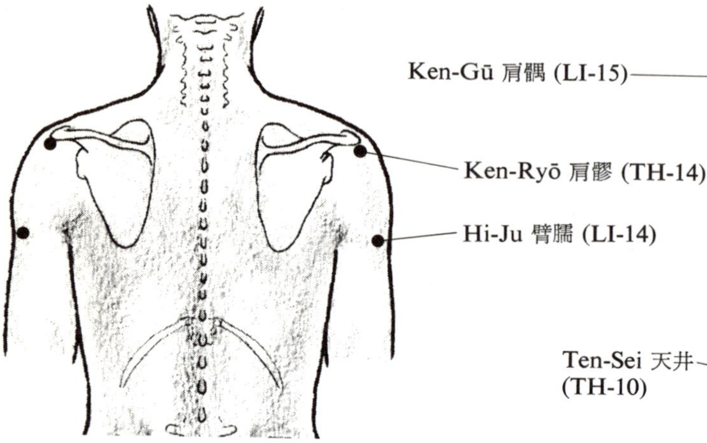

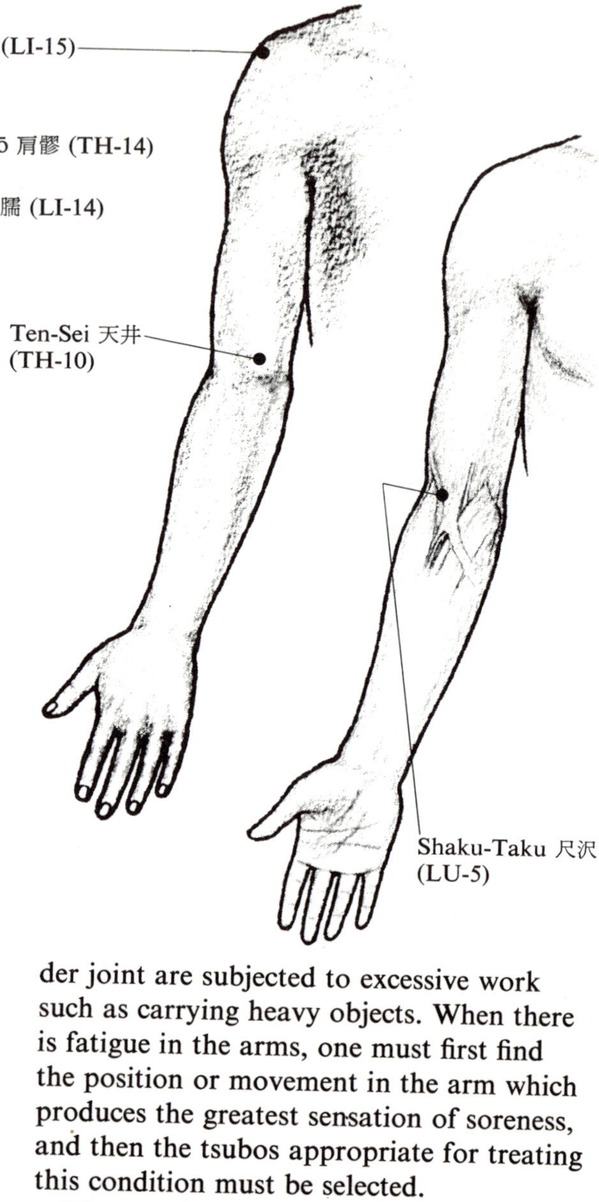

In anatomical terminology the upper arms, from the shoulders down to the elbows, are called the brachium, while the forearms, from the elbows down to the wrists, are called the antebrachium. Even in cases of simple fatigue of the arms, the symptom of soreness usually appears predominantly in either the upper arm or the forearm. The common type of fatigue in the arms which everyone feels now and then is fatigue in the upper arm. It goes without saying, that this is the typical situation where sore arms result because the muscles around the shoulder joint are subjected to excessive work such as carrying heavy objects. When there is fatigue in the arms, one must first find the position or movement in the arm which produces the greatest sensation of soreness, and then the tsubos appropriate for treating this condition must be selected.

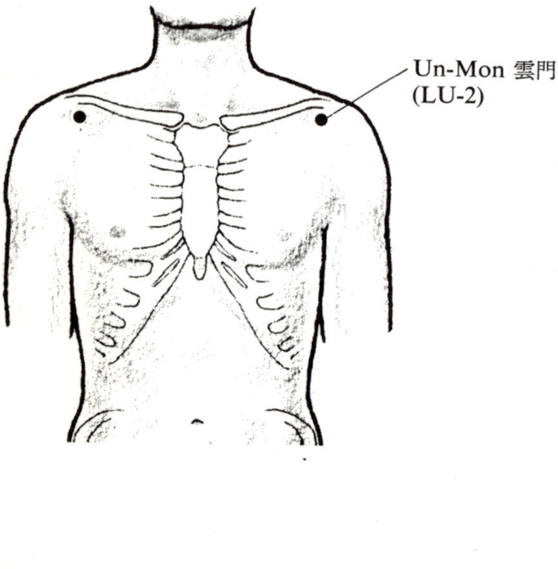

The sore feeling in the arms which occurs most commonly is that which can be felt when the arm is raised to the side. In this case the tsubos Hi-Ju 臂臑 (LI-14) and Ken-Gū 肩髃 (LI-15) discussed before need to be treated. As already stated, the arm is lifted out to the side by the action of the deltoid muscle, and Hi-Ju and Ken-Gū work to restore the function of the deltoid muscle.

If the feeling of soreness occurs when the elbow is extended, Ken-Ryō 肩髎 (TH-14) and Ten-Sei 天井 (TH-10) should be treated. Both these tsubos are located around the origin of the muscles which extend the elbow. Ken-Ryō is slightly to the back of the tip of the shoulder, while Ten-Sei is on the back of the upper arm in the hollow place just above the elbow. These tsubos are known as being effective for pain and numbness extending from the base of the neck down to the shoulders and arms, as well as for chilling of the arms.

Finally, for soreness which occurs when bending the elbow, treat Un-Mon 雲門 (LU-2), just under the outer end of the clavicle, and Shaku-Taku 尺沢 (LU-5) on the inside of the elbow to the outside of the thick tendon of the biceps brachii muscle. It is easy to understand how these tsubos restore the function of the biceps brachii muscle which work to bend the elbow because this muscle bulges up right between these tsubos when the elbow is flexed. Un-Mon, in particular, is a vital tsubo from an anatomical perspective because it is located over a complex network of nerves and blood vessels.

The treatment of these tsubos need not consist only of finger pressure. Grasping successively down the muscle instead, to cover the whole area between the tsubos can also be quite effective. Do not forget to also exercise these parts by moving the shoulders up and down, and forward and backward, as well as by flexing and extending the elbows.

B. Arm cannot be reached around to back——Ken-Tei 肩貞 (SI-9)

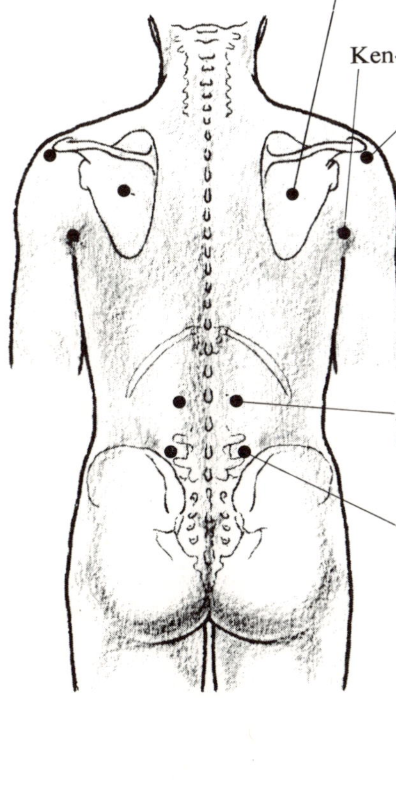

In Japan there are many businessmen who change into traditional house robes to relax, as soon as getting home from work. Sometimes, when these men try to tie the belt of their robes, which tie around at the back, they find themselves unable to do this. This could be a sign that the person is middle-aged, because this is a symptom of "frozen shoulders," very common among the middle-aged. This problem is a real nuisance to the Japanese in particular because things are quite often carried on one's back, and babies and little children as well are commonly carried on the back with the arms.

As already mentioned many times before, "frozen shoulders" is a problem in the shoulder joint which results from aging. On the other hand, if this same symptom appears the day after overexertion, such as carrying some heavy object, it is fatigue in the latissimus dorsi muscle which covers the back from the lumbar vertebrae and goes over the scapulae to reach the armpits. In either case, the specially effective tsubos used to treat this condition are Ken-Tei 肩貞 (SI-9), to the back of the shoulder above the vertical crease of the armpit, Ken-Ryō 肩髎 (TH-14), slightly to the back of the tip of the shoulder, Ten-Sō 天宗 (SI-11), right in the middle of the scapula, Jin-Yu 腎兪 (UB-23), to the side of the point below the second lumbar vertebra, and Dai-Chō-Yu 大腸兪 (UB-25), to the side of the point below the fourth lumbar vertebra.

Along with finger pressure on each tsubo, rub down the area between Ken-Ryō and Dai-Chō-Yu using the palms or just the thumbs. Also, do not forget to provide grasping pressure down the arms. You can feel the latissimus dorsi muscle by grasping the muscle on the backside of the armpit. Grasping a large area of this muscle and massaging it in this way will speed the recovery. Although one should grasp the muscle firmly, care must be exercised not to grasp too strongly. Fatigue in the latissimus dorsi muscle should be relieved completely when the simple exercise of making a fist and moving the arm up around to the back is performed in addition to the tsubo therapy.

All of the tsubos mentioned are very important ones, but Ken-Tei in particular should be kept in mind. The best way to locate this tsubo is to relax both shoulders and let the arms hang down by one's side. There is a crease which forms to the back of the armpit between the arm and the chest, and Ken-Tei can be found just above the top of this crease.

C. Arm cannot be raised forward——Un-Mon 雲門 (LU-2)

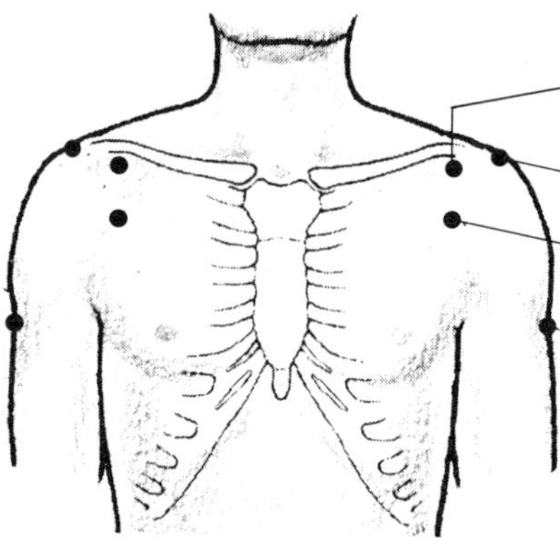

There are people in their mid-forties who experience a slight dull pain from the tip of their shoulder down to their arm in the morning, and they also experience difficulty in lifting their arm forward. This is where a person cannot extend the arms straight out to the front. This condition is commonly referred to as "frozen shoulders." In these cases, there is usually an immediate cause such as the person having done something to overexert his arms such as playing golf. In other words, it is fatigue which comes from sudden strenuous loads being placed on the muscles of the shoulders and upper arms. Finger pressure or massage as described below is very effective in bringing relief.

As already stated, the muscle which works to raise the arm out to the side is the deltoid muscle which lies over the shoulder and ends in the upper arm. The big muscle which bulges up when the arm is flexed is called the biceps brachii muscle. The specially effective tsubos for restoring the function of these muscles, as already mentioned, are Ken-Gū 肩髃 (LI-15) and Hi-Ju 臂臑 (LI-14). Ken-Gū is particularly effective when pressed alternately on both shoulders, and provides relief after one's shoulders have become stiff from too much work or study. Quite often people pound on their shoulders with their fists when it becomes stiff and sore, but pressing Ken-Gū patiently is much more effective.

The next thing to do is to work off the fatigue accumulated in the pectoralis minor and coracobrachialis muscles which work to raise the arm forward. The specially effective tsubos for this purpose are Chū-Fu 中府 (LU-1) and Un-Mon 雲門 (LU-2). Keeping one arm straight down by your side, gently press upward with the other hand in the groove between the muscles of the torso and the muscles of the arm. You will reach a point in the depression under the clavicle about two finger widths below it which is hard and feels tender when pressed. Un-Mon and Chū-Fu are located above and below this point. Both these tsubos, aside from symptoms in the shoulders and arms, are used to treat nose colds and sore throats.

As mentioned briefly when Un-Mon was introduced before, this point lies over a complex network of nerves and blood vessels. Seen from this perspective, it is easily understandable how Un-Mon and Chū-Fu are vital tsubos indispensable for treating symptoms in the arms.

D. Arm cannot be raised to other shoulder——Chū-Fu 中府 (LU-1)

Raise your arm up to your side and then move it to your front; if there is any pain from the tip of your shoulders down to your arm, or if the shoulder joint does not move smoothly, this is a sign that the muscles in the shoulder and upper arm are quite fatigued. Next, without lowering the elbow, take your arm from the straight ahead position and grab the left shoulder with the right hand, or otherwise, grab the right shoulder with the left hand. Sometimes the arm feels heavy or painful when doing this. This condition is also caused when middle-aged office workers strain their arms while golfing on a holiday.

In specialized language, this condition

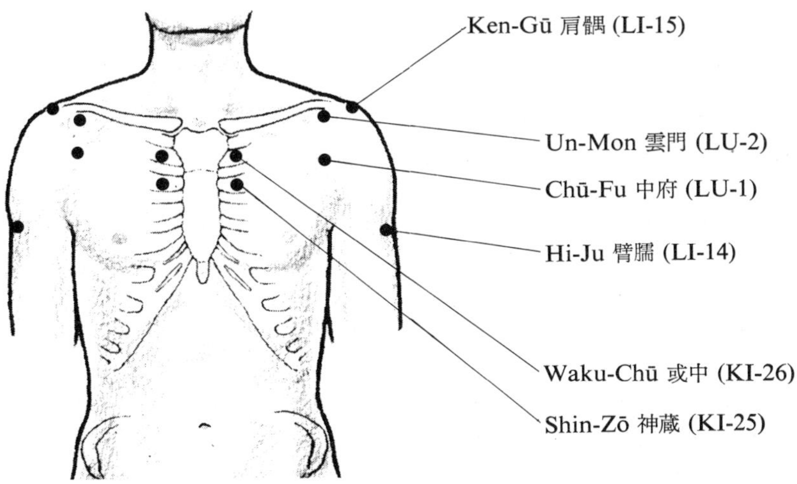

where the arm cannot be raised to the shoulder is termed a problem in the adduction of the shoulder joint. The direct cause is usually fatigue in the pectoralis major and pectoralis minor muscles which work to move the arm forward. Any tension or hardening in these muscles can be felt by grasping the muscle in front of the right armpit with the left hand while extending the right arm straight out in front and moving it toward the left, keeping it level. The pectoralis major is the muscle which can be felt on the top, and the pectoralis minor is the muscle under this.

There are four tsubos related to the function of these muscles that are located right around these pectoral muscles as if to surround them. These are Un-Mon 雲門 (LU-2) and Chū-Fu 中府 (LU-1), right under the clavicle as explained in the previous section, Waku-Chū 彧中 (KI-26), just to either side of the sternum in the second intercostal space, and Shin-Zō 神蔵 (KI-25), similarly located in the third intercostal space. Also, since the deltoid muscle is very much involved in the adduction of the shoulder joint, the tsubos Ken-Gū 肩髃 (LI-15) and Hi-Ju 臂臑 (LI-14) can be supplemented.

When there is pain in the shoulder joint in these cases, the treatment should consist of strong finger pressure on each of the tsubos mentioned. When the pain is very slight, however, it is not so important to be exact about the location of the tsubo. Simply rub down the area around the tsubos with the palm of your hands and massage the area in small circles. Add to this the exercise of moving the shoulders up and down (shrugging) as well as forward and back. Smooth movement of the shoulder joint can be regained when such measures are taken before the condition becomes very serious.

E. Fatigue from elbow to wrist——Shaku-Taku 尺沢 (LU-5)

Man is about the only animal that can throw things for any distance. To throw something like a ball, one's arm has to be extended as far as it will go. A ball cannot be thrown just by extending the arm, however. First the arm has to be drawn back fully to provide a spring-like action. It is obvious that great freedom in movement of the arm is an unique physical characteristic of man. For this reason, the muscles in the forearm for moving the wrist and fingers are especially developed in man. The more developed a muscle is, the softer and more pliable it is, and this also makes it more susceptible to fatigue. Carrying heavy objects, for example, causes fatigue in the forearms very quickly.

In order to alleviate such fatigue, first treat those tsubos on the inside (palmar) surface of the arm. This is because all the flexor muscles, or the muscles which flex the wrist and fingers, are located on the inside of the forearm. The specially effective tsubos for fatigue on the inside of the forearm are Shaku-Taku 尺沢 (LU-5), on the inside of the elbow, and Kan-Shi 間使 (HC-5), four finger widths above the wrist. Shaku-Taku, in particular, is a focal point of a meridian for the flow of *ki* energy and blood as spoken of in Oriental medicine. It is regarded as a vital point which can cause pain and numbness down the arm when energy becomes blocked here. Acupuncture and moxibustion are performed on this tsubo to treat pain caused by neuralgia of the median nerve which travels from the upper arm down into the palm of the hand.

Naturally, when one's arm is fatigued, the muscles in the back of the arm also become tired. The muscles on the back of the fore-

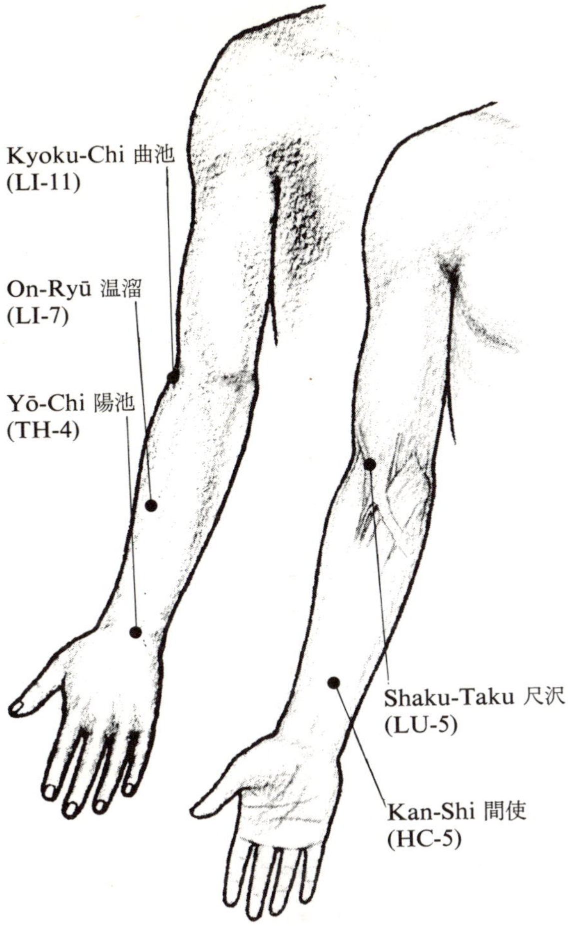

arm work to extend the wrist and fingers. Even better results can be obtained for fatigue in the forearms, when in addition to treating Shaku-Taku and Kan-Shi, also Kyoku-Chi 曲池 (LI-11), just to the outside of the crease in the elbow when it is fully bent, On-Ryū 温溜 (LI-7), on the midpoint of the forearm between the outside of the elbow and the wrist, and Yō-Chi 陽池 (TH-4), in the middle of the wrist on the back, are treated. Yō-Chi has been discussed in detail before, and *Yō-Chi* (yang pond) and *On-Ryū* (collect heat) both mean a place where harmful energy collects, as their names imply. In Oriental medicine, if for example, harmful energy (pathogenic factor) like wind sets in to cause an illness, treating the tsubos where this harmful energy collects is sufficient to dispell and prevent the occurrence of a disease.

The fatigue in the muscles of the forearm can be alleviated by gently pinching up and massaging the muscles along the lines connecting the tsubos mentioned.

F. Elbow cannot be fully extended——Ten-Sei 天井 (TH-10)

Sometimes, after we carry some heavy object for a long time, we get a numb feeling which extends from our shoulders down to our upper arms. In this case, we are unable to extend our elbows fully when reaching for something on a high shelf, and quite often this causes pain in the upper arms. This condition often occurs when a person walks a long distance carrying a heavy suitcase while traveling. The function of extending our elbow is performed by the triceps brachii muscle which extends from the shoulder down to the elbow on the back of the arm. When something heavy is carried for any length of time, the triceps brachii muscle is kept in the extended state for the whole duration, so it is only natural that the circulation slows down in the arm and the ability to extend the arm is weakened.

The specially effective tsubos for restoring the condition of the triceps brachii muscle are Ken-Ryō 肩髎 (TH-14), slightly to the back of the tip of the shoulder, and Ten-Sei 天井 (TH-10), which is in the hollow place directly above the back of the elbow. When the arm is in very poor condition, also treat Ken-Gū 肩髃 (LI-15), slightly to the front of the tip of the shoulder, and Shō-Reki 消濼 (TH-12), at the middle of the back of the upper arm. The method of treatment is exactly the same as that applied for the symptoms discussed in previous sections, and that is to lightly massage and press along the lines connecting the tsubos.

After people become middle-aged, sometimes upon waking up in the morning, they find that they have a heavy stifling sensation over their neck and shoulders, as well as fatigue in the arm and difficulty in moving the fingers. This is called "cervicobrachialgia," and one of the leading causes is an abnormality in the intervertebral disks of the cervical vertebrae which serve as a cushion between the vertebrae. The displacement of these disks puts pressure on the nerves and blood vessels going to the shoulders and arms to produce the above mentioned symptoms.

When the symptoms are quite mild, applying hot compresses like towels or hot packs between the neck and shoulders is enough to relieve the symptoms little by little. When the symptoms become heavier, however, the stiffness and pain cannot be alleviated by hot compresses alone. Even modern medicine does not have a good method for treating this condition. The best results are obtained with physiotherapy like acupuncture and moxibustion. The specially effective tsubos always used in acupuncture are the above mentioned Shō-Reki and Ten-Sei.

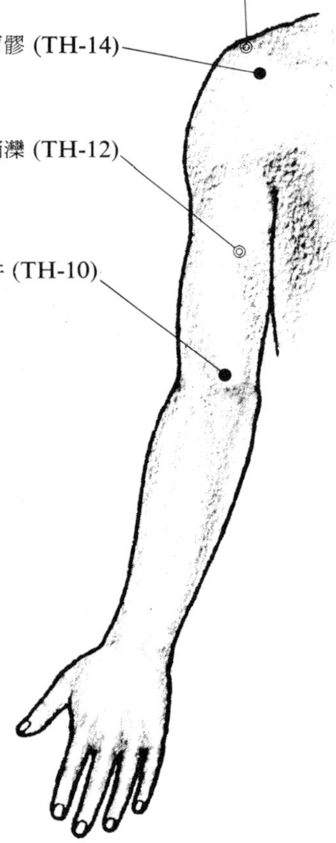

G. Elbow cannot be fully bent——Shaku-Taku 尺沢 (LU-5)

Sometimes a condition opposite to that discussed in the previous section where the elbow cannot be fully bent occurs when working around the house on weekends and performing manual labor which one is not accustomed to. Just try doing some push-ups. After a certain point your arms will get weak and the elbows will become harder to bend.

The muscle that bulges up when a person flexes his arm, as mentioned before, is the biceps brachii muscle which has the function of flexing the arm. The pectoralis major and minor muscles are also operative in bending the arm at the elbow. These muscles are some of the most developed in the body, and since they get a large amount of use, they are that much more prone to fatigue.

The specially effective tsubos Chū-Fu 中府 (LU-1) and Shaku-Taku 尺沢 (LU-5) are used in this case to relieve muscular fatigue. The biceps brachii muscle lies between these two tsubos, and this muscle should be grasped and massaged gently with the thumb and four fingers, or otherwise, rub down the front of the arm and then press each tsubo just strong enough not to cause pain. This will relax the biceps brachii muscle and the elbow will bend fully once more. If the elbow still does not bend well, give light finger pressure between Hi-Ju 臂臑 (LI-14) and Ten-Pu 天府 (LU-3), and massage between these tsubos.

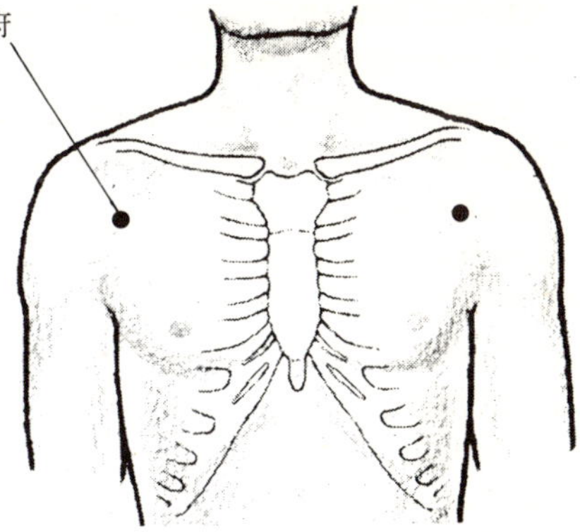

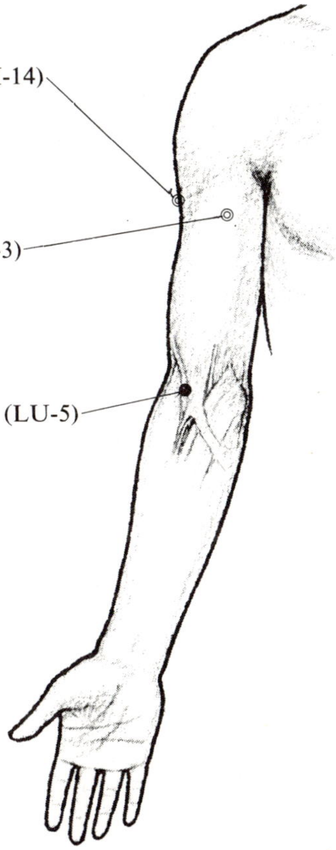

Sometimes, when people carry a heavy backpack over a long distance when backpacking or climbing a mountain, they experience a numbness between the shoulders and the upper arms. When this happens, on occasion, the elbow cannot be bent fully. This is sometimes called "backpacker paralysis," and it is one type of "brachial plexus paralysis" which results from the nerve going to the arm through the supraclavicular fossa being compressed for a long time by the straps of a backpack. There is no need for concern because usually a person recovers from this condition naturally in a few days. When you want to obtain relief from these symptoms as soon as possible, this can be done just by covering the area between the neck and arms with towels soaked in hot water, and blowing hot air on it with a hair drier. The heat and wind pressure serve to relax the tension in the muscles.

H. Fatigue in wrists——Yō-Kei 陽谿 (LI-5)

The flexor and extensor muscles which stretch from the elbow to the tips of the fingers are the muscles responsible for moving the wrist and the fingers. Therefore, when a person works a long time at a job which requires one to use mostly the fingers, before the fingers become tired, the wrists become fatigued. This is a condition which often occurs among writers and editors, and those in other professions which require that a person write a great deal. Fatigue in the wrists is also a type of "occupational disability" for those who have to use their fingers constantly on the job such as key punchers and typists.

As explained before, the flexor muscles

which bend the fingers and wrists are on the inner (palmar) side of the forearm, while the extensor muscles which extend the fingers and arm are on the back side of the hand. In Oriental medicine, the arm to the inside, on the side of the palm is regarded as yin and the back of the arm is regarded as yang. For the purpose of alleviating fatigue in the wrist, the tsubos on both the yin and yang sides of the arm are used. There is a saying which goes, "Yin and yang complement one another," and using tsubos on both surfaces of the body is an important rule in Oriental diagnosis.

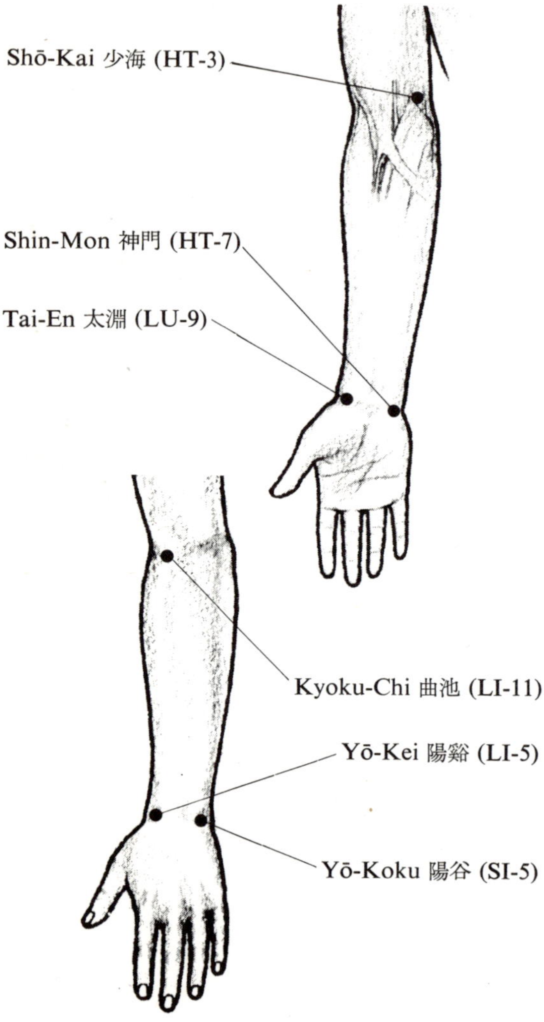

On the side of the wrist toward the palm, there is a tsubo called Tai-En 太淵 (LU-9) at the base of the thumb, and to the base of the little finger there is Shin-Mon 神門 (HT-7). Also, on the back of the wrist there is Yō-Kei 陽谿 (LI-5) which is at the base of the thumb, and Yō-Koku 陽谷 (SI-5) which is in line with the little finger. There are tsubos on the inside of the elbows where a big crease forms in the skin, and the tsubo on the end of this crease in line with the little finger is Shō-Kai 少海 (HT-3), and the tsubo on the opposite side of this crease in line with the thumb is Kyoku-Chi 曲池 (LI-11). The best way to treat these effective tsubos for fatigue in the wrists is to press firmly with the thumbs.

Each of the names of these tsubos above include a character meaning chasm, ravine, valley, sea and pond, respectively, and they are thus conceived as places where harmful energy tend to collect. Nevertheless, these tsubos are not meant only to be troublesome places where the flow of energy becomes blocked up. The amount of harmful energy collected around each tsubo is useful in Oriental medicine for diagnosing the overall condition of the body. The specially effective tsubos are then selected according to the symptoms, and these tsubos are treated in order to clear out the harmful energy and facilitate the flow of energy throughout the body.

l. Chilling of hands——Rō-Kyū 労宮 (HC-8)

It is normal for one's fingers to get chilled in the cold seasons, but there are those who complain of their hands being cold even in milder weather. At times, people even experience unusual sensations like numbness in the tips of their fingers, which causes them to worry if this is an insidious sign of some serious disease. It is true that sometimes such symptoms of chilling and numbness appear in the initial stages of degeneration in peripheral nerves, but the large majority of cases are simply caused by fatigue, and the symptoms are a result of poor circulation of blood from the heart to the hands and the tips of the fingers.

What needs to be done in this case, therefore, is to improve the circulation, and the specially effective tsubos for this purpose are Nai-Kan 内関 (HC-6) and Rō-Kyū 労宮 (HC-8) located toward the palm of the hand, and Yō-Chi 陽池 (TH-4) and Gō-Koku 合谷 (LI-4) on the back of the hand. Rō-Kyū, located in the middle of the palm of the hand between where the middle and the ring fingers touch, is a tsubo for alleviating fatigue in the upper half of the body. Nai-Kan is a tsubo for curing acute symptoms appearing below the elbows. When the wrist is bent backward, two thick tendons can be felt in the center of the forearm to the inside. Nai-Kan is located between these tendons, three finger widths (the index, middle and ring fingers) above the wrist. This tsubo is very effective for chilling of the hands which comes from overwork, as well as for pain and numbness in the shoulder and forearm. Whenever your hands feel cold give strong thumb pressure on these tsubos using your right hand to treat your left hand, and your left hand to treat your right. This should improve your circulation and your hands will even begin to feel warm.

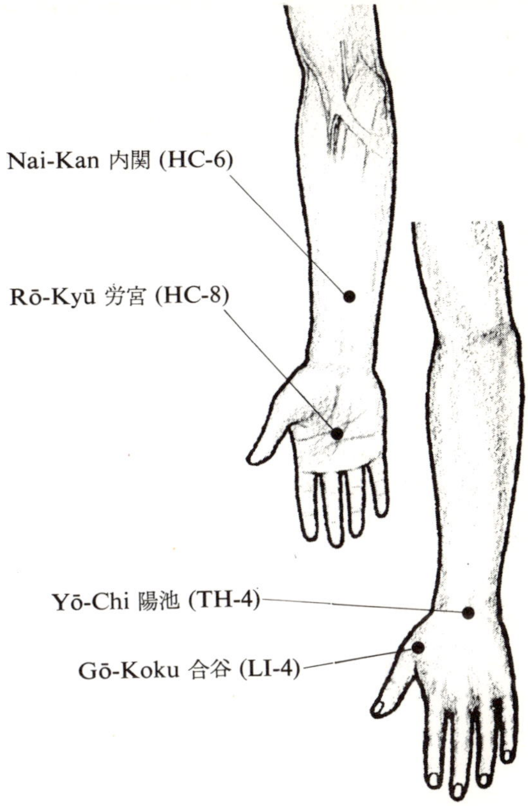

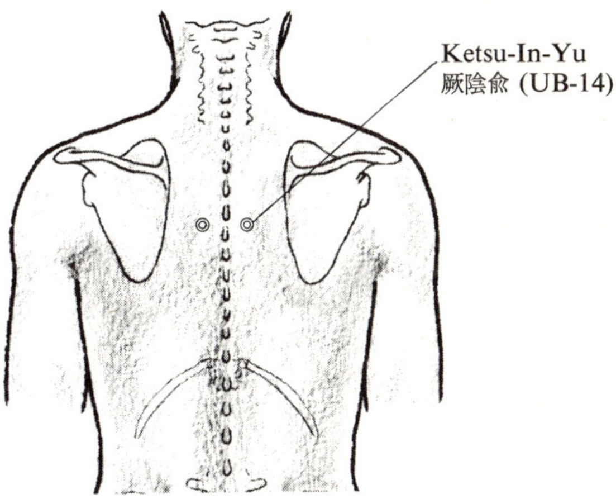

If possible, it would be even more effective to have someone apply gentle pressure on Ketsu-In-Yu 厥陰兪 (UB-14) which is on the back, and to also massage the area slowly in a circular pattern. Ketsu-In-Yu is a vital tsubo for improving circulation throughout the whole body, so it is very good to keep in mind for those who tend to get chilled easily. There are also those who tend to have high blood pressure, or otherwise, low blood pressure, who often feel chilled in their hands. In this case, just giving a good massage on both sides of the hand is sufficient to improve circulation, and one's hands will eventually warm up. At the same time, this treatment will serve to keep a person's blood pressure normal.

J. Hotness in hands——Gyo-Sai 魚際 (LU-10)

Sometimes, when people stay up late many nights in a row working or studying, and they become exhausted both physically and mentally, their hands become hot and feverish in the palms. In Oriental medicine this is referred to as "heat in the palms," and is regarded as a typical sign of overwork and exhaustion. In very simple terms, it is a symptom which results from abnormalities in the autonomic nerves which control circulation in the hands.

As you are well aware, the temperature of our skin surface changes constantly along with changes in our environment such as in temperature and humidity. Change in our skin temperature is also brought about by the difference in the amount of circulation in the hands which is controlled by the constriction, or dilation of blood vessels. The dilation of peripheral blood vessels is controlled by the parasympathetic nerves and constriction is controlled by the sympathetic nerves, both of which belong to the autonomic nervous system which normally cannot be controlled consciously. When a person becomes physically exhausted, the control of the parasympathetic nerves becomes dominant to cause the dilation of blood vessels in the hands which produces a sensation of heat. Conversely, when the function of the sympathetic nerves become hyperactive, the blood vessels in the hand constrict and this causes chilling of the hands as was discussed in the previous section.

In the case of hotness in the palm of the hand, it means that blood circulation is coming more to the hands at the expense of circulation to other parts and organ systems. Therefore, to prevent the exhaustion from causing a more serious disease, the feeling of heat in the hands must be treated right away. When there is any feverishness in

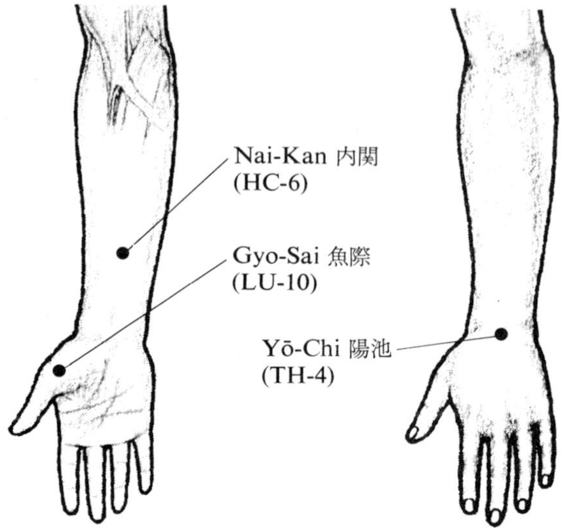

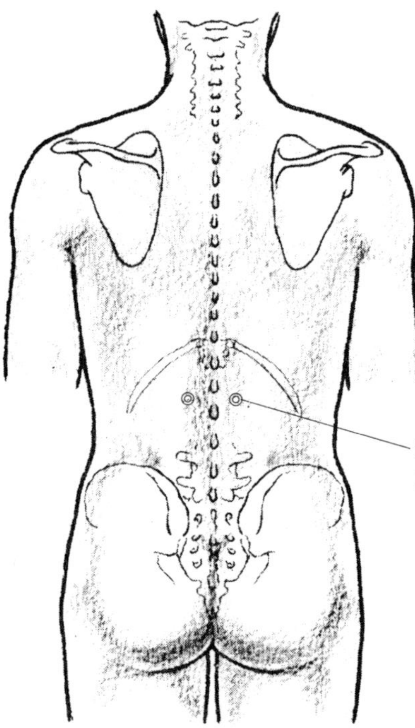

the palms, give thorough pressure on the tsubos Nai-Kan 内関 (HC-6), Gyo-Sai 魚際 (LU-10) and Yō-Chi 陽池 (TH-4) as shown in the figure. This will normalize the circulation and hotness in the hands should be alleviated. Since the tsubo Nai-Kan and

Yō-Chi have already been discussed in detail, Gyo-Sai will be explained.

The mound in the palm of the hand at the base of the thumb is called the thenar region in anatomy, and in Oriental medicine it is called *Gyo-Fuku* 魚腹 (fish belly). The area which feels tender near the bottom of this mound when pinched up lightly is Gyo-Sai. It has been said from the olden days in Japan that if there was intestinal trouble, blue veins appeared on the "belly of the fish." Thus, Gyo-Sai has been used to treat people that have overindulged in food or drink, as well as people who have diarrhea. Also, in this case, it is best to apply finger pressure to the tsubo San-Shō-Yu 三焦兪 (UB-22) that is thought to regulate the temperature through the whole body, which is located on either side of the point below the first lumbar vertebra.

K. Trembling in fingers——Rō-Kyū 労宮 (HC-8)

When a person tries to do exacting work such as writing, after having been lifting heavy objects, one's fingers often tremble and cannot be coordinated. In our bodies the arterioles and venules, as well as capillaries, form a fine meshed network in our muscles. The small muscles in our fingers are no exception to this. When we carry heavy objects, these small blood vessels are compressed and the circulation is reduced. When this happens, the supply of oxygen and nutrients necessary for muscular activity is insufficient, and furthermore, the elimination of the cellular waste products such as lactic acid also does not proceed smoothly. As a result, muscular activity is impaired and the fingertips begin to tremble, or otherwise, there is a disturbance in their sensitivity and they feel cold.

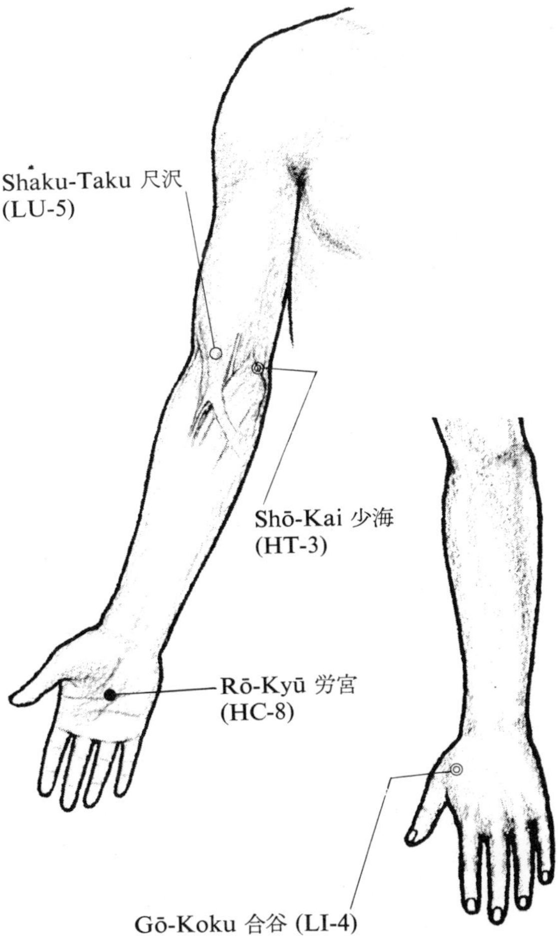

As mentioned many times earlier, the specially effective tsubo for improving circulation in the hand and alleviating fatigue is Rō-Kyū 労宮 (HC-8), in the middle of the palm of the hand. Pressing Rō-Kyū on the left hand firmly with the right thumb, or vice versa, will effectively prevent trembling in the fingertips after carrying heavy objects. Often we find ourselves pressing the center of our palms without thinking about it when our fingers have become sore from writing too much. This unconscious action actually serves to alleviate fatigue in the hands and fingers.

Another thing which must be noted about carrying heavy objects is that the fingers are not the only place where the circulation is impaired. Naturally, similar symptoms of poor circulation also appear in the palms and the backs of the hands, as well as from the wrist to the elbow. When this happens, aside from trembling in the fingers, often the whole arm below the elbow feels tense and begins to shake. Therefore, in this case it is also recommended that rather strong pressure be applied on the tsubos Shō-Kai 少海 (HT-3), Gō-Koku 合谷 (LI-4) and Shaku-Taku 尺沢 (LU-5).

Gō-Koku, as mentioned before, is located on the back of the hand on the web between the thumb and the index finger. It is also called *Ko-Kō* (tiger's mouth) because the hand looks much like a tiger's head with an open mouth when a shadow is cast with the thumb downward.

L. Weakening of fingers——Shō-Kai 少海 (HT-3)

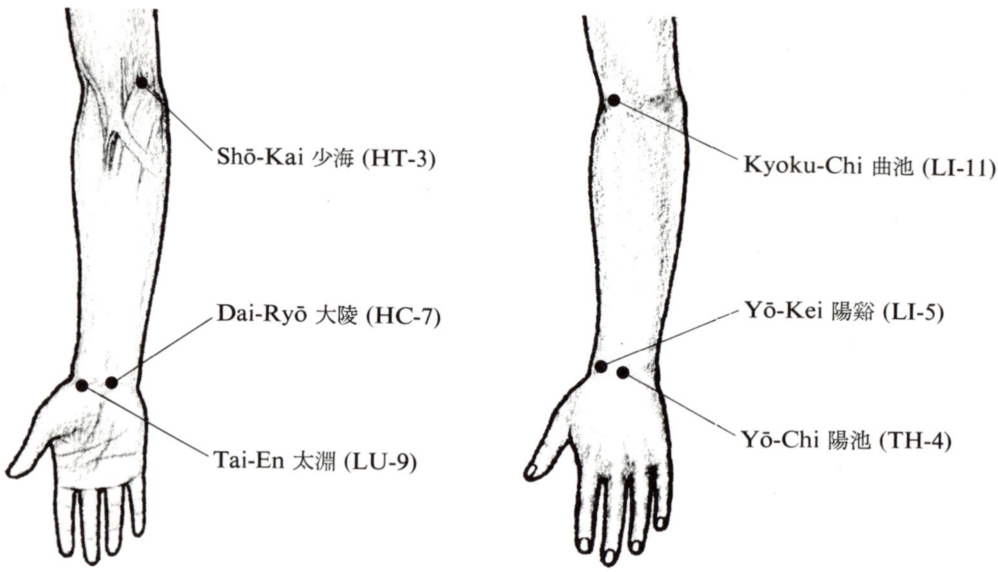

Fatigue in the forearm or the fingers is manifested by soreness in the wrists and trembling in the fingers, just as discussed previously. Another related symptom is where one loses strength in the fingers. Many people come to our clinic with such complaints, and the majority of them are typists and key punchers, or otherwise have jobs that require constant use of the fingers. Nevertheless, symptoms in the fingers are not limited to people in such job classifications, because these symptoms are a common occurrence among ordinary individuals as well.

As explained briefly before, the muscles of the arm which extend the fingers begin at the elbow on the same side as the thumb and go to the back of the hand, while the muscles which bend the fingers start from the elbow on the side of the little finger and pass under the palm of the hand to reach the tip of the fingers. In order to treat the symptoms mentioned above, whenever there is a loss of strength in a hand, you must determine whether it is weak while extending the fingers, or weak when bending the fingers. The tsubos must be used selectively according to what you find. When the fingers are weak when extending, treat the tsubos Kyoku-Chi 曲池 (LI-11), Yō-Kei 陽谿 (LI-5), and Yō-Chi 陽池 (TH-4), on the back of the arm. When the fingers are weak in bending and one has difficulty in grasping things, the important tsubos for treatment are Shō-Kai 少海 (HT-3), Tai-En 太淵 (LU-9), and Dai-Ryō 大陵 (HC-7), on the inside of the arm. Most of these tsubos have been discussed before, so Dai-Ryō which has been mentioned for the first time will be explained.

Dai-Ryō is located right in the middle of the inside of the wrist, between the two big tendons which appear when the wrist is flexed toward the inside. It is written in the classics of Oriental medicine that "the organ which is the most yang among all yang parts of the body is the heart, and its source comes out at Dai-Ryō." It is thus inferred that whenever a person has symptoms associated with heart problems, Dai-Ryō most often becomes sore or painful to the touch.

The way to treat these tsubos mentioned above is to use finger pressure, but massaging along the lines connecting these tsubos is also very good. When giving a tsubo treatment, first warming the area for about twenty minutes with a hot towel or a hot pack will increase the effects tremendously. Give a thorough massage to the areas around each tsubo after warming it up.

M. Hotness in hands and chilling of feet——Rō-Kyū 労宮 (HC-8)

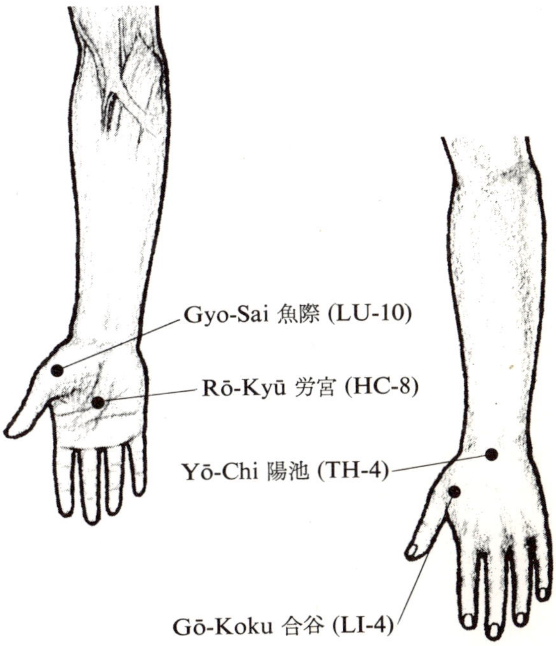

The physiological norm of skin temperature for a healthy individual is about 34°C on the average. In terms of various parts of the body, the skin temperature for a healthy person is around 34°C on the forehead, 32°C on the arms and legs, and 30°C to 32°C at the feet. When a person becomes tired, however, most often the hands begin to feel hot and the feet start to feel chilled. Oriental medicine attaches great importance to such "hotness" or "chilling." Feeling heat in the hands as discussed previously is a sign of overwork and exhaustion. Also, when circulation in the organs of the lower abdomen, or the pelvic region, become impaired, this causes chilling of the feet. In both cases the function of the autonomic nervous system controlling peripheral circulation is adversely affected and causes a marked loss of circulation in one part of the body, while increasing the amount of circulation in another part.

In order to treat this condition, before pressing the tsubos, first warm up the waist area. This is because the major blood vessel supplying the legs branches into both legs at the height of the fourth lumbar vertebra, approximately where the belt goes across on the waist. Warming this area will serve to warm up the entire leg right down to the tips of the toes. The tsubos to treat in this case are Gyo-Sai 魚際 (LU-10), Rō-Kyū 労宮 (HC-8), Yō-Chi 陽池 (TH-4) and Gō-Koku 合谷 (LI-4). Just pressing each tsubo

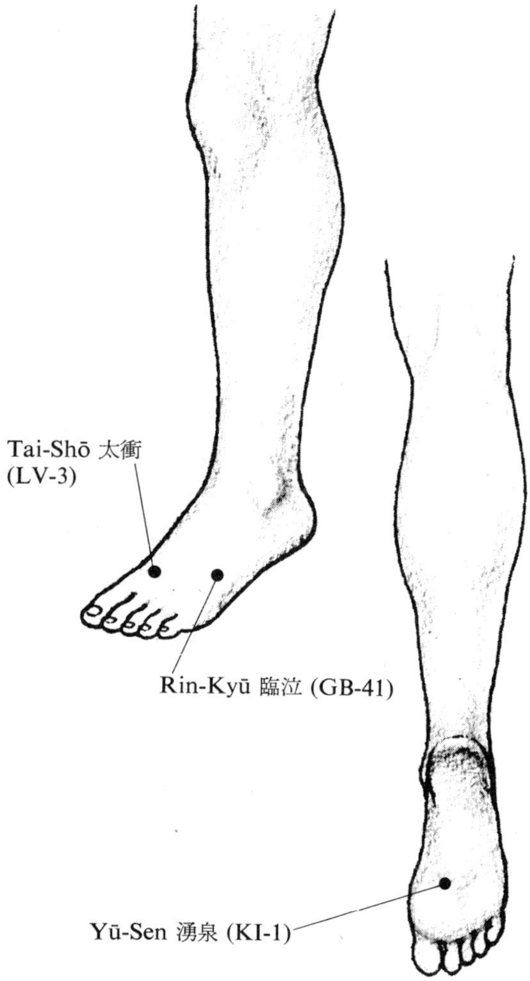

with a slight kneading action is quite effective. Generally, kneading and poking around a tsubo is not considered as being a very refined approach, but it is actually quite effective from the standpoint of actual physical benefits.

The specially effective tsubos for warming up the feet are Tai-Shō 太衝 (LV-3), Rin-Kyū 臨泣 (GB-41) and Yū-Sen 湧泉 (KI-1). The part of the feet which usually becomes chilled is the area below the Achilles tendon, or the entire area covered, by socks. Firmly grasping the area above each tsubo on the foot therefore gives good results.

Another method which is simple and very effective is alternately soaking the feet in hot and cold water. The best way to do this is to fill one basin or bucket with hot water between 42°C and 45°C, and to fill another basin with cold water. Start by soaking your feet for about three minutes in the hot water and then soak them in the cold water for about a minute. Repeat this about three times in a row and then rub down the feet vigorously with a dry towel. This will make the feet feel warm and glowing. Also, in addition to warming up the feet, amazingly enough, this will serve to reduce the heat in the palms of one's hands.

N. Fatigue in front of thigh——Fuku-To 伏兎 (ST-32)

No matter how healthy a person may be, walking for longer distances than one is used to, or otherwise going on hikes up and down steep mountain trails, causes fatigue in the lower half of the body, and makes one's thighs feel heavy and tired. This is only a natural physical reaction to strenuous exercise, but the reason fatigue appears in this fashion can be understood by examining the structure of the muscles in the thighs. Firstly, to the front of the thighs, there is the quadriceps femoris muscle which starts from the front of the pelvic bone (iliac) and goes into the knee where it attaches firmly on the back of the kneecap. This muscle attaches to the pelvic bone in four different places, and since it is a very large muscle, it starts out as thick and hard tendons. Whenever we visit physicians, they check our reflexes by hitting a point right below our kneecap with a special hammer, and this tendon is actually an extension of the quadriceps femoris muscle. The muscles of the thighs are thus very deeply related with the workings of the knee. The quadriceps femoris muscle works to extend the knee completely with great force. This is the reason our knees begin to feel unsteady when the muscles in our thighs are sore and tired.

When this happens, slowly extend the knees and give firm grasping pressure from the bottom of the knee up to the thigh, placing the thumbs toward the inside of the leg and the four fingers toward the outside. Also, while doing this, press the following three tsubos; Kyo-Ryō 居髎 (GB-29), below the most prominent part of the pelvic bone to the front, Kan-Chō 環跳 (GB-30), just to the front of the protuberance (greater trochanter) on top of the thighs to the outside of the leg, and Fuku-To 伏兎 (ST-32), right in the middle of the front of the thighs straight above the kneecap. The name *Fuku-To* (laying rabbit) comes from the bulge in the muscles on the front of the thighs being likened to the rounded back of a rabbit.

It would be ideal if the area immediately around the knee could also be treated. There are two hollow places to either side of the leg just under the kneecap. The hollow place to the inside is called *Nai-Shitsu-Gan* 内膝眼 (inside knee eye) and that to the outside is called *Gai-Shitsu-Gan* 外膝眼 (outside knee eye). These extra tsubos got this name because the hollow places under the kneecap looks somewhat like eyes. Both of these are important tsubos for treating fatigue in the muscles of the thighs. Press these tsubos firmly with the thumbs of both hands, and massage over these tusbos by moving the fingers back and forth while pressing. The muscles of the thighs should begin to feel much better after this treatment.

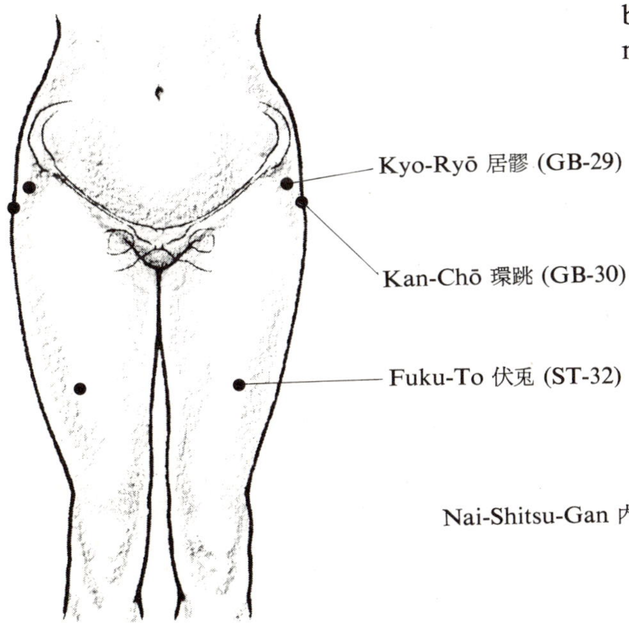

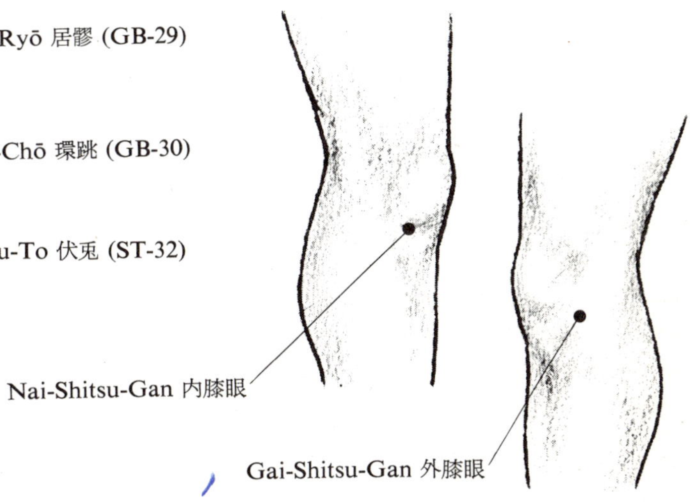

O. Fatigue in back of thigh——Shō-Fu 承扶 (UB-50)

Another condition which results from overworking the legs is one where the opposite side of the legs from that discussed in the previous section is affected, and the back of the thighs become heavy and sore, and also the legs become difficult to fully extend. Flex

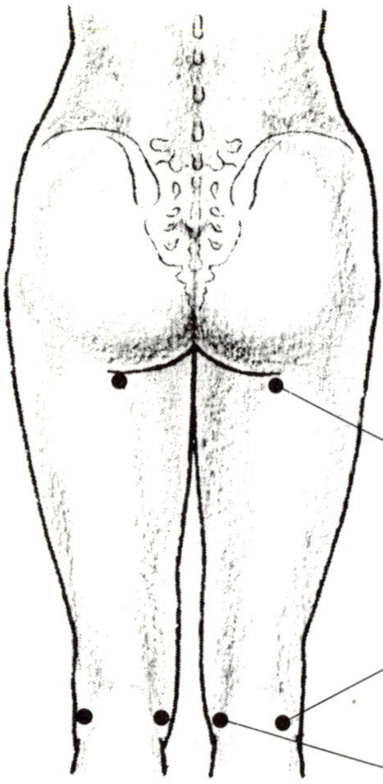

your knee and feel the back of your thigh from the bottom of your hip down. You should be able to feel two large muscles to the outside and the inside of the thigh. The muscle to the outside is called the biceps femoris muscle, and it works to flex the knees with great force, in opposition to the quadriceps femoris muscle which extends the knee joint. Generally, the reason the back of one's thighs feel sore and tired is because this muscle is fatigued.

The method of grasping down the thighs is used to treat this condition also. Begin grasping from just under the hips and work downward until you reach the place where the biceps femoris muscle divides into two tendons at the inside of the knee. This muscle should be grasped firmly between the thumb and four fingers to be kneaded around. The specially effective tsubos to be pressed at this time are Shō-Fu 承扶 (UB-50), I-Yō 委陽 (UB-53), and In-Koku 陰谷 (KI-10).

Shō-Fu is noted as being a specially effective tsubo for sciatica, which is a pulling pain which radiates from the back of the thighs down to the foot. When there is a sharp pain in the back of the legs like sciatica, fatigue and soreness also result in the muscles of the hips because they work harder to avoid pain. In the case of fatigue in the back of the thighs, there are also symptoms in the hip muscles, although not to a great an extent as in sciatica. When a person stands straight up, two horizontal creases form under the buttocks on both sides. Shō-Fu is located in the middle of this horizontal crease. I-Yō is in the back of the knee on the outside, while In-Koku is on the inside. After giving thorough finger pressure to the above three tsubos, it is important to follow this up with firm grasping pressure down from Shō-Fu to I-Yō and also from Shō-Fu to In-Koku.

Usually when one's thighs become fatigued, it is very rare for only the front, or the back to become fatigued. The muscles to the thighs are interlinked by flexion and extension movements, so the knees are not really affected until fatigue has affected both the front and back of the thighs. When the back of the thighs feel particularly sore and tired, use the tsubos listed above, and supplement these with treatments on the tsubos discussed in previous sections.

P. Shaking in the knees——Ryō-Kyū 梁丘 (ST-34)

Sometimes it happens that someone who rarely participates in sports is compelled to play in a baseball or volleyball game with his company or neighborhood group, where after exercising vigorously, his knees buckle under him and he cannot stand up for a while because his knees shake so badly. In Japan, shaking in the knees is sometimes

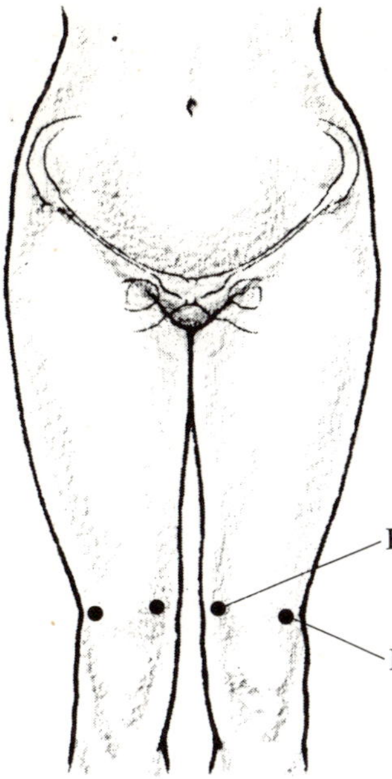

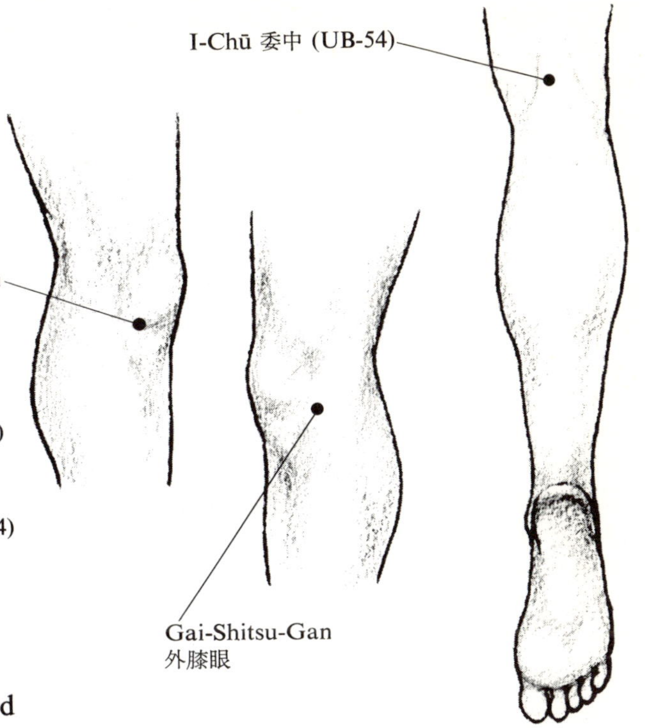

called "the knees laughing." This is an interesting expression since the knees could be "laughing" at the person because he is so out of condition. As touched on earlier, shaking in the knees is a symptom which results from weakness in the muscles on the front of the thighs. In other words, shaking knees, rather than being fatigue in the knees itself, is caused by fatigue and impairment in the muscles which flex and extend the knee joint. This is why treating only the points around the knee is generally not effective.

There is a slight groove on the outside of the leg right above the kneecap (outer edge of quadriceps femoris muscle) when the knee is fully extended, and the tsubo Ryō-Kyū 梁丘 (ST-34) is five to six centimeters above the top of the kneecap, around where this groove ends. In a similar manner, there is a groove above the inside of the kneecap (inner edge of quadriceps femoris muscle), and the tsubo Kek-Kai 血海 (SP-10) is located at the top end of it. Press these tsubos on the opposite sides of the leg.

Next, bend the knee at a 90 degrees angle and use both thumbs to press Nai-Shitsu-Gan 内膝眼 (extra tsubo), in the hollow place just below the knee to the inside, and Gai-Shitsu-Gan 外膝眼 (extra tsubo), in the hollow place to the outside. The tsubo I-Chū 委中 (UB-54), in the center of the crease in the back of the knee is also important, and it is particularly effective for pain in the knees after sitting a long time in an uncomfortable position.

To treat shaking in the knees, aside from using tsubos around the knee, it is also important to use those on the thigh. Fatigue down the whole leg can be alleviated by supplementing the above treatment with that described in the sections for fatigue in the front and back of the thighs, and this will also serve to cure shaking in the knees. The important point is to always treat fatigue in the knees as being a consequence of fatigue in the leg as a whole.

Q. Fatigue in the shin area——Ashi-San-Ri 足三里 (ST-36)

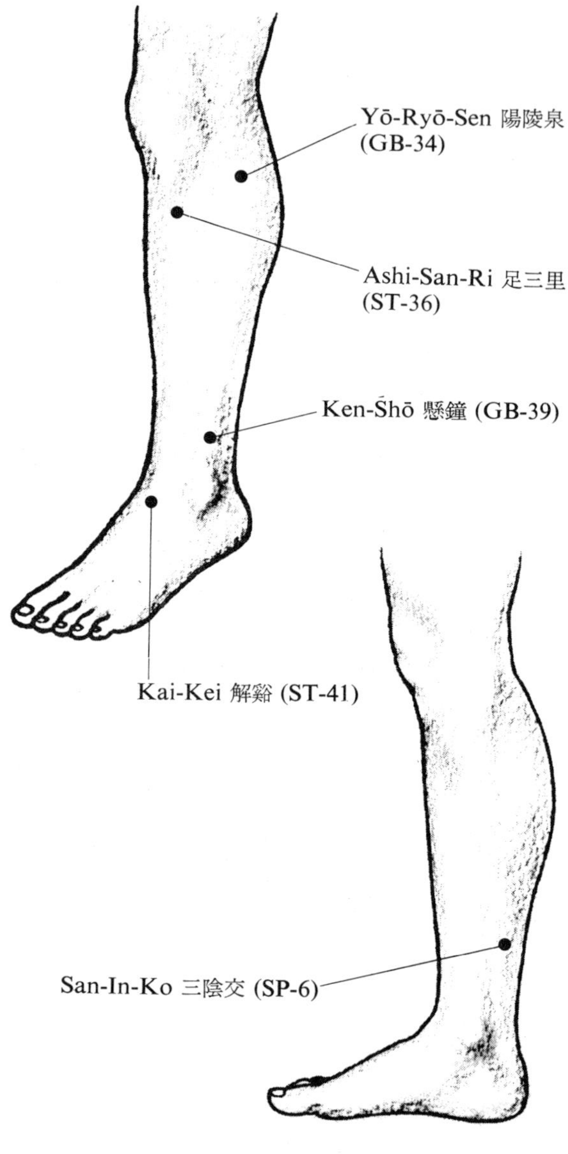

The feeling of fatigue in the shin area usually results from using one's legs too much in strenuous exercise which one is not accustomed to, or otherwise, from walking long distances. The front of the lower leg has two different muscles and they are the extensor hallucis longus muscle to the inside which flexes the ankle joint and extends the big toe, and the extensor digitorum longus muscle to the outside which extends the toes. Fatigue in the shin area is simply fatigue in these two muscles.

To alleviate fatigue in the shin area, first massage vigorously from the knee down to the ankle using the inside of the wrists. Often, people goad or poke the muscles in their shin area with their thumbs, but this is not very effective. The reason for this being that the muscles of the shin area, compared to the calf muscles, are harder because they serve to hold and support the joints. Hard muscles are generally weaker than soft muscles and the more the shin area is goaded, the more it will hurt, and eventually the ankles will become very weak. This is why, no matter how tired and sore it may feel, it is better not to goad or to poke the shin area with one's fingers. Fatigue in the shin area can be eliminated just by giving vigorous massages down the front of the legs, and applying firm pressure along with circular movements on the specially effective tsubos using the index or middle fingers.

The specially effective tsubos for fatigue in the shin area are Ashi-San-Ri 足三里 (ST-36) and Kai-Kei 解谿 (ST-41). There is a thick tendon to the front of the ankle in line with the big toe, and Kai-Kei is located just to the outside of this in a hollow place where the bone can be felt underneath. Aside from the above tsubos, also treat Yō-Ryō-Sen 陽陵泉 (GB-34), just below and to the front of the head of the fibula, Ken-Shō 懸鐘 (GB-39), four finger widths above the outer ankle bone, and San-In-Kō 三陰交 (SP-6), the same distance above the inner ankle bone.

It often happens that the shin area becomes tense after breaking in a new pair of shoes. This occurs because new shoes feel different than usual, and without knowing it we put more strength in our feet to maintain our balance. It is easy to understand why fatigue builds up in this way, once you become aware of the role of muscles in the shin area.

R. Fatigue in the calves——Shō-Kin 承筋 (UB-56)

Often we see people in the office sitting at a desk who are rubbing and massaging their calf muscles without really being aware of it. Somehow it is ingrained in us to first give our attention to this area whenever our legs feel tired. Originally our legs were designed for kicking or pushing backward, and this is very apparent when we observe the movements of four-legged animals such as dogs and cats. Four-legged animals move forward by extending their front legs and pushing backward with their hind legs. Man has assumed an upright posture, but still there is no difference from other animals in that we must push backward with our legs to move forward. As you already may know, the muscles that work to push the lower leg backward are the calf muscles. The calf muscles extend from the back of the knees to the heels and attach firmly on the heel with the Achilles tendon. Muscles of the calf also terminate at the base of the big toe and the little toe to provide three points of support which hold the leg straight and play a vital role in holding the body erect.

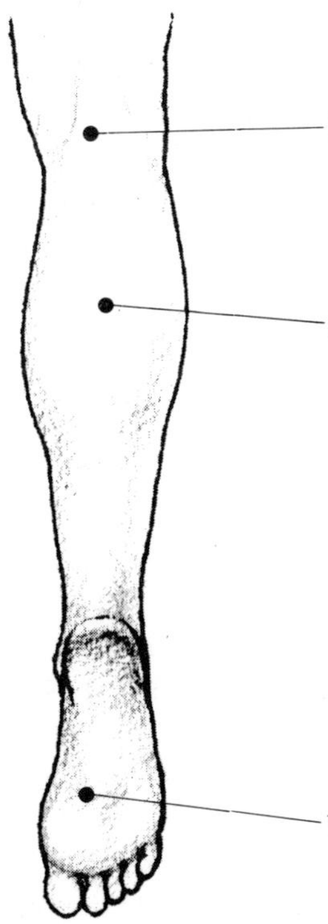

The tsubos effective for fatigue in the calves are, firstly I-Chū 委中 (UB-54), in the middle of the back of the knee, secondly Shō-Kin 承筋 (UB-56), in the middle of the calf muscle at the highest point, and thirdly Yū-Sen 湧泉 (KI-1), in the middle of the back of the foot. The important point about treating these tsubos is never to use too much force when pressing Shō-Kin and I-Chū. Gently stroking these tsubos is usually enough. Only Yū-Sen needs to be given firm thumb pressure with enough force to cause a penetrating sensation.

Another approach which should not be overlooked when giving tsubo treatments is to grasp down the calf muscle with the thumb and four fingers. Begin just below the knees and work your way slowly down to the Achilles tendon. The treatment to alleviate fatigue in the calves can be considered complete when, in addition to this, the heels and the bases of the big toes and little toes are thoroughly massaged with both thumbs.

S. Fatigue in Achilles tendon——Shō-Zan 承山 (UB-57)

Mr. Yazawa, a professional baseball player in Japan who plays for the Chūnichi Dragons, wears spikes which almost look like boxing shoes that go up to the calves. The reason he wears these special shoes is because once in a mishap on the field his Achilles tendon was severed, and such an injury can put an end to the career of a professional ball player. If this happens again, it could retire him permanently, so Yazawa received special permission from the baseball commissioner to wear specially designed spikes. It is an obvious point that the Achilles tendon plays a crucial role, not only in the lives of professional athletes, but in the day to day activities of all of us.

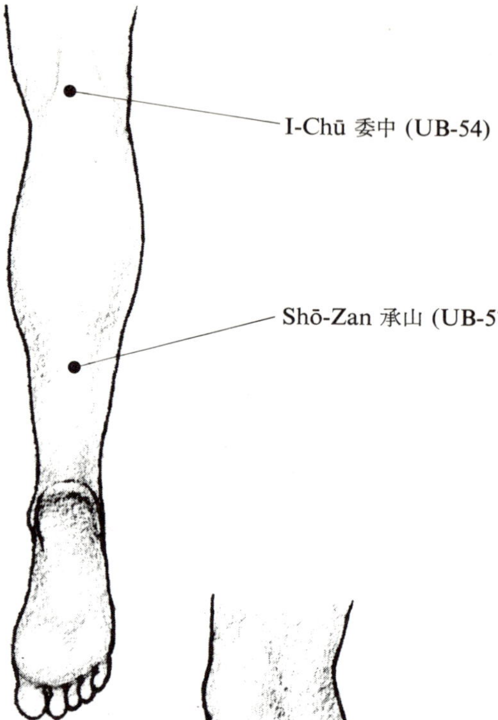

The Achilles tendon forms the bottom end of the triceps surae muscle of the calf which forms a hard tendon just above the heel. Occasionally, when a person engages in vigorous exercises, especially like kicking very hard even though one's calf muscles are very fatigued, the Achilles tendon will break. Of course, the Achilles tendon is very thick, and is attached very firmly to the heel bone, so it does not usually break unless an inordinate amount of force is brought to bear on it.

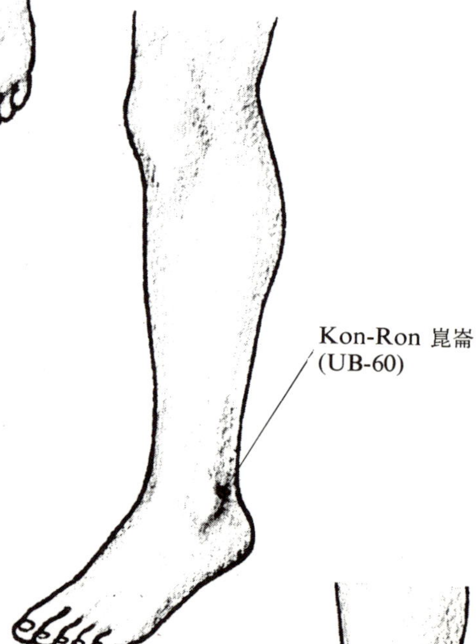

When people work standing up for extended periods, fatigue accumulates in the calves and in the Achilles tendon, and this increases the tendon's susceptibility to such lesions. Alleviating the fatigue in these muscles is therefore the best way to strengthen one's legs. The treatment recommended for this purpose is to alternately immerse the legs in hot and cold water as explained earlier. The alternate stimulation of heat and cold will cause the blood vessels in the feet to expand and contract, and this will improve the circulation and alleviate the fatigue surprisingly fast.

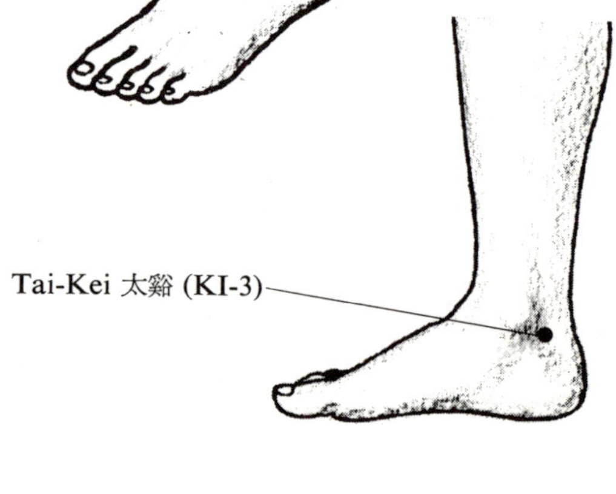

After alternately soaking the legs in hot

and cold water, give thorough finger pressure to I-Chū 委中 (UB-54), in the back of the knee, Shō-Zan 承山 (UB-57), to the bottom of the calf muscle, Kon-Ron 崑崙 (UB-60), right behind the outer ankle bone, and Tai-Kei 太谿 (KI-3), just to the back of the inner ankle bone. The tsubos Kon-Ron and Tai-Kei are especially noted as being good for strengthening the area where the Achilles tendon attaches to the heel. Since the Achilles tendon is an extension of the triceps surae muscle of the calf it is easy to understand why, in order to strengthen the Achilles tendon, the tsubos on the calf muscle require attention.

7. Fatigue in ankles——Yū-Sen 湧泉 (KI-1)

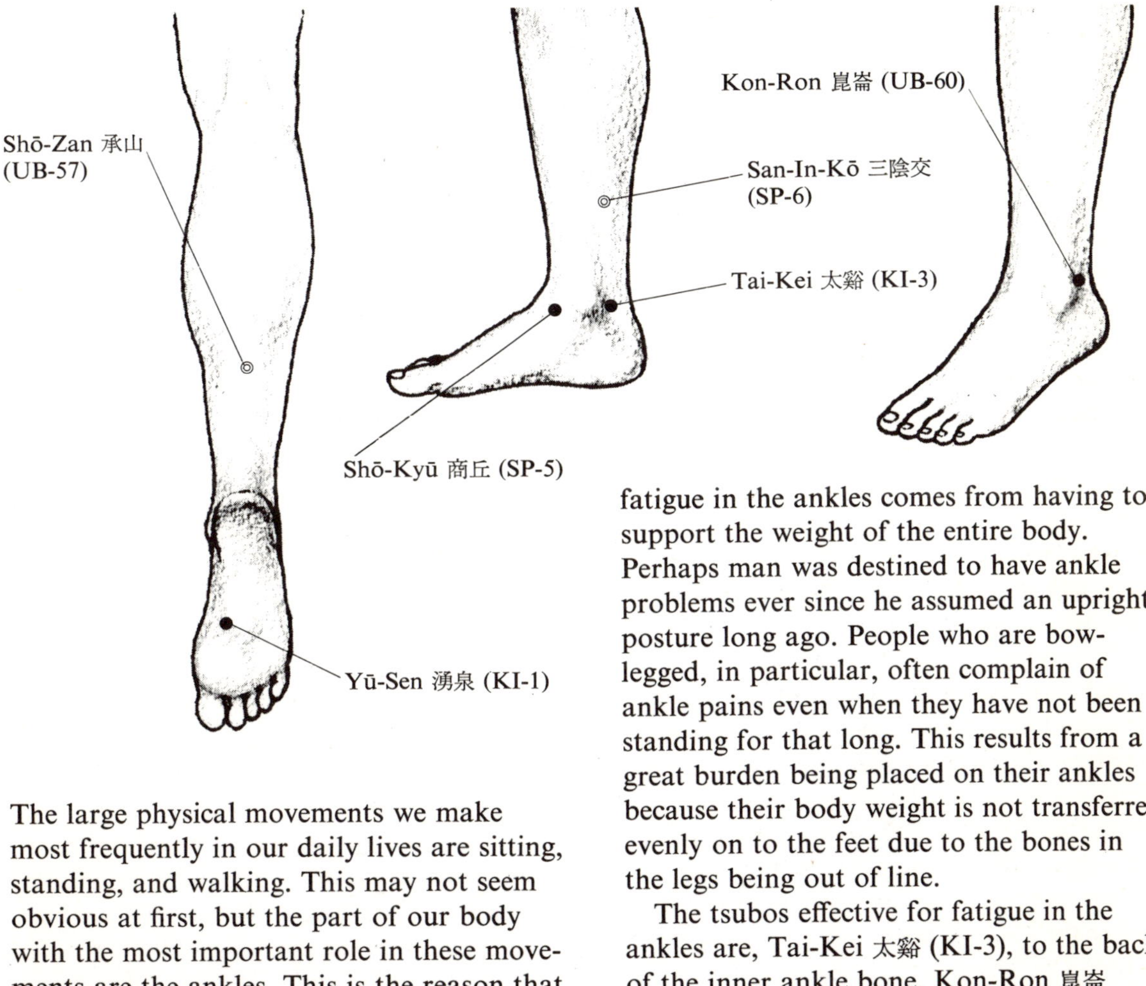

The large physical movements we make most frequently in our daily lives are sitting, standing, and walking. This may not seem obvious at first, but the part of our body with the most important role in these movements are the ankles. This is the reason that whenever we stand for a long time or carry heavy objects a large load is placed on our feet and the ankles are left fatigued. It is unthinkable that one's ankles should become sore when one is bed ridden, and thus, fatigue in the ankles comes from having to support the weight of the entire body. Perhaps man was destined to have ankle problems ever since he assumed an upright posture long ago. People who are bow-legged, in particular, often complain of ankle pains even when they have not been standing for that long. This results from a great burden being placed on their ankles because their body weight is not transferred evenly on to the feet due to the bones in the legs being out of line.

The tsubos effective for fatigue in the ankles are, Tai-Kei 太谿 (KI-3), to the back of the inner ankle bone, Kon-Ron 崑崙 (UB-60), to the back of the outer ankle bone, Shō-Kyū 商丘 (SP-5), to the front of the outer ankle bone, San-In-Kō 三陰交 (SP-6), four finger widths above the inner ankle bone, and Yū-Sen 湧泉 (KI-1), on the back of the foot. Yū-Sen is of particular importance among these tsubos. As explained earlier, man maintains an upright posture by evenly distributing his weight over the tripod formed by the heels and the balls (base) of the big toe and the little toe. Yū-Sen is located approximately in the center of these three points, and just from this, it can be understood why finger pressure on Yū-Sen is so effective.

In addition to this, the tsubo Shō-Zan 承山 (UB-57) should not be overlooked because fatigue in the ankle is also related to problems in the Achilles tendon. When one's ankles become tired and sore, often hard lumps of tension appear around Shō-Zan and San-In-Kō. When this happens, massage and work out the tension around Shō-Zan gently so as not to cause undue pain. Also, since the ankles are not a very muscular area and there are a large number of tsubos here, gently massaging around the ankles and softly massaging between the tendons using the thumb or middle finger, is almost as effective as pressing each and every tsubo individually.

U. Fatigue in arches of feet——Yū-Sen 湧泉 (KI-1)

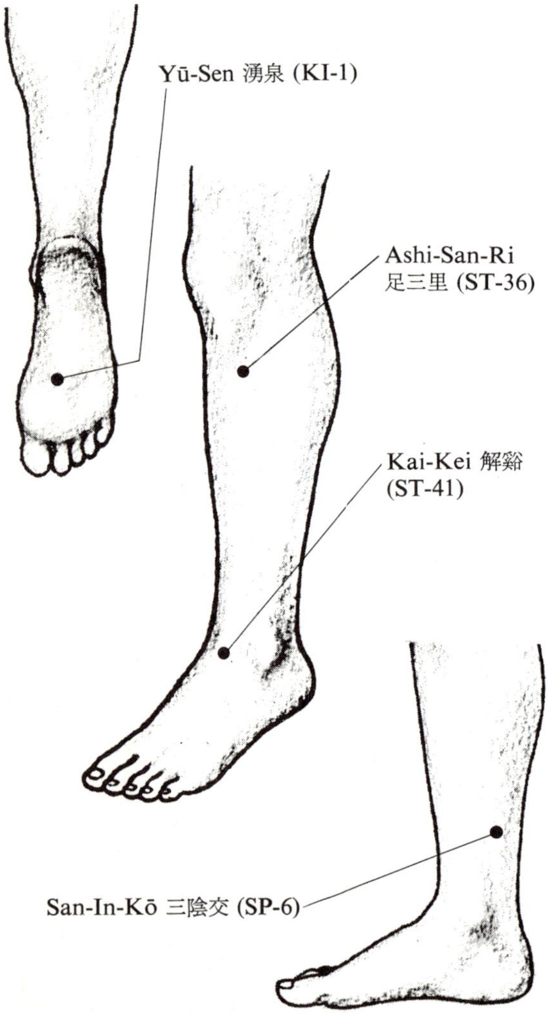

Recently in Japan there are a few elementary schools which have adopted the policy of having their students go barefoot during physical education classes. No doubt, the aim is to develop the arches of their students' feet, and to improve their physical fitness in general. It is true that flat-footed people tend to tire more easily, and that generally they are less capable of vigorous exercise. Why is it that people seem to tire more easily when their arches are underdeveloped? As explained before, human beings stand erect by support from the three points of the heel and the balls of the big toe and the little toe. In other words, normally the arches of the feet should remain clear of the ground and span the three points. The three points of support are thereby able to accurately relay information concerning the state of a person's balance. When a person is flat-footed, however, the distribution of weight to the three points becomes unclear. The brain receives various conflicting signals from the soles of the feet, and naturally this causes great fatigue both mentally and physically. And furthermore, the fatigue in the ankles extends up to the calves and the shins, as well as the thighs.

The soles of our feet were originally meant

to be a great source of power and vitality. The importance of the soles is inferred by skin cancer often starting from the bottom of the feet, and it being very difficult to cure. This is just one indication of how this area is central in maintaining health and vigor. It is no coincidence that the tsubo Yū-Sen 湧泉 (KI-1), from where life energy is said to "well up," is located in the center of the soles of the feet. Yū-Sen can therefore be listed first as the specially effective tsubo for relieving fatigue in the arches of the feet, and otherwise the tsubos Kai-Kei 解谿 (ST-41), San-In-Kō 三陰交 (SP-6), and Ashi-San-Ri 足三里 (ST-36) may be raised. Give thorough finger pressure to each of these tsubos and the balls of the big toe and the little toe, as well as beneath the heel.

Also, using special devices for foot massage, or walking barefooted on uneven surfaces is quite effective for relieving fatigue in the feet. The main point is to restore the arches of the feet to the ideal condition, where the weight of the body goes on the three points of support evenly. If you do not have a special device for foot massage (in Japan people step on pieces of bamboo split in half), you can get the same effect by sitting in a chair and rolling a beer bottle under your foot. The maximum benefit can be obtained by always finishing such foot massages with finger pressure on Yū-Sen.

V. Hotness in feet——Yū-Sen 湧泉 (KI-1)

There are people who come to my clinic with complaints like "My feet always feel hot and sweaty, and it bothers me." I always reply, "You have nothing to worry about; hot feet are much better than cold feet, and besides, it is a sign of health." There are some people, however, whose feet become hot as soon as they get into bed, and sometimes the heat in their feet is so excessive, even in the wintertime they cannot sleep without sticking their feet out from under their covers. People like this always have a couple of things in common. One is that the soles of their feet are hard and lacking in resiliency. Ideally, the soles of one's feet should be soft and resilient. Also, these people do not have enough flesh on the balls of their big toes and little toes.

The specially effective tsubo for reducing the sensation of heat in the feet is Yū-Sen 湧泉 (KI-1) in the sole of the foot. The best results can be obtained by also treating Kon-Ron 崑崙 (UB-60), behind the outer ankle bone, Tai-Kei 太谿 (KI-3), behind the inner ankle bone, San-In-Kō 三陰交 (SP-6), four finger widths above the inner ankle

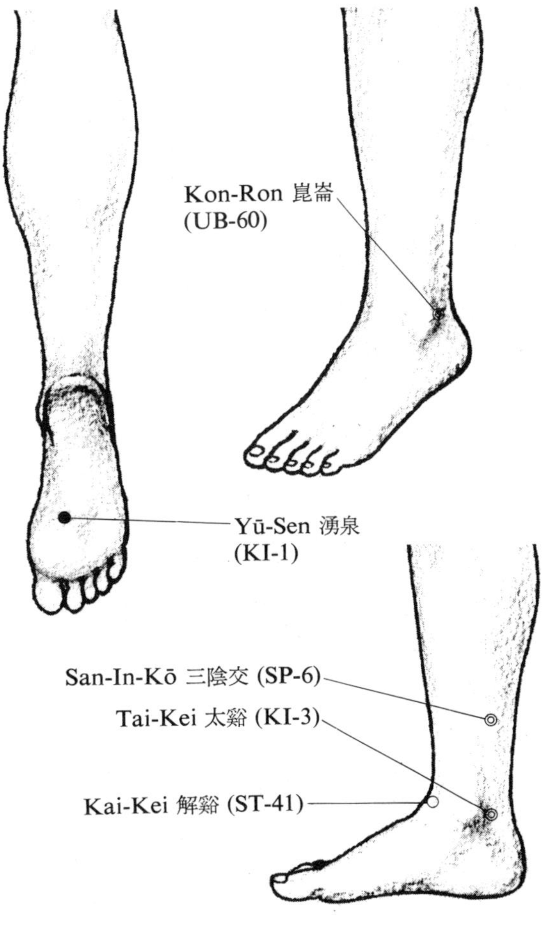

bone, and Kai-Kei 解谿 (ST-41), on the front of the ankle. The best way to treat these tsubos is to apply firm pressure on them, and the most important thing in giving shiatsu is to find just the right amount of pressure for the maximum effect.

Heating or chilling of the feet is a sure sign that there is some problem in the autonomic nervous system which regulates the flow of blood through the vessels in the feet. For heating or chilling of the feet, aside from treating various tsubos, there is another effective method. As already explained before, it is simply to immerse the feet alternately in hot and cold water. The effectiveness of this method has been proven even in modern medical practice, and this same method is applied in physiotherapy to treat symptoms of heating or chilling in the lower limbs. This is a very simple method that can be applied at home, so it is highly recommended.

W. Chilling of feet——Tai-Shō 太衝 (LV-3)

Many people complain that their feet begin to feel cold and uncomfortable when they become tired. This is caused most often by a disturbance in the functional condition of the autonomic nervous system which controls peripheral circulation to drastically reduce the amount of blood flow to the feet. A person's feet can begin to feel either hot or cold when the function of the autonomic nervous system becomes impaired. Since both symptoms can result from a decline in the functional state of the autonomic nervous system, only a fine line separates the sensation of heat in the feet from that of chilling. The feeling of the feet becoming cold, however, seems to be the most commonly experienced symptom.

When chilling of the feet becomes a problem, in addition to the tsubos listed in the previous section for alleviating the sensation of heat, find Tai-Shō 太衝 (LV-3) on the foot between the big toe and the second toe, as well as Rin-Kyū 臨泣 (GB-41) also on the foot between the bones of the fourth and fifth toes, and give firm pressure on these tsubos. Even greater effects can be obtained when pressing tsubos on the foot by first warming up the feet with such things as hot pads, paraffin baths, or alternately immersing the feet in hot and cold water.

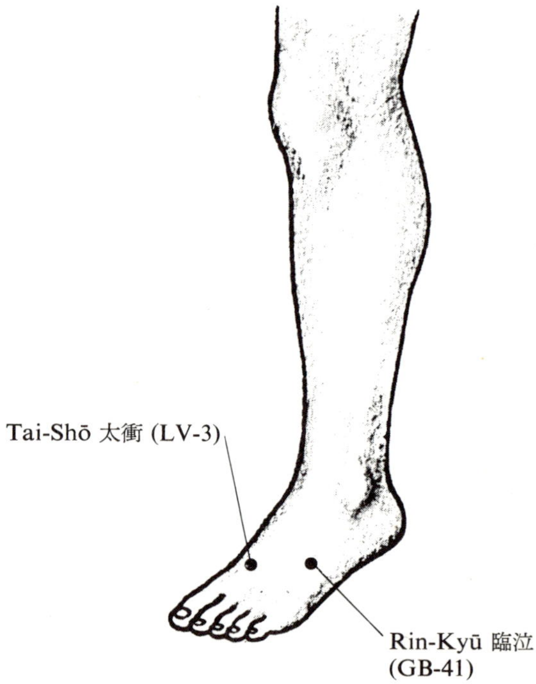

Chilling of one's feet is rarely just a problem in the feet. As explained briefly before, the abdominal artery divides into two branches at the level of the fourth lumbar vertebra and supplies the legs. It has been verified through numerous studies conducted by acupuncture specialists that acupuncture points or tsubos are located in great numbers around the places where blood vessels divide near the skin surface.

This means that if the function of the autonomic nervous system is facilitated by stimulating the tsubos which are closely connected to the dividing points of the blood vessels, the blood flow from below that area can be greatly improved. This explains why points on the back can be important for curing chilling of the feet.

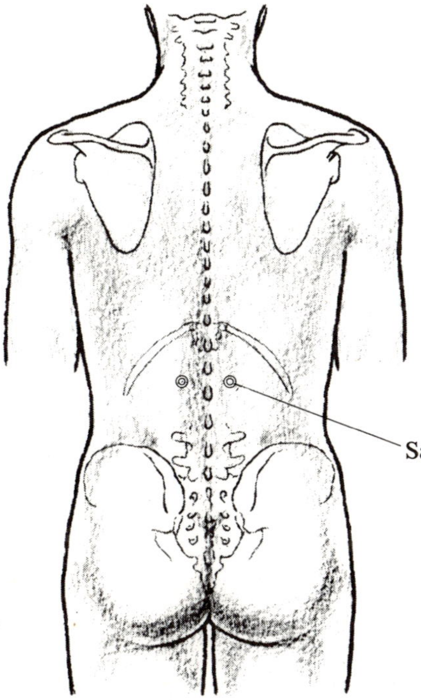

The tsubo specially effective in this case is San-Shō-Yu 三焦兪 (UB-22) to either side of the point below the first lumbar vertebra. It has been known from the olden days as an important tsubo for controlling the temperature of one's body below the waist. There is another tsubo effective for chilling of the feet which may seem rather unlikely, and this is Yō-Chi 陽池 (TH-4) in the middle on the back of the wrist. Yō-Chi has always been known as being effective for regulating circulation in the upper half of the body, but it is also related to circulation of blood in the feet.

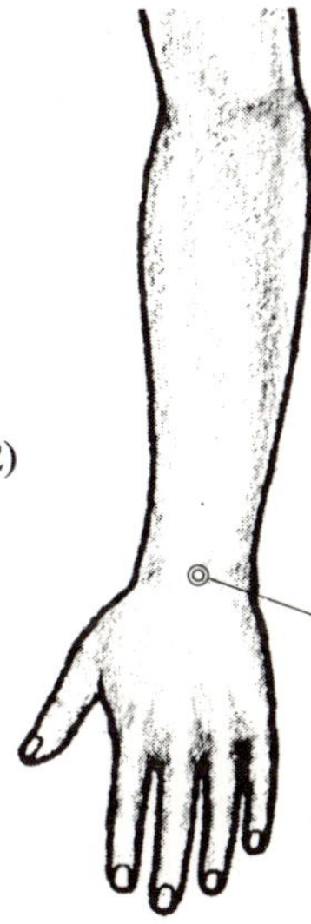

X. Swelling of feet——Ashi-San-Ri 足三里 (ST-36)

When people wear tight fitting shoes all day long, sometimes their feet begin to feel somewhat swollen in the evening. It also happens that people removing their shoes while working at a desk, later find their feet do not fit back into their shoes very easily. When people become fatigued, their feet almost always become swollen to some extent. This condition also results from the accumulation of fatigue in the muscles. The blood that is pumped by the heart reaches all parts of the body through a network of arteries, and returns to the heart once again via a network of veins. Be that as it may, blood does not flow by the pumping action of the heart only. The expansion and contraction of the muscles all over the body assist the work of the heart and facilitate the return flow of blood.

When we maintain the same posture for a long time, or otherwise, remain standing for some length of time, our muscles become

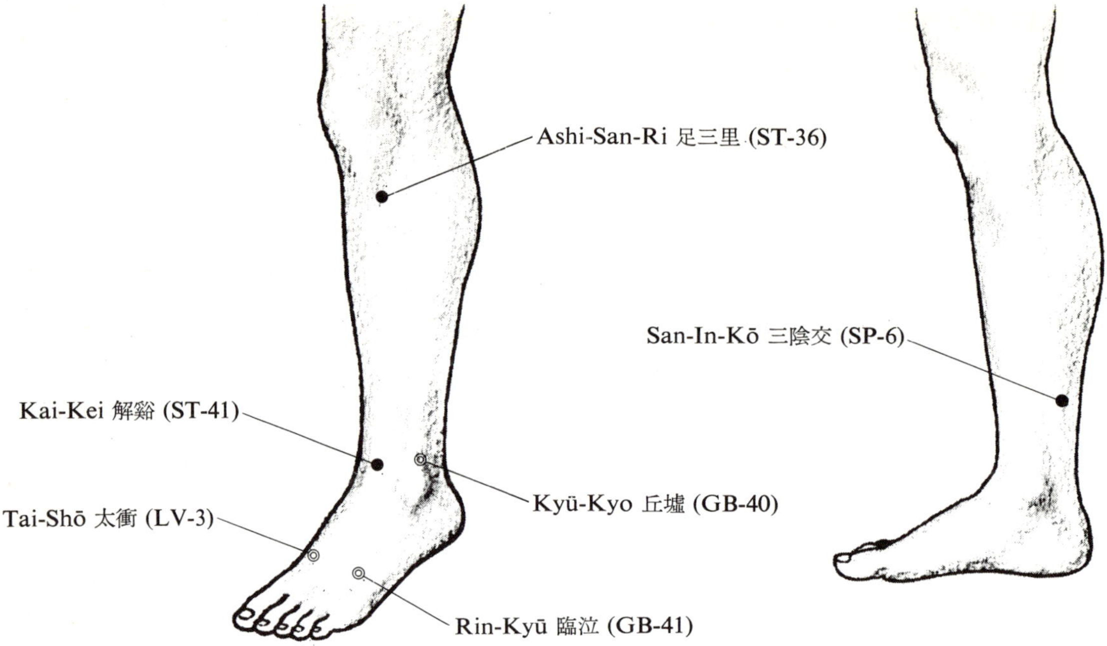

fatigued and the number of movements begins to decrease. When this happens, the blood that has reached our hands and feet cannot return to the heart as easily as before. In other words, the fresh blood which once reaches the muscles through arterioles and capillary networks to supply oxygen and nutrients is unable to return to the heart through the blood vessels or lymphatic system. Thus, fluid from venous blood begins to collect in between the muscle tissues. This is what causes swelling, or edema, in the hands and feet.

Six tsubos can be listed here as being effective for swelling of the feet and they are Ashi-San-Ri 足三里 (ST-36), Kai-Kei 解谿 (ST-41), San-In-Kō 三陰交 (SP-6), Kyū-Kyo 丘墟 (GB-40), Tai-Shō 太衝 (LV-3), and Rin-Kyū 臨泣 (GB-41). These tsubos will not be discussed here because each one has been explained in previous sections.

Applying thorough pressure on these tsubos should make the swelling go down. When the amount of swelling is very slight, just massaging the shin area, the calf muscles, the ankles, and the arches of the feet will reduce the swelling fairly quickly.

Swelling, or edema, in soft tissues such as under the skin of the face is generally regarded as being a sign of kidney disfunctions, while edema in harder tissue like that of the hands and feet are considered to be a sign of a weak heart. Not too seldom, however, perfectly healthy individuals just become fatigued and experience some swelling in their feet. Therefore, one need not worry about heart problems as soon as the feet become a bit swollen. So long as other symptoms such as palpitations and shortness of breath do not exist, the majority of edema in the feet can be thought of as being caused by accumulated fatigue.

5. Treating Disorders of Visceral Organs and Stress Related Symptoms

A. Heavy and distended feeling in stomach——I-Yu 胃兪 (UB-21)

The condition where one's stomach often feels distended even though one has not eaten that much is sometimes referred to as "gastrasthenia," which means a weak stomach. This condition is not so serious as to be called a disease. Most middle-aged men who have an accumulation of stress seem to experience such symptoms from time to time. As long as this is not a long-standing problem stemming from a weak physical constitution, such stomach symptoms can be alleviated through tsubo therapy.

The most important tsubos for distention in the stomach is I-Yu 胃兪 (UB-21) and Hi-Yu 脾兪 (UB-20). In Oriental medicine, the spleen and stomach are regarded as being an interconnected organ system, but a person does not need to know this to realize that these two tsubos on the back are important, because there is a certain discomfort and tension that is felt in the middle of the back when the stomach feels heavy and distended.

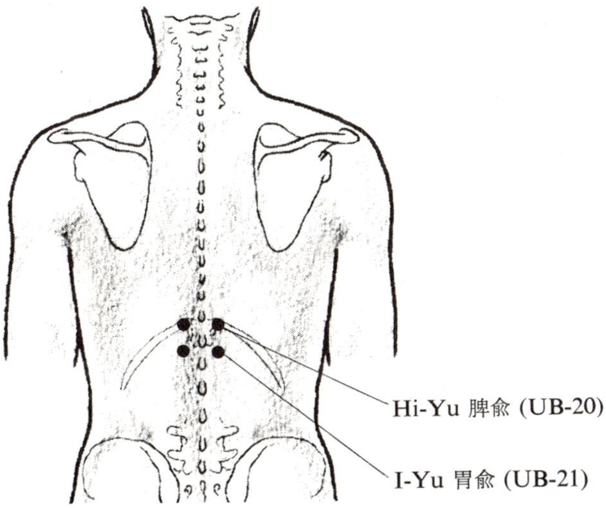

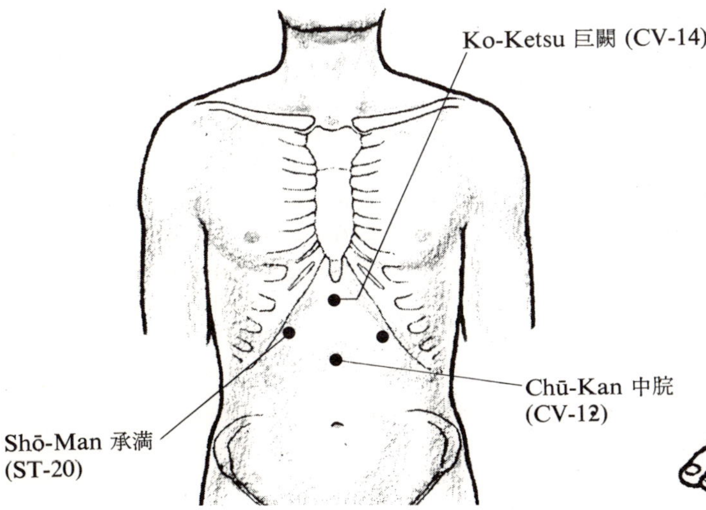

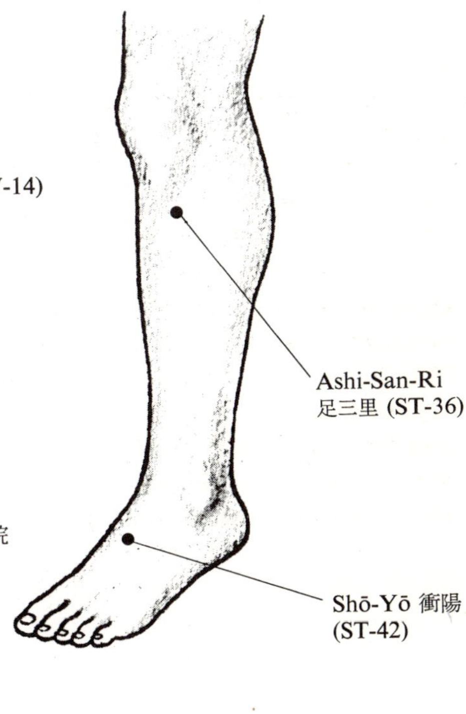

Another tsubo that should not be missed when one has a distended stomach is Ko-Ketsu 巨闕 (CV-14), a little below the pit of the stomach. Ko-Ketsu is indispensable for those who have high blood pressure and frequent palpitations, while also being very effective in cases of chronic gastritis. Another effective tsubo in this case is Shō-Man 承満 (ST-20), slightly below and to the side of Ko-Ketsu. Finger pressure on this point just under the ribs serves to improve one's digestion. Chū-Kan 中脘 (CV-12) is yet another important tsubo for this purpose which is located directly over the stomach.

Furthermore, there are other effective tsubos on the legs as well. The old favorite, Ashi-San-Ri 足三里 (ST-36), is the main one. It may seem strange that a point on the leg controls the function of the stomach, but Ashi-San-Ri happens to be a focal point along the pathway of energy deeply connected with the stomach. There is another tsubo on the back of the foot on the hump between the second and third metatarsals. When a person has stomach problems, the area around Shō-Yō 衝陽 (ST-42) often becomes hard and sore. There are even those who use a sharp object like the tip of a ball point pen to goad this point on the back of the foot, but few of them realize that the real problem lies with their stomach. The reciprocal feedback mechanism between the skin and organs is truely amazing because such massaging or prodding serves to stimulate the function of the stomach.

B. Feeling nauseous——Tan-Yu 胆兪 (UB-19)

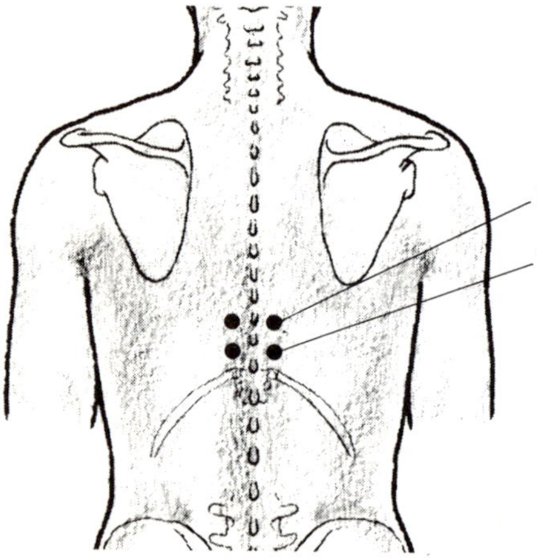

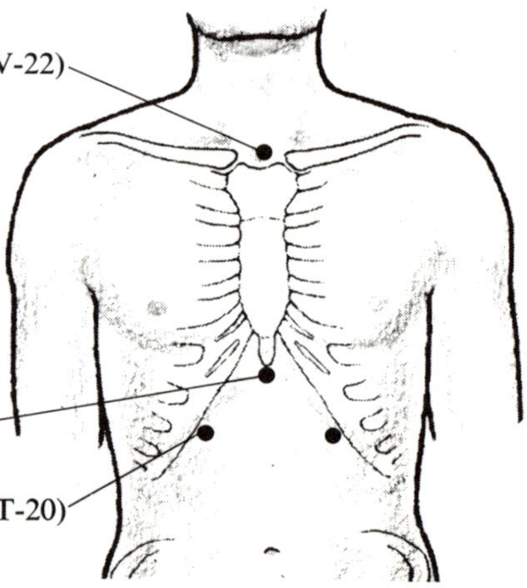

It is quite fascinating how practically the human body is designed. Vomiting after drinking too much alcohol is one example of this. It may seem like something repulsive, but getting sick is nothing other than a red light from the physiological mechanism of a person saying in effect, "Your body will not be able to maintain normal functions if you drink any more." One may say that the body assumes control in place of its master who is becoming unconscious.

When our body discovers something wrong with what we have drunk or eaten before it reaches the stomach, our natural defense mechanism comes into play and the offending substance is expelled out the mouth. Obviously a similar defense mechanism operates even when the unwanted substance gets beyond the stomach to reach the small intestine and the large intestine. In this case, the body expels the substance in the form of diarrhea. So as long as there is nothing drastically wrong, the human body is able to expel or otherwise render harmful substances harmless by its powers of natural accommodation.

In Oriental medicine the therapeutic method of cooperating with the body's power of natural recuperation is expressed as *Kan-Do-Ge-Wa* 汗吐下和. These characters refer to natural physical reactions of sweating, vomiting, diarrhea, and neutralizing. For example, when a person has a cold and a fever, this is purged from the body by sweating. Nausea is often a symptom which arises from fatigue in the digestive system, and the tsubos such as Kan-Yu 肝兪 (UB-18) and Tan-Yu 胆兪 (UB-19) which have a detoxifying effect also work to relieve nausea.

When a person is nauseous, or getting sick, it means that there is some unwanted substance in the body, so instead of using tsubos related to the stomach function like I-Yu 胃兪 (UB-21) and Hi-Yu 脾兪 (UB-20), the tsubos Kan-Yu and Tan-Yu associated with detoxifying the body become important. In addition to these, the tsubos effective in relieving nausea include Kyū-Bi 鳩尾 (CV-15), at the tip of the xiphoid process below the sternum, Shō-Man 承満 (ST-20), useful for retention of food in the stomach, and Ten-Totsu 天突 (CV-22), effective in alleviating the feeling of nausea from deep down.

People who are used to taking care of their drunk buddies sometimes reach their arms around the drunk person from behind to press in the pit of his stomach. This commonsense method actually conforms with the approach in tsubo therapy.

C. Heartburn——Shō-Man 承満 (ST-20)

When I conduct oral examinations for the acupuncture licensing board, one of the often asked questions is "what are the symptoms of chronic gastritis?" The answer almost always comes back automatically as "belching, heartburn, and distention of the stomach." In Oriental medicine heartburn is called *Don San* 呑酸 (swallow acid), and since it is like a burning sensation in the middle of the chest when very sour drinks are taken, it is a very appropriate description. All three of the symptoms mentioned above are those which the majority of us experience from time to time. Sometimes heartburn is related to diseases in the digestive system, but only occasional heartburn usually results from fatigue in the digestive organs due to overeating, or drinking too much.

The specially effective tsubo for heartburn and poor digestion is Hi-Yu 脾兪 (UB-20) on the back which is good for alleviating

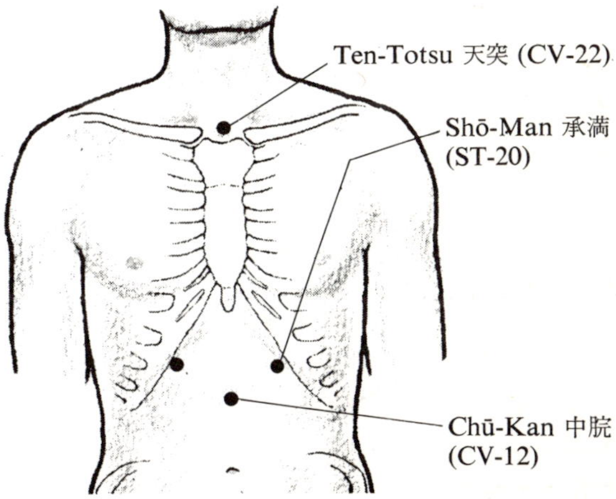

general fatigue. Also, since heartburn is a symptom resulting from a weakened digestive system which causes the retention of food in the stomach that ferments and produces acid which irritates the nerves in the esophagus, the first thing that needs to be done is to improve the digestive function. The best tsubo for this purpose is Shō-Man

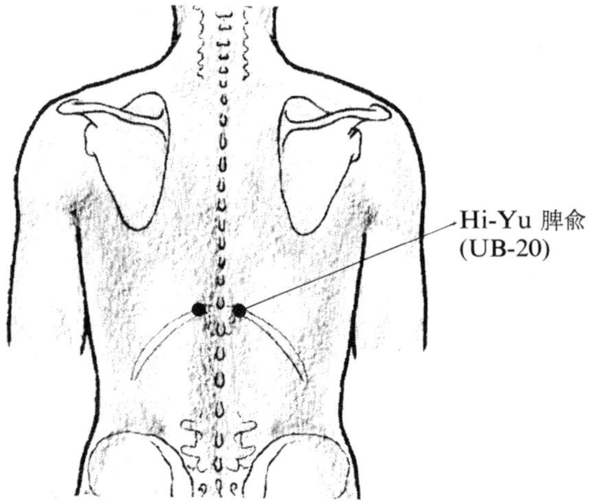

承満 (ST-20), located on the abdomen at the tip of the eighth rib.

Furthermore, Chū-Kan 中脘 (CV-12), right between the pit of the stomach and the navel, is an important tsubo for this purpose. The stomach has three important points called Jō-Kan 上脘 (CV-13: top opening), Chū-Kan 中脘 (CV-12: middle of opening), and Ge-Kan 下脘 (CV-10: bottom opening), and Chū-Kan is the most important tsubo among these. It can be understood how vital this tsubo is when it is noted that Chū-Kan is located directly over the solar plexus of the autonomic nervous system which works to regulate the function of the digestive organs.

The symptom of heartburn should gradually subside by firmly pressing and moving the fingers back and forth slightly on each of these tsubos. Nevertheless, if an uncomfortable sensation still remains at the base of the throat as if regurgitating some acid, also give pressure to Ten-Totsu 天突 (CV-22).

When the symptom of heartburn becomes a chronic condition it becomes very hard to cure by tsubo therapy alone. When this is the case, chronic gastritis, peptic ulcers, or duodenal ulcers may be indicated, so it is best to consult a specialist for a thorough examination.

D. Lack of appetite——Chū-Kan 中脘 (CV-12)

In the summertime even healthy people tend to lose their appetite. This is because there is greater blood circulation close to the skin surface in the summer, and the function of the visceral organs, especially that of the stomach, slows down. When autumn comes around, blood circulates more completely once again to supply the organs, and usually one's appetite returns. When fatigue or physical exhaustion from the summer lingers on, however, one's appetite remains poor. Lack of appetite is also caused by other factors such as overwork, psychological stress produced by being overly concerned or anxious, and otherwise, by the presence of gastritis, ulcers, or parasitic worms. When there are diseases in the digestive organs, of course, it is necessary to consult a physician, however, loss of appetite stemming from

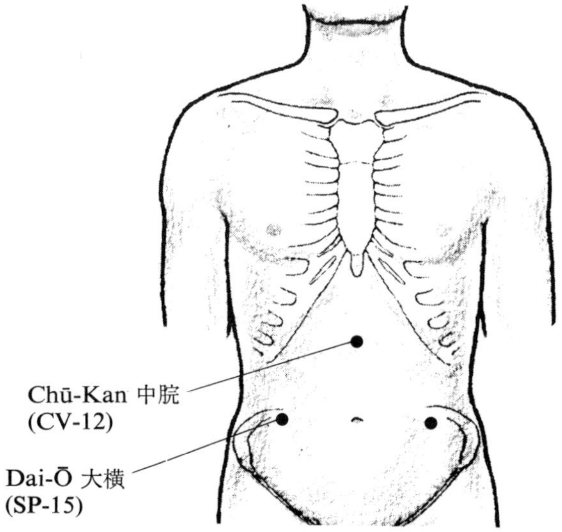

physical and mental fatigue can be restored by applying tsubo therapy.

Two tsubos mentioned many times already, Kan-Yu 肝俞 (UB-18), to the side

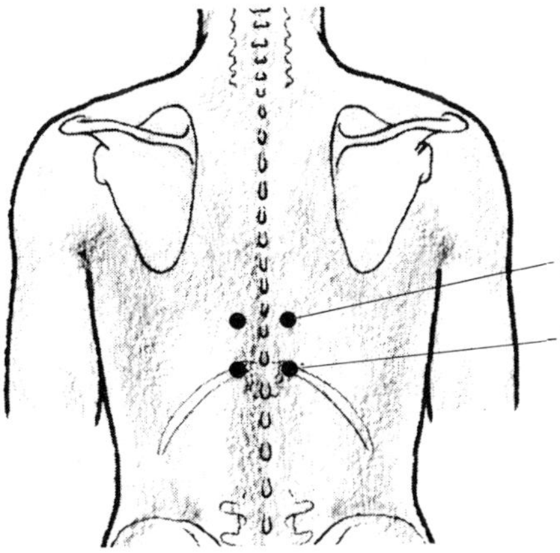

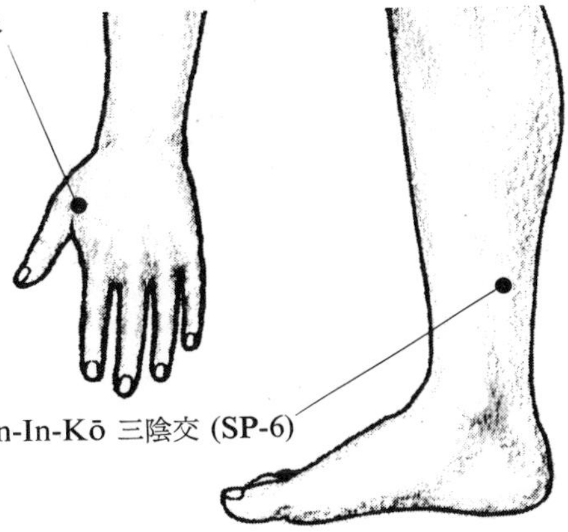

of the ninth thoracic vertebra, and Hi-Yu 脾兪 (UB-20), a little below this, should be treated. Also, Chū-Kan 中脘 (CV-12), between the pit of the stomach and the navel, and Dai-Ō 大横 (SP-15), to the side of the navel in line with the nipple, should be pressed. In addition, Gō-Koku 合谷 (LI-4) on the back of the hand, and San-In-Kō 三陰交 (SP-6), above the inner ankle bone, are important tsubos which serve to regulate the function of the digestive organs, and they may be treated for even better results.

One thing which has to be borne in mind when pressing the above tsubos is not to press as strongly as when trying to relieve symptoms of tension in the shoulders or back. The best way to get positive results is to give just the right amount of pressure according to each symptom, and to take time and press only strong enough to where it feels good. Continuing with such tsubo therapy over time should make a person's appetite return.

There are some people who think that it is not good to skip meals even though they have no appetite, but this attitude only serves to make them anxious and lose their appetite even more. The best thing to do is to keep a relaxed attitude about it and find ways to stimulate the appetite by arranging food in an appetizing manner and to select foods which are easy to digest.

E. Constipation——Dai-Ko 大巨 (ST-27)

The symptom common to middle-aged people who complain of being in poor physical shape with tension in their shoulders, aches and pains all over, and general fatigue, is constipation. When these symptoms become chronic, the constipation also becomes a constant problem, and this is generally accompanied with headaches. In the case of women, there are even more complications, and the amount of nutrition to their skin decreases so that makeup does not go on their faces the way it should. It is said that 70 percent of Japanese women

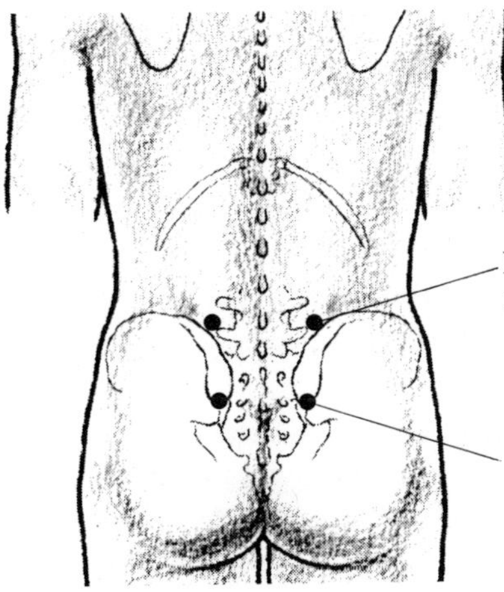

are constipated to some extent, so it is no overstatement to say that constipation is a real enemy of women.

When people come to our clinic complaining of poor hearing and tinnitus, I make it a rule to ask if they are constipated, and in fact, almost all of them are. This is why, when a patient receives treatment for constipation, quite often they return to happily report that their appetite has improved and that the ringing in their ears has stopped. Therefore, one should keep in mind that constipation has a very negative overall effect on the body.

Quite often constipation is caused by the lack of exercise. The internal organs, especially the stomach which digests food, does not move very well unless a person's body is exercised. The stomach is always in motion with a steady rhythm, extending, contracting, and extending again. The food which comes from the mouth is mixed together thoroughly and broken down to reduce it to a readily digestible form. When this peristaltic action of the stomach becomes weak, a person becomes constipated. It goes without saying that the presence of mental and physical stress coupled with the lack of exercise makes the situation even worse.

The tsubos Dai-Chō-Yu 大腸兪 (UB-25) and Shō-Chō-Yu 小腸兪 (UB-27) on the back should be pressed when a person is constipated. These tsubos are right over the spinal nerve centers related to the function

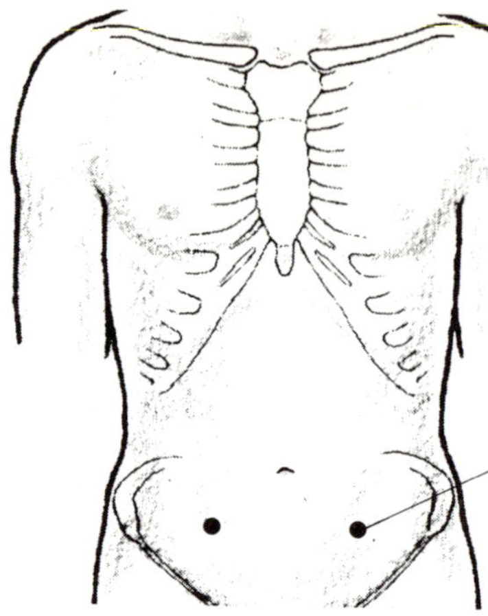

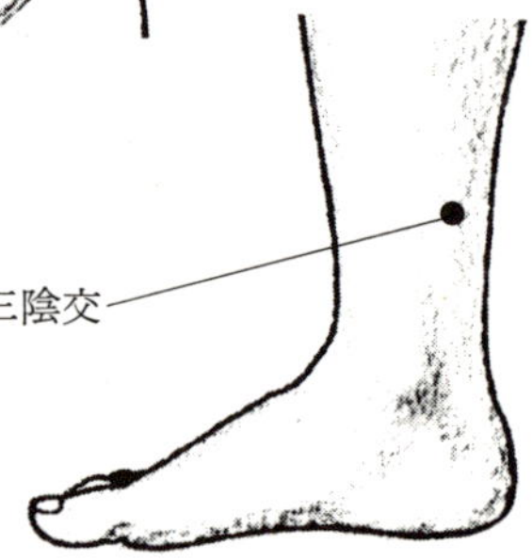

of elimination. Also, press the tsubo Dai-Ko 大巨 (ST-27), located between the navel and the protrusion of the pelvic bone to the front, and give special emphasis to that on the left side. In addition to this, give finger pressure to San-In-Kō 三陰交 (SP-6).

Pressing both sides of the lower spine with the four fingers while sitting on the toilet seat will make bowel movements much easier. Also, do not forget to give yourself thorough massages over the abdomen on a daily basis.

F. Diarrhea——Dai-Chō-Yu 大腸兪 (UB-25)

I have a friend who likes to go out drinking so much that he is constantly in trouble with his wife. His coming home late every night, however, is not the only reason for his wife's dismay. It also seems to have something to do with his going to the toilet the next morning. As soon as this man wakes up, he rushes to the bathroom and moves his bowels which are always on the loose side. It is easy to see why his wife who cleans the bathroom becomes upset at having to put up with this day after day. In the case of this man, rather than his drinking being the cause of diarrhea, psychological stress and a disorderly life-style are more likely the cause. There seem to

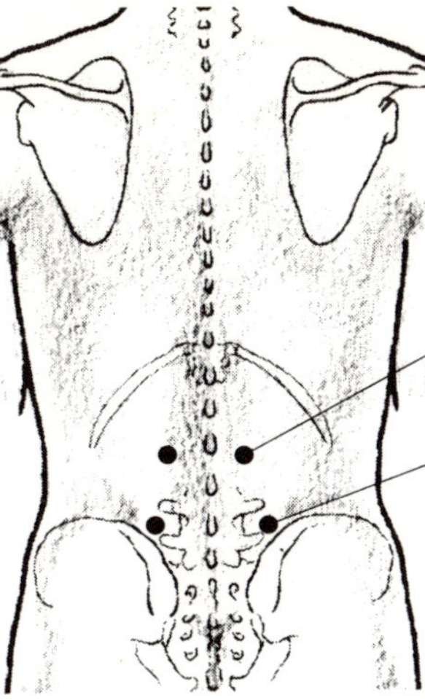

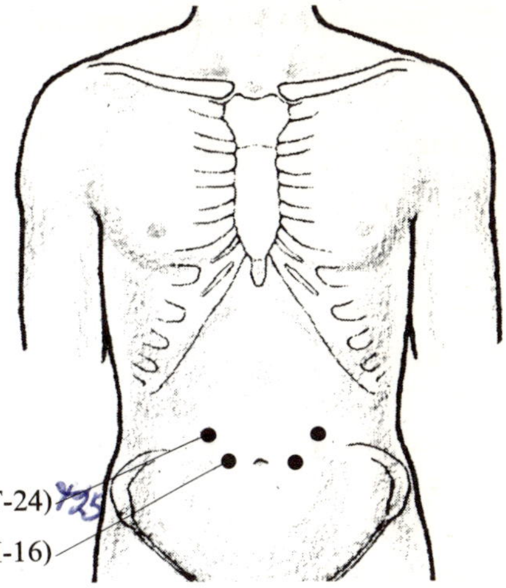

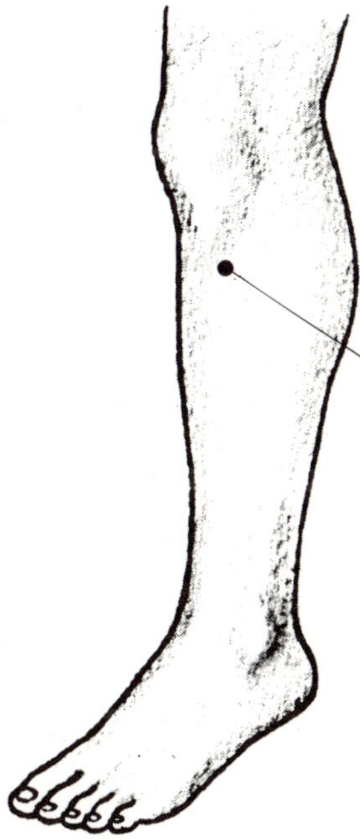

be many men with positions of responsibility in companies with similar problems since they have to drink with their business associates.

Some say that tsubo therapy is not so effective for stopping diarrhea, and since constipation can be treated with better results, the tsubos used in both cases turn out to be pretty much the same. First of all, Jin-Yu 腎兪 (UB-23) and Dai-Chō-Yu 大腸兪 (UB-25) on the lower back are used, and next, Kō-Yu 肓兪 (KI-16), right next to the navel, is the important tsubo. When a person's physical condition deteriorates, even light pressure on Jin-Yu and Kō-Yu reveals pressure sensitivity, or an abnormal painful reaction. Such pressure sensitivity serves as an indicator of the decline in a person's physical state. Be sure to provide thorough treatments whenever there are such tender areas.

Just above Ten-Sū 天枢 (ST-25) which is three finger widths to the side of the navel is Katsu-Niku-Mon 滑肉門 (ST-24), a tsubo with a very important function, so be sure to treat this tsubo also.

People who tend to have loose stools generally have weak constitutions and they also tend to get constipated when they are in a bad physical state. For these people, finger pressure on Ashi-San-Ri 足三里 (ST-36) proves effective. When one treats this tsubo patiently to remove fatigue in the legs and improve the condition of the stomach, the occurrence of diarrhea should gradually stop.

In any case, no one who is really healthy gets diarrhea just from fatigue or exhaustion. Therefore, the main point in preventing diarrhea is to maintain one's body in good shape on a constant basis.

G. Menstrual irregularity——Hō-Kō 胞肓 (UB-48)

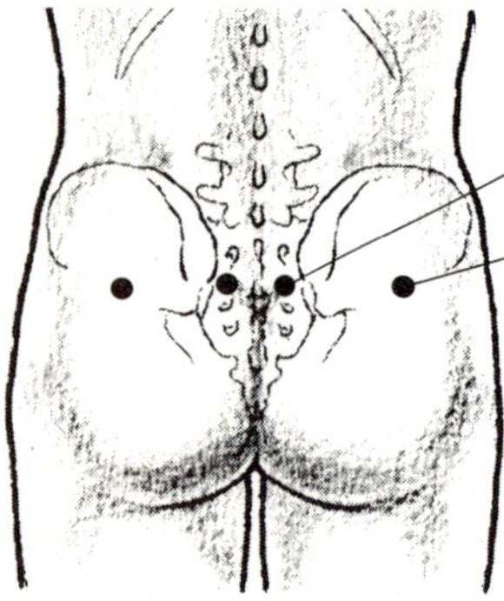

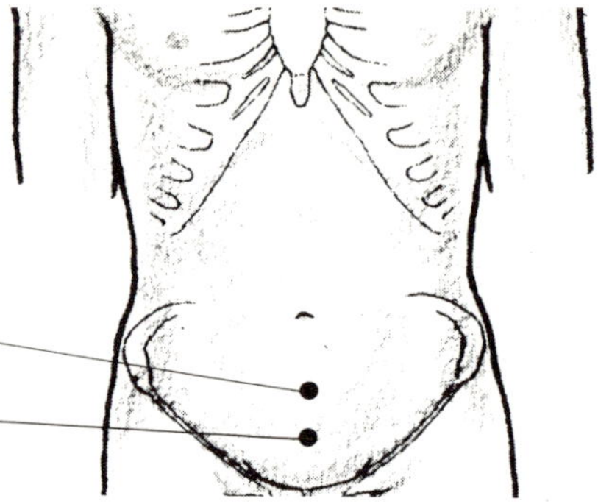

Women normally have their period once every four weeks, and although many women always have their period right on time, there are those who have tremendous irregularities in their period with only slight changes of mood, or periods of emotional instability. Such menstrual irregularities are caused by the emotions affecting the thalamus, lying between the right and left hemispheres of the brain, that controls the excretion of hormones and regulates the menses in women. The menstrual irregularity discussed here will focus on the physical causes rather than psychological ones. The occurrence of menstrual irregularities does not necessarily mean that a woman has serious physical problems, but instead, it is often experienced among healthy women when fatigue accumulates. The main physical symptom appearing in this case is fatigue and soreness in the lower back area.

The specially effective tsubos for menstrual irregularities are Ji-Ryō 次髎 (UB-32) and Hō-Kō 胞肓 (UB-48) on the lower back, and Kan-Gen 関元 (CV-4) on the lower abdomen four finger widths below the navel. Kan-Gen is regarded in Oriental medicine as being the tsubo which regulates the level of congenital energy that is present from birth, and it is known to be effective for loss of vitality, high blood pressure, chilling in the extremities, and diseases having to do with the reproductive organs. The tsubo Chū-Kyoku 中極 (CV-3), two finger widths below Kan-Gen, is also a very important tsubo which is considered to be effective for disease of the urogenital system, especially gynecological disorders. This is a bit off the subject, but these tsubos below the navel are also effective for symptoms typical to elderly men who have an enlarged prostate gland that causes difficulty in urination along with the feeling of urine retention.

Pressing these tsubos mentioned will not rectify the problem immediately when a woman has menstrual irregularities. The most important thing is to continue these treatments patiently over a long period of time. It is also important to pay special attention to keeping the area around the waist warm. The underwear of women seem to be getting thinner and thinner these days, and even middle-aged women who used to wear woolen underwear seem to be getting by with only one thin pair of panties. The best way to improve circulation to the organs in the pelvic cavity is to keep the area under the waist warm and to prevent it from becoming chilled. It is alright to keep with styles, but thicker underwear is recommend in colder weather. This is the best way to guard against menstrual irregularities.

H. Heavy feeling in lower abdomen——Chū-Kyoku 中極 (CV-3)

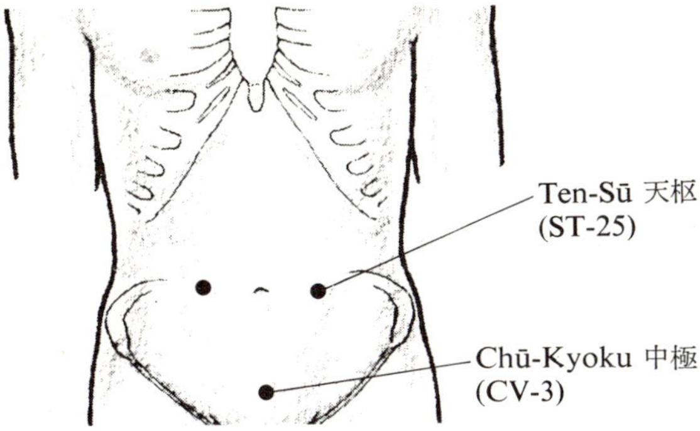

When women have their period they undergo various changes both physically and psychologically. In terms of psychological changes, they may become irritated for no apparent reason, or become angered over the slightest incident. Physically, their feet may feel as cold as ice, and they experience a dull pain with a pulling sensation in the lower abdomen. In addition to this, sometimes there is a feeling of tension in the lower abdomen which feels somewhat heavy. Such symptoms are quite common in women during the onset of their period.

Many women suffer from these symptoms especially when they have a great deal of work to do during their period, or otherwise, when they have many worries and accumulate mental and physical fatigue. These are obviously symptoms which come from functional disorders of the organs in the pelvic region. The important point in tsubo treatments is to normalize the function of these organs and restore a healthy menstrual cycle.

The specially effective tsubos for this purpose, interestingly enough, forms a circle around the body at the level of the second sacral vertebra. The sacrum is the bone composing the back wall of the pelvis along with the coccyx (tailbone) at its tip. When an imaginary line is drawn connecting the protrusion of the pelvic bones (iliac) on the top at both ends, and then an inverted triangle is formed by connecting the ends of this line to the tip of the coccyx, the second sacral vertebra is located just about in the center of the triangle. The important tsubos for treating pain in the lower abdomen is Ji-Ryō 次髎 (UB-32), just to either side of the second sacral vertebra, Bō-Kō-Yu 膀胱俞 (UB-28), more to the outside, and Hō-Kō 胞肓 (UB-48), a little more to the outside, as well as Chū-Kyoku 中極 (CV-3) which is around to the front side on the center line of the lower abdomen just above the pubic symphysis. These are all very beneficial tsubos for women so they are well worth keeping in mind. An additional tsubo for adjusting imbalances between the upper half and lower half of the body is Ten-Sū 天枢 (ST-25), located three finger widths to either side of the navel.

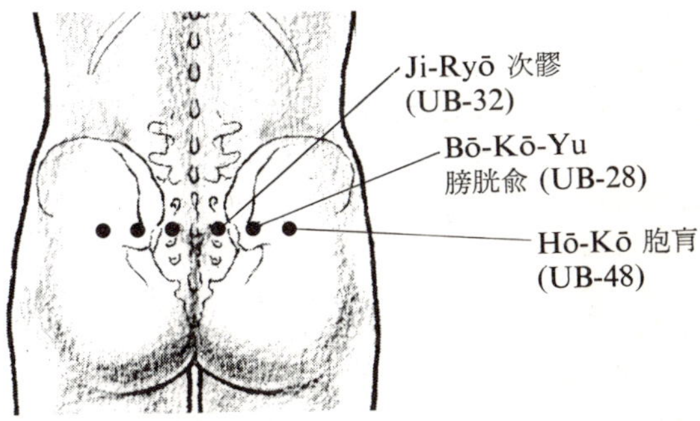

The symptoms in the lower abdomen should be relieved considerably after each one of these tsubos are pressed thoroughly and light massage and finger pressure is provided along the lines connecting these tsubos. Another method which is very simple and almost as effective as pressing and massaging the tsubos is to warm up the area below the waist. In the old days women in Japan used to take what were called "waist baths," where they would soak themselves in a bathtub just from the waist down so that only the lower half of their body was heated up. This was a very effective approach considering the location of the tsubos that are effective for normalizing disfunctions in the organs of the pelvic region.

/. Strong menstrual cramps——Bō-Kō-Yu 膀胱俞 (UB-28)

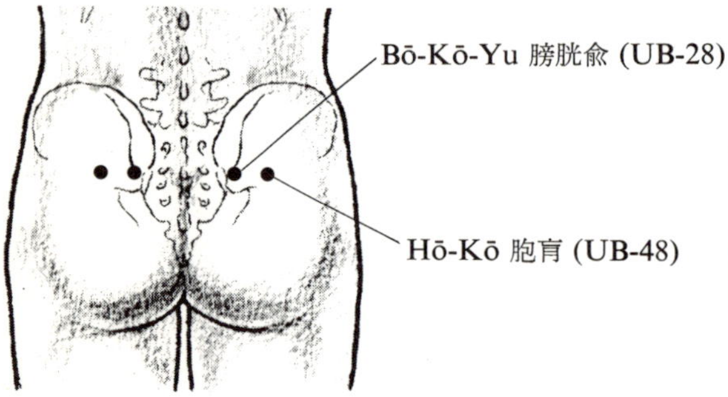

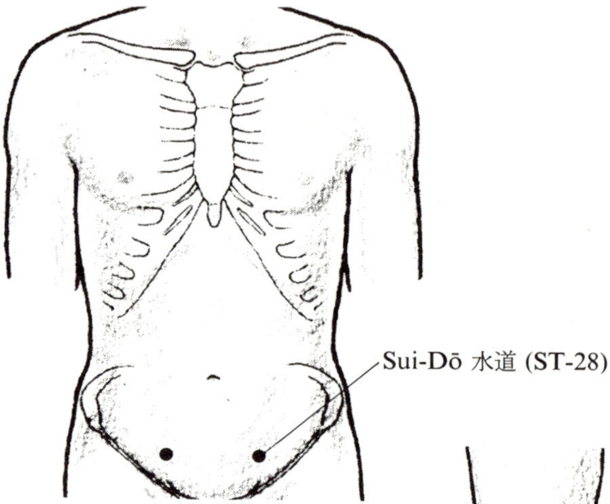

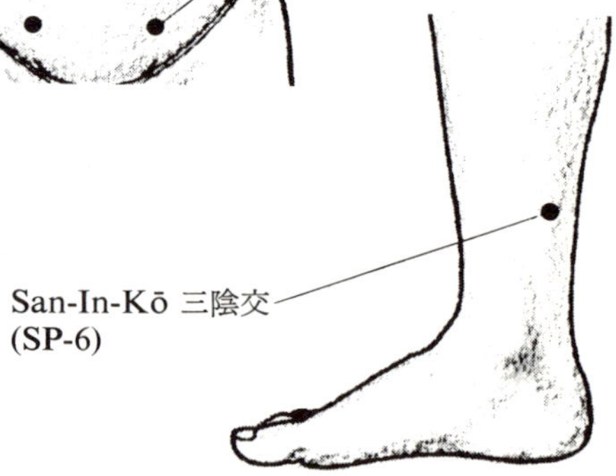

The general symptoms accompanying menses for some women include fatigue, lassitude, headaches, heaviness in the head, dizziness, lack of appetite, insomnia and anxiety. Naturally, some women are entirely unaffected by their period and continue to work and take part in regular activities such as exercising. Nevertheless, a large number of women experience such symptoms along with their period although there is considerable difference in the extent of these symptoms.

Menstrual cramps are among these symptoms, and similar to what was discussed before about menstrual irregularities, the severity of such cramps becomes considerably worse when a woman is exhausted from backpacking and overnight trips, or otherwise, when psychological stress has piled up due to family problems and the like.

The tsubos effective for such bad menstrual cramps are Bō-Kō-Yu 膀胱俞 (UB-28), Hō-Kō 胞肓 (UB-48), Sui-Dō 水道 (ST-28), and San-In-Kō 三陰交 (SP-6). The occurrence of menstrual cramps can be roughly divided into that before and during the period, but the above tsubos are effective in both cases. Also, women who have menstrual cramps most often have cold feet. Therefore, do not forget to also treat the tsubos Tai-Shō 太衝 (LV-3), Rin-Kyū 臨泣 (GB-41), and Yū-Sen 湧泉 (KI-1) listed under the section for chilled feet. No matter what the treatment consists of, these symptoms will not disappear with just one or two treatments. These tsubos listed can all be treated by oneself, so continue to treat them persistently. Treatments over a long period will first alleviate chilling in the feet, and this will be followed by relief from shoulder tension and headaches. Menstrual cramps really disappear only after this.

Although this may be slightly off the subject, a symptom often experienced by women who are infertile is insomnia. In one report, there were cases where treatments using tsubos similar to those listed above proved effective in alleviating menstrual cramps, and the lower half of their body became warmer and the women began feeling warmth around their waist. Eventually some of the infertile women even became pregnant and gave birth to healthy babies.

It is good to remember that symptoms such as low back pain and chilling of the feet in women are usually related to menstrual problems in one way or another.

J. Palpitations and shortness of breath——Geki-Mon 郄門 (HC-4)

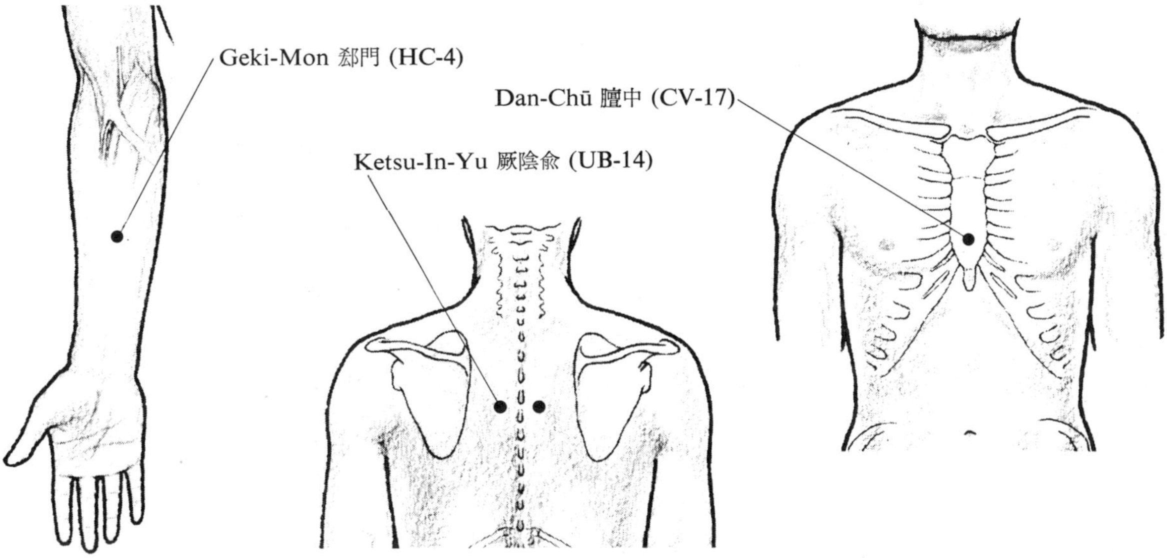

The presence of palpitations and shortness of breath is often used to judge whether a middle-aged person is healthy or not, but even healthy individuals have palpitations and get short of breath after vigorous exercise. Nevertheless, when these remain long after the physical effort, and when just climbing a short flight of stairs causes strong palpitations and panting, or otherwise, when people wake up in the middle of the night with their heart wildly pounding, there is a strong possibility of disorders in the circulatory system so it is wise to consult a specialist. If there are no problems in the circulatory system, these symptoms obviously are a result of overwork and fatigue, and in this case one can treat oneself with tsubo therapy.

Ketsu-In-Yu 厥陰兪 (UB-14) is a tsubo introduced several times before, and it is located to either side of the point below the fourth thoracic vertebra. Begin the treatment by applying soft finger pressure on this tsubo, and then add a slight circular movement. Ketsu-In-Yu is also good for poor circulation and when a person feels a general loss of vigor.

Follow this with firm finger pressure on Dan-Chū 膻中 (CV-17) located on the sternum between the nipples. Moving the finger slightly back and forth on this tsubo will cause a sharp piercing sensation. Dan-Chū is also effective in relieving palpitations and shortness of breath by finger pressure alone. In addition to the above points, also treat Geki-Mon 郄門 (HC-4), located in the middle of the inside of the forearm right between the elbow and the wrist. The name of this tsubo means a crevice or cleft between bone and muscle. People with angina pectoris often have a sharp pain which travels from their middle finger up to the tendon next to this tsubo.

Since Ketsu-In-Yu cannot be reached by oneself because it is located on the upper back, the following method should be used. As soon as you feel palpitations or shortness of breath, sit down in a chair and assume a comfortable posture. Have someone give rather strong pressure around Ketsu-In-Yu which is between the shoulder blades, and at the same time, put pressure on Dan-Chū yourself. After this, give strong pressure with a kneading action to Geki-Mon on both arms. The palpitations and shortness of breath will gradually ease and the heart rate and breathing will return to normal.

K. Mild fevers——Hai-Yu 肺兪 (UB-13)

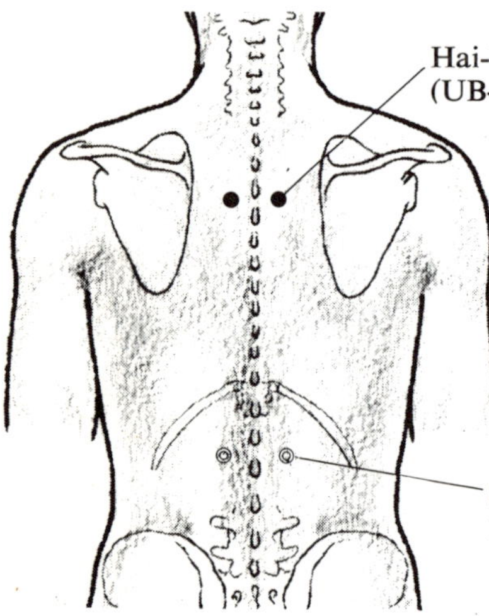

People with a weak constitution from childhood who lack stamina, and those who catch colds very easily such as during the change in seasons, as well as those with a chronic case of bronchial asthma, used to be called "willow types." In Japan the willow is used to illustrate something weak and yielding in contrast to the strength of a pine. When a person is healthy, it is very rare for fatigue alone to cause even a slight fever. This symptom occurs when people who have a weak constitution along with some functional disorder perform excessive manual labor or physical exercise.

In Oriental medicine a slight fever is regarded as being a symptom associated with the respiratory system, so the specially effective tsubo used most often to cure this is Hai-Yu 肺兪 (UB-13: lung *yu* point) two finger widths to either side of the point below the third thoracic vertebra. When lightly stroking, pinching or pressing this area reveals the presence of tension or sensitivity, it means that the function of the lungs is abnormal. Chū-Fu 中府 (LU-1) which is located a little below the outside tip of the clavicle is also an important tsubo, and various indications are said to appear here when the lungs are afflicted. Rek-Ketsu 列欠 (LU-7) is also a tsubo used when there is a chronic symptom associated with the respiratory system, and it is located just

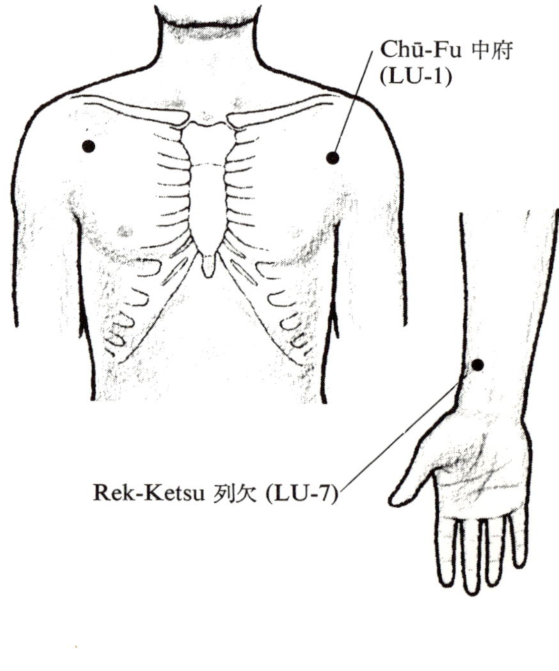

two finger widths above the inside of the wrist in line with the thumb.

When a person gets a slight fever, tension always seems to accumulate on the shoulder blades, and one often feels short of breath. The specially effective tsubo Chū-Fu is above the nipples on the chest, and this area should be treated thoroughly first. Some other symptoms common to this condition is chilling or heating of the hands. The tsubos to be used in this case are the same as those mentioned in the sections covering these symptoms.

Another tsubo which should be mentioned here is San-Shō-Yu 三焦兪 (UB-22) on either side of the point below the first lumbar vertebra. This tsubo has been mentioned many times before, and it is regarded to be a tsubo for regulating the overall temperature of the body.

Whatever the case may be, the most important thing that is needed is to strengthen one's physical condition. Instead of relying solely on tsubo therapy, one should remember to make an effort to improve one's overall physical condition. Whenever you feel tired, you should be sure to give your body a rest and get plenty of sleep.

L. Bad hangovers——Kan-Yu 肝兪 (UB-18)

People are able to recover completely from a night of heavy drinking with just a good nights sleep only up until their early thirties. Once people get beyond their mid-thirties, even moderate drinking can cause one to have bad hangovers the next morning with a pounding headache and an oppressive feeling in the upper abdomen along with nausea. Many quick cures have been proposed for hangovers such as drinking a little more alcohol, or various other concoctions (in Japan some people consider *miso* soup effective), but none of these methods are completely effective in eliminating a hangover. About the only thing a person can do for a bad hangover is to take a day off from work and soak in a warm bath. Nevertheless, most people cannot afford to take a day off from work just because of a hangover. For this reason, tsubo treatments effective for hangovers will be discussed here.

The biggest priority when one has a hangover is to restore the function of the liver, so the effective tsubo is Kan-Yu 肝兪 (UB:18: liver *yu* point) on either side of the ninth thoracic vertebra, and Ki-Mon 期門 (LV-14) at the tip of the ninth rib. Kan-Yu

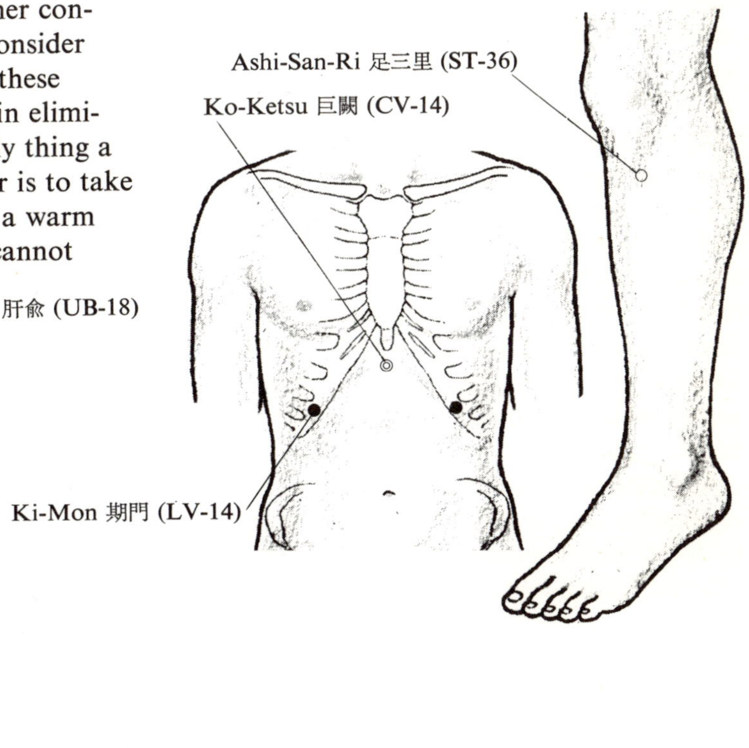

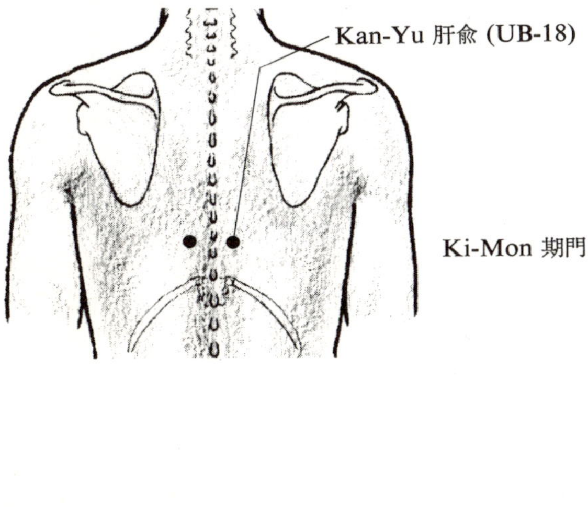

has been discussed before, and Ki-Mon is another tsubo effective for functional disorders in the liver. Pressing lightly on this tsubo in a slightly upward direction while breathing deeply will usually cause quite a bit of pain when a person is hangover. This is evidence that the liver is congested, and massaging around Ki-Mon will also provide considerable relief. When a person also has the symptoms of a flushed face and a heavy head, pressing the tsubos of Ketsu-In-Yu 厥陰俞 (UB-14), on either side of the point below the fourth thoracic vertebra, and Ashi-San-Ri 足三里 (ST-36) is very beneficial.

One more simple massage technique good for hangovers will be introduced here. Get an old sitting cushion which is quite firm; fold it in half and lie face up on the cushion and adjust it so that it is right between the base of your neck and the bottom of your shoulder blades. Then press firmly along the bottom of the rib cage with your thumbs from Ko-Ketsu 巨闕 (CV-14) to Ki-Mon while exhaling. Then use the four fingers to slowly press in under the rib cage going from Ko-Ketsu to Ki-Mon, and farther out to your side. This is a simple method, but it is actually very effective for relieving symptoms of hangovers. Of course, it goes without saying that even before depending on tsubo therapy, the best thing to do is to practice moderation.

M. Decline in sexual performance——Jin-Yu 腎俞 (UB-23)

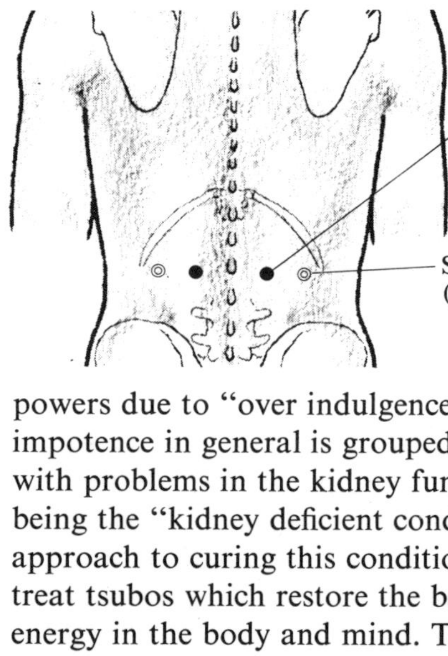

There is nothing more depressing to middle-aged men than impotence, or the inability to have sex. Some men sadly resign themselves to the "inevitable," while others purchase all manner of aphrodisiacs like ginseng to try and revive their sexual potency in any way they can. Impotence is caused by functional impairment in the penis, and injury to the central nervous system which includes the brain and the spinal cord, as well as by alcoholism, addiction to amphetamines, and diabetes. The large majority of cases, however, are caused by mental stress. Psychological tension affects the function of the sexual apparatus which is particularly susceptible to such influences, and produces psychosomatic impotence. The quickest way to restore the sexual function is to remove the cause of stress and to calm down. After doing this, try the tsubo treatments suggested in this section. The cases of impotence with a physical cause have to be referred to a specialist, but tsubo therapy can be unexpectedly effective for those cases caused by stress which are largely psychosomatic.

In Oriental medicine, the loss of sexual powers due to "over indulgence," and impotence in general is grouped together with problems in the kidney function, as being the "kidney deficient condition." The approach to curing this condition is to treat tsubos which restore the balance of energy in the body and mind. The tsubos used for this purpose are Jin-Yu 腎俞 (UB-23) and Shi-Shitsu 志室 (UB-47) on the back, and Kō-Yu 肓俞 (KI-16) right next to the navel. When a person becomes impotent, the area on either side of the second lumbar vertebra becomes tense and rigid, and hard spots form on either side of the navel. The specially effective tsubos for impotence lie right over these areas of tension. Other tsubos important for this condition are Chū-Kyoku 中極 (CV-3), just above the pubic symphysis, Dai-Kaku 大赫 (KI-12), to either side of this, and San-In-Kō 三陰交 (SP-6), above the inner ankle bone. Dai-Kaku, especially, is known to have a powerful effect in reviving sexual potency, such that it is even said to turn the male sex organ red.

When you feel that your sexual performance has been on the decline, press and massage around each of the tsubos mentioned. Once your body becomes soft and pliable, your mind will also relax and mental stress will disappear, and the impotence will eventually be sure. The most important thing in treating impotence, however, is to keep a relaxed attitude about the whole situation.

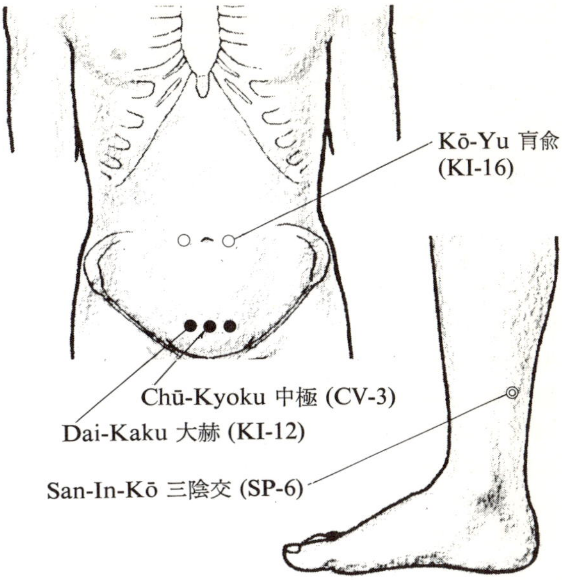

N. Irritability and impatience——Kyū-Bi 鳩尾 (CV-15)

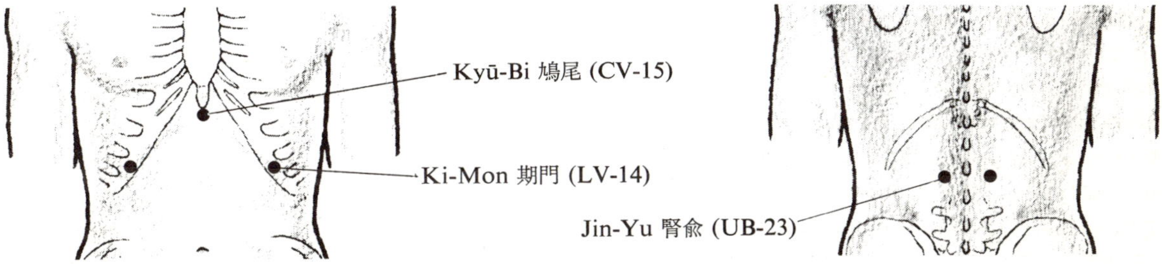

In the *Yōjōkun*, a book written by Kaibara Ekiken (1630–1714) concerning how to live a long and fruitful life, there is a rule for longevity of "drink only enough to become mellowed, eat only 80 percent of your stomach's capacity, practice moderation in sex, and keep your mind calm and serene." This implies that a long life is possible for all of us providing we do not eat or drink in excess, we temper our sexual desires, and avoid accumulating stress. Nevertheless, putting these simple rules into practice is just about impossible for people today. The issue of eating, drinking, and sex aside, today's society is brim full of conditions which produce stress, such that people who are calm and undisturbed are the exception and they even seem to be the abnormal ones.

Irritability and impatience in physiological terms are symptoms caused by imbalances in the function of the cerebral cortex, and this may lead some people to think that tsubos on the head are used in this case. Actually, however, Jin-Yu 腎兪 (UB-23) on the back, Ki-Mon 期門 (LV-14) on the abdomen at the tip of the ninth rib, and Kyū-Bi 鳩尾 (CV-15) below the sternum are the specially effective tsubos in this case. The reason tsubos on the back and stomach are used to calm a person down when they are irritated is because in Oriental medicine, not the brain, but the internal organs are thought to control a person's emotions. This

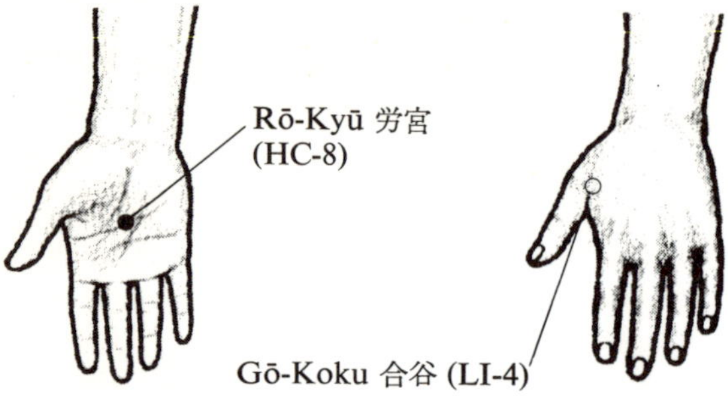

aspect of Oriental medicine has been discussed in preceding sections of this book. This may seem like a strange idea to those who are accustomed to the concepts of modern medicine, but this is not so hard to understand when we give it a little thought.

When one loses his mental equilibrium or emotional balance, there are always attendant physical symptoms such as palpitations, shortness of breath, heating or cooling of the hands and feet, digestive problems and lack of appetite. When one's physical condition is improved through the stimulation of the appropriate tsubo, one's irritability will also cease as a result. In this manner, first treating physical symptoms even when there are psychological problems can be called one of the special characteristics of Oriental medicine.

The method of treating the tsubos listed above is to have someone press Jin-Yu with plenty of force, and give gradual finger pressure on Kyū-Bi and Ki-Mon yourself while exhaling. When you are extremely tired, the effects will be greatly enhanced if finger pressure could also be given to Rō-Kyū 労宮 (HC-8) and Gō-Koku 合谷 (LI-4) on the hand.

O. Difficulty in getting to sleep——Kaku-Yu 膈兪 (UB-17)

This may just be a reflection of our busy times, but there are a great many patients who come to our clinic complaining of various types of insomnia including difficulty in getting to sleep, inability to sleep deeply, and waking up very early in the morning. Insomnia sometimes is caused by high blood pressure, or disorders in the digestive organs, but the large majority of cases are caused by psychological factors. It is quite common even for healthy individuals, when they are mentally exhausted, to have insomnia. The advice of a medical specialist should be sought for insomnia caused by serious diseases so that the root cause of the problem can be treated. Conversely, for insomnia stemming from various psychological causes, quite dramatic results are possible through tsubo therapy.

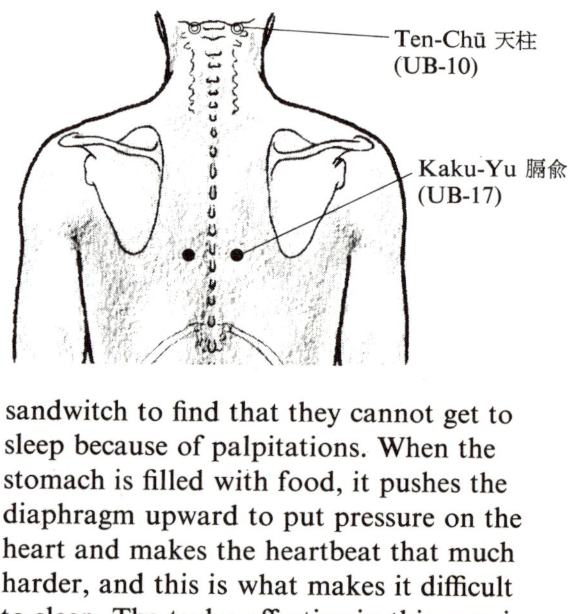

The most common case of insomnia among otherwise healthy individuals is where they feel hungry right before going to bed and end up eating something like a sandwich to find that they cannot get to sleep because of palpitations. When the stomach is filled with food, it pushes the diaphragm upward to put pressure on the heart and makes the heartbeat that much harder, and this is what makes it difficult to sleep. The tsubo effective in this case is Kaku-Yu 膈兪 (UB-17), to either side of the point below the seventh thoracic vertebra. As discussed before, Kaku-Yu lies right between the level of the *yu* points controlling the functions of the organs in the chest

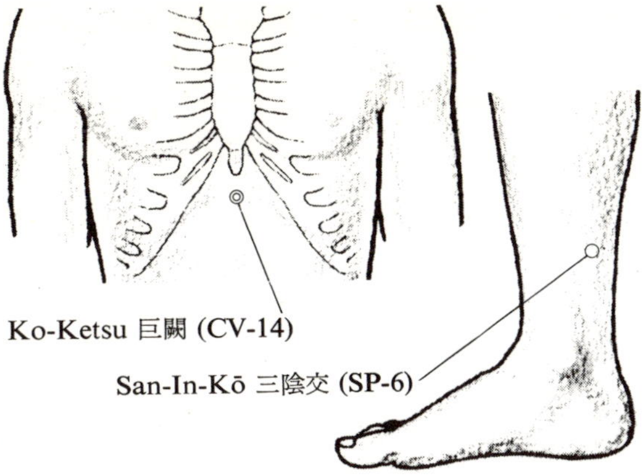

cavity, and those of the abdominal cavity. For this reason Kaku-Yu is considered to be effective against symptoms on both sides of the diaphragm, including the entire range of respiratory, circulatory, and digestive disorders. Apply thorough pressure on this tsubo, and since one's head often feels muddled when having trouble getting to sleep, also give finger pressure to Ten-Chū 天柱 (UB-10).

People with insomnia almost always have considerable tension in the pit of their stomach and in their back. There is no need to worry about the location of each tsubo when giving treatments to relieve tension down the back. The tension should gradually go away if you can get someone to press both sides of your spine with care.

The tsubo for relieving tension in the pit of the stomach is Ko-Ketsu 巨闕 (CV-14). Often when a person has difficulty in sleeping, there is a heavy or stifling sensation here. When this is the case, press in slowly along the bottom of the rib cage from Ko-Ketsu out to the side while exhaling. Once the tension in the back and the pit of the stomach disappears, the insomnia also should be cured.

Furthermore, since warming one's feet has an effect in helping insomnia, pressing San-In-Kō 三陰交 (SP-6) on the foot should make the treatment complete.

P. Too many dreams (shallow sleep)——Kaku-Kan 膈関 (UB-41)

There are many people that are able to get to sleep, but who suffer from nightmares and sometimes wake up startled by their own voice to find themselves drenched with sweat. When classifying problems having to do with sleep, insomnia discussed in the previous section is a problem in getting to sleep. Not being able to sleep soundly and being disturbed by too many dreams are problems of "shallow sleep." These symptoms of "shallow sleep" are common to hypersensitive individuals who tend to be anxious about things, as well as those who have weak constitutions and feel lingering effects from fatigue. The cause of "shallow sleep" is usually psychological, so the tsubos used to help this condition are naturally very similar to those used for insomnia.

Usually a great deal of tension can be

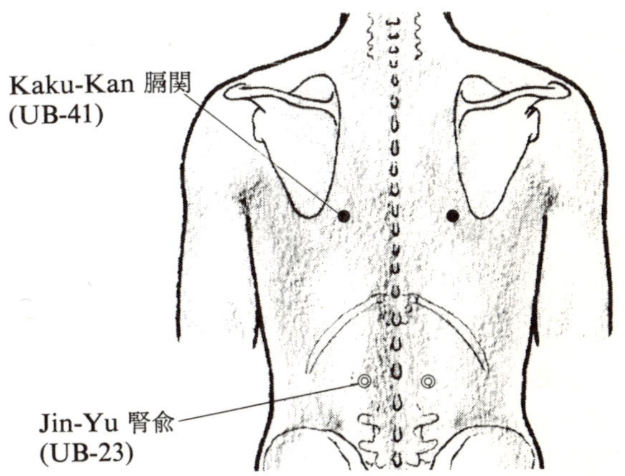

detected along the spine when feeling down the back of a person who has problems with sleeping soundly. The best tsubo for removing such tension is Kaku-Kan 膈関 (UB-41). This tsubo is located to the outside of Kaku-Yu 膈兪 (UB-17), and is used often to treat nausea and stifling sensations in the chest. The tension in the back will gradually be relieved by giving strong pressure to Kaku-Kan, and by pressing and massaging down both sides of the spine from Kaku-Kan to Jin-Yu 腎兪 (UB-23). There may also be tension and pressure sensitivity under the rib cage from Ko-Ketsu 巨闕 (CV-14) out toward the side, so slowly press along this line also. As the tension and tenderness in these areas begin to disappear, the person should become able to sleep soundly.

This was covered already in previous sections, but the trick in applying finger pressure, especially to points just under the rib cage, is to press in slowly while exhaling. This may be an extreme example, but in Japanese martial arts such as *karate* or *kendō* (sword fighting), the secret of an effective blow is to strike just at the opponent has finished exhaling. The logic behind this is that our body becomes tense when inhaling, and relaxes while exhaling.

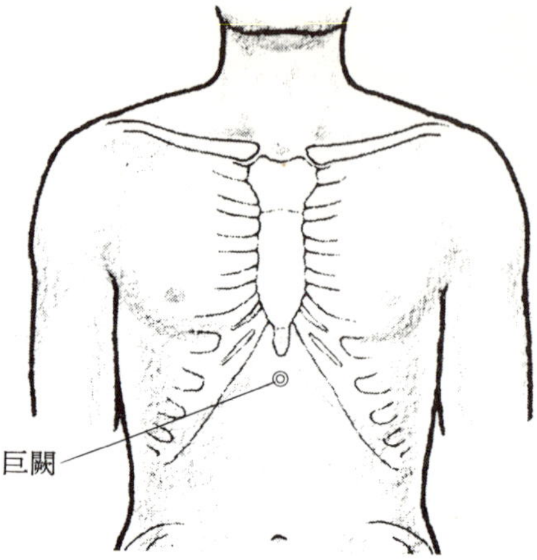

It does little good to apply pressure or force on the body when it is in a state of tension.

In *Tai-Chi* exercises, which have become very popular in Japan recently, one basic movement involves slowly exhaling while rhythmically drawing a circle in the air with one's hands about eighteen times a minute. This feature of exhaling while making a movement relates to the secret of effective shiatsu or finger pressure treatments.

Q. Difficulty in waking up——Ten-Chū 天柱 (UB-10)

There are some people who can sleep in any position, even while standing up, but the majority of us can sleep only in the

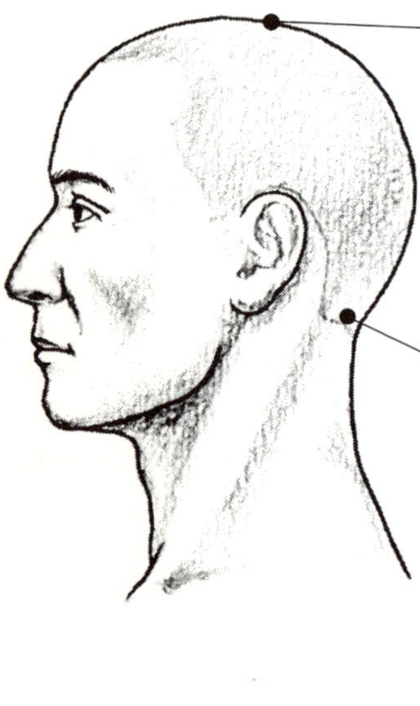

reclined position. Why is it that we are able to sleep best when lying down? This is, of course, because we are able to relax all of our muscles completely. When we are awake, various stimuli are transmitted to our central nervous system from all the muscles in our body, and this stimuli serves to facilitate the function of the sympathetic nerves which keep the life functions of respiration and heartbeat at a high level. On the other hand, once we lie down and all our muscles relax, the stimuli to the central nervous system decreases, and along with this the respiration and heart rate also decline, and one enters sleep. When a person's body is fatigued, however, one moves the body unconsciously trying to find a more comfortable position. This causes tension in the muscles, however slight, and this sends stimuli to the central nervous system which disturbs one's sleep. As a result, the next morning after waking up, one's head feels foggy and unclear, and one has difficulty in really waking up. This is another symptom typical to people who are overworked and exhausted.

The first thing that needs to be done in this case, obviously, is to clear up one's head. The specially effective tsubos for this purpose are Hyaku-E 百会 (GV-20) and Ten-Chū 天柱 (UB-10). These tsubos can be pressed while still in bed, so place the index and middle fingers of both hands together on Hyaku-E and give strong pressure. Next press Ten-Chū toward Hyaku-E and move the fingers in a small circular pattern.

Generally, when a person does not feel rested upon waking up in the morning, the person's digestive organs are in a poor condition. Therefore, press Chū-Kan 中脘 (CV-12), between the navel and the pit of the stomach, by using the tips of the fingers with one hand over the other to press in deeply while exhaling. Once your head feels clear and the condition of your stomach has improved, sit up in bed and give a strong massage to Yū-Sen 湧泉 (KI-1) on the back of the foot to dispel fatigue in the legs. The above mentioned treatment covers every angle for times when you wake up, but drowsiness does not go away. You should be able to jump up out of bed after doing this treatment on yourself.

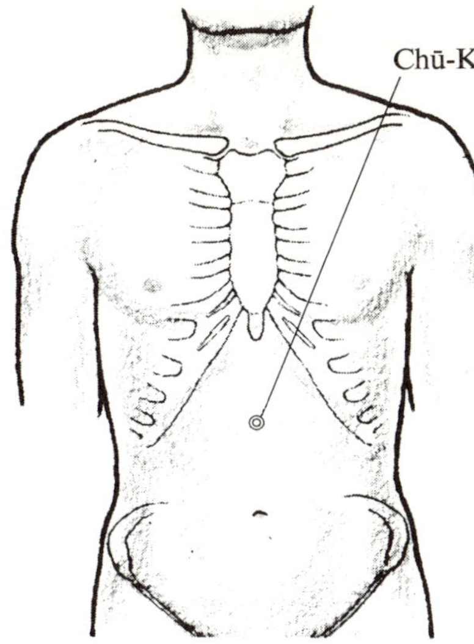

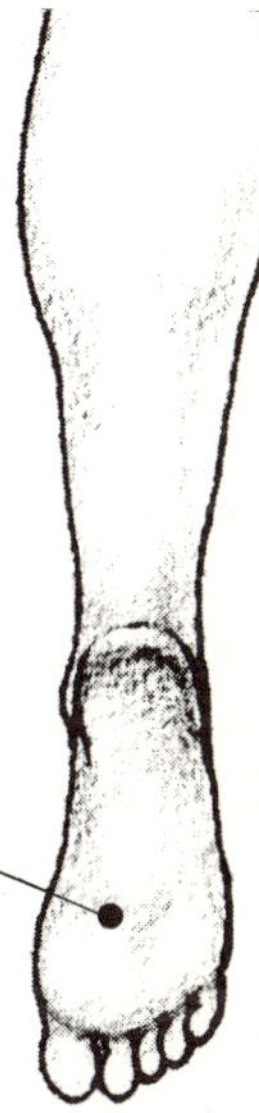

R. Feeling tired and yawning all day long——Tai-Yō 太陽 (extra tsubo)

In recent years, there seems to be an increasing number of young office workers afflicted with the "drowsiness syndrome," where they become very drowsy during the day. It is said that disease like diabetes are often responsible for this, but more commonly, it can be regarded as a symptom resulting from overwork and general fatigue. The human body is of a very ingenious design, and whenever people become tired, they always begin to feel drowsy. So the eyelids feeling very heavy when one is tired can even be regarded as a self-defense mechanism of sorts. The best way to recover from this fatigue is to get some sleep. There are cases, however, where a person feels drowsy despite getting an ample amount of sleep. This may be thought of as a disturbance in the autonomic nervous system resulting from exhaustion.

As discussed previously, the autonomic nervous system is divided into the sympa-

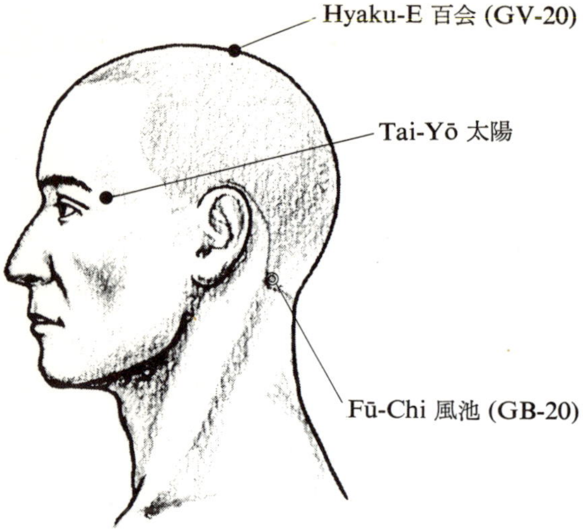

thetic and parasympathetic nerves. During the daytime the sympathetic nerves are active and control the functions of respiration and circulation, as well as the workings of various organ systems and muscular activity. Conversely, at night the parasympathetic nerves become dominant to slow down life processes considerably, and one goes to sleep. When a person becomes very fatigued, the balance between the two sectors of the autonomic nervous system becomes upset. This condition is called "autonomic ataxia," and getting very drowsy in the middle of the day happens to be one of its manifestations.

The tsubos to be treated in this case, first of all the clear up one's head, consists of Hyaku-E 百会 (GV-20), located on the very top of the head, Tai-Yō 太陽 (extra tsubo), a little behind the point between the outer corner of the eye and the eyebrow, and Fū-Chi 風池 (GB-20), in the back of the head. All of these tsubos have been discussed before, so they will not be explained here. Providing stimulation to these tsubos by massage and finger pressure facilitates the activity of the sympathetic nerves and revitalizes the function of the brain.

When the above treatment does not remove the drowsiness completely, and your body still feels languid, give strong pressure on the tsubo Nai-Kan 内関 (HC-6) located about six centimeters up from the inside of the wrist in the middle of the forearm. When this tsubo is pressed strong enough to make a sensation travel down to the wrist and the fingers to cause a numbing sensation in the middle finger, your body will feel awake once more, and the drowsiness should disappear completely. If the familiar tsubo of Gō-Koku 合谷 (LI-4) is also goaded and pressed strongly this should be sufficient to keep you alert.

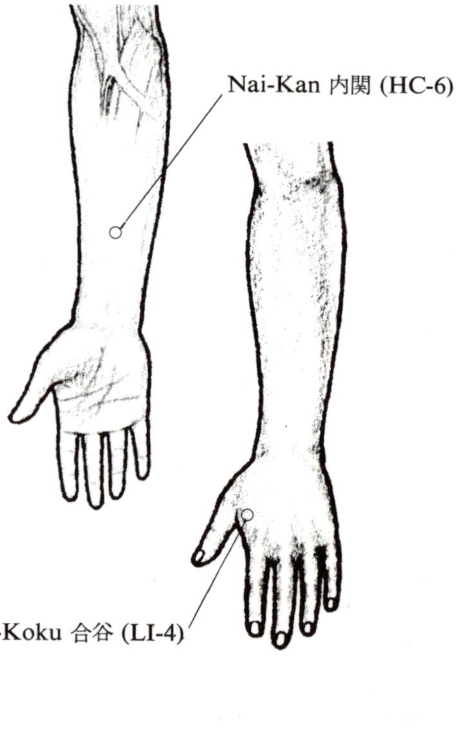

Index